NATURAL SUPPLEMENTS
FOR DIABETES

Also by Frank Murray

100 Super Supplements for a Longer Life (English and Chinese)

The Big Family Guide to All the Minerals

Program Your Heart for Health

Gingko Biloba

All About Menopause

Acidophilus and Your Health

Remifemin: Herbal Relief for Menopausal Symptoms

Happy Feet

NATURAL SUPPLEMENTS FOR

DIABETES

*Reduce Your Risk and Lower Your
Insulin Dependency with Natural Remedies*

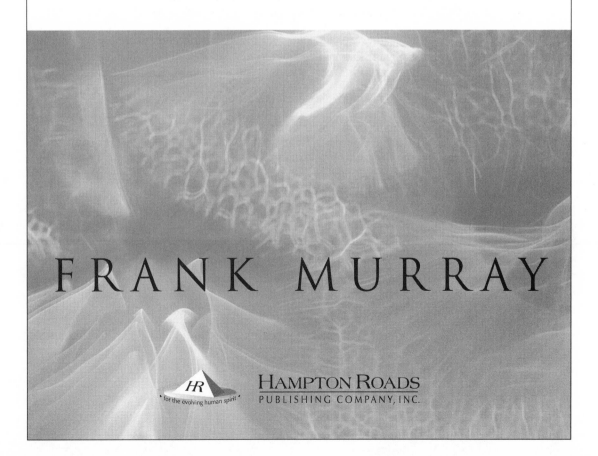

FRANK MURRAY

HAMPTON ROADS
PUBLISHING COMPANY, INC.

HR
for the evolving human spirit

Cover design by Steve Amarillo
Cover art/photographic image ©2003 Loyd Chapplow

Hampton Roads Publishing Company, Inc.
1125 Stoney Ridge Road
Charlottesville, VA 22902

434-296-2772
fax: 434-296-5096
e-mail: hrpc@hrpub.com
www.hrpub.com

If you are unable to order this book from your local
bookseller, you may order directly from the publisher.
Call 1-800-766-8009, toll-free.

Library of Congress Cataloging-in-Publication Data

Murray, Frank, 1924-
    Natural supplements for diabetes : reduce your risk and lower your
insulin dependency with natural remedies / Frank Murray.
        p. cm.
Includes bibliographical references and index.
    ISBN 1-57174-327-8 (trade pbk. : alk. paper)
    1. Diabetes--Alternative treatment. 2. Dietary supplements. I.
Title.
RC661.A47M87 2003
616.4'620654--dc21

                                            2003007483

                    ISBN 1-57174-327-8

                    10 9 8 7 6 5 4 3 2 1

            Printed on acid-free paper in Canada

Disclaimer

This book is written as a source of information to educate the reader. It is not intended to replace medical advice or care, whether provided for by a primary care physician, a specialist, or a licensed alternative medicine professional. The author took a great deal of time and energy to support the information contained in this book with published documentation from scientific and clinical research; however, this research is not meant to be used as justification for any of the recommendations contained in the book. When supplements are recommended, dosages are given in ranges for the average adult and are to be used as generalized guidelines only. Effects from any supplement can vary a great deal from person to person and applications must be adjusted to meet individual requirements.

The author has no financial ties to any of the supplements, clinics, services, or medications cited in the text. Specific products and medications are recommended solely to help the reader get better results.

Neither the author nor the publisher shall be liable or responsible for any adverse effects arising from the use or application of any of the information contained herein, nor do they guarantee that everyone will benefit or be healed by these techniques and are not responsible if they are not. Please consult your doctor before beginning any new medications, diet, nutrients, or any form of health program.

Contents

Foreword

There is an alarming increase in the incidence of diabetes. Neither the billions of dollars spent on medical research nor the arsenal of pharmaceutical drugs and medical devices that have subsequently emerged have been able to curb this epidemic. Too many people are suffering, and we cannot sustain the skyrocketing costs that support these therapies. Fortunately, there is a better way.

Americans are becoming proactive about their health. We are also entering an exciting integrative era that is blending the best of conventional and alternative medicine with the ancient wisdom of indigenous healing systems. Never before in our history have we had the opportunities that are possible today. We are in the process of changing from a "disease care" into a "health care" medical model. Our focus is shifting to optimizing health by preventing disease and promoting wellness. Lifestyle enhancement and the use of natural therapies are emerging as powerful tools that can achieve these goals.

While we all recognize and highly value the achievements of modern technology, we are becoming less dependent on the "miracles" of high-tech medicine. Despite its technological brilliance, modern medicine has not solved the epidemic of chronic diseases; its lack of safety has become a frightening reality, and it has become unaffordable for too many of us. There are just too many health problems, and too few solutions.

Natural Supplements for Diabetes addresses everything you need to know to prevent or manage every aspect of diabetes. This rich compendium of extensively referenced information is practical, effective, safe, and affordable—put simply, you can use it. Frank Murray's commonsense wisdom inspires confidence so that you can take responsibility and realistically expect to optimally manage, or even prevent, diabetes for yourself and for your loved ones.

Murray begins by providing an easy to understand view of what diabetes is and highlights the importance of identifying risk factors that predispose one to its development or progression. Medical statisticians have estimated that more than 50 million Americans suffer from the so-called Syndrome X, or "metabolic syndrome," which many experts feel is the prelude to the development of overt diabetes. Murray reviews this condition and offers strategies that can minimize its effects, and possibly even prevent its onset. He also devotes individual chapters to the impact of obesity, hypertension, cholesterol, homocysteine, smoking, diet, and exercise on diabetes. Valuable information that will help protect the target organs that are particularly vulnerable to the complications of diabetes—heart, brain, eyes, feet, kidneys, and thyroid gland—is presented in detail.

Murray's strategies go far beyond mainstream medical approaches to help reverse the underlying problems leading to the development of diabetes. Natural therapies that promote healing and allow the body to help restore normal physiology are offered. As they reverse the severity of the diabetic state, these insights also enhance overall health. Although these simple and effective tools are fully compatible with pharmacological drugs, typically, dosages can be dramatically reduced, or in some instances, entirely eliminated.

The value of specific vitamins, minerals, and supplements is addressed in the second half of this book. The science behind their use is thoroughly documented, and a strong rational basis for using them is established. There is an enormous database of modern, cutting-edge biochemical research supporting the concept that many complications of diabetes are related to increased oxidative stress—the chemical damage of vital structures within the cell that results in premature aging. Reducing oxidative stress is certainly one of the major keys that can not only slow the development of aging, but also improve health and vitality. Murray proposes novel ways that these simple and powerful natural substances can be used to prevent and repair oxidative stress.

While it is wise to include your health care practitioner in the decision-making process when considering changes in therapy, *Natural Supplements for Diabetes* makes it possible for you to begin the process of creating your own program to minimize the manifestations of diabetes and maximize health.

Today's health care is transforming into a collaborative process in which dialogue between patients and physicians is the norm. We are learning that the best way to ensure good health comes from taking responsibility for making our own decisions about our individual health care needs while considering the advice of our health care practitioners. Now that information is so readily available from the news, books, magazines, and the Internet, it is realistic to partner with your practitioner and contribute the potentially important information that emerges from your research.

Len Saputo, M.D.,
Co-Founder and Medical Director,
Health Medicine Institute
Lafayette, California

Introduction

Diabetes mellitus—once called "sugar diabetes"—has plagued mankind for centuries. As explained in this book, there are two basic types of the disease: Type 1, or insulin-dependent diabetes, and Type 2, or non-insulin-dependent diabetes. In Type 1, patients must be given insulin, since the pancreas does not produce enough of the hormone to control glucose (sugar) in the bloodstream. In Type 2, the body may produce enough insulin, but the body does not process and distribute it correctly.

When you eat, your body turns your food into glucose to use as fuel. In healthy people, insulin helps the glucose get into the cells. But for Type 2 patients, the cells simply ignore what insulin is being produced.

When blood sugar is too high, you may experience a headache, blurry vision, dry, itchy skin, or have to make frequent trips to the bathroom. In Type 1 diabetics, especially, harmful ketones or waste products build up in the blood and cause ketoacidosis. If untreated, this can lead to a diabetic coma and even death.

High blood sugar levels can damage eyes, kidneys, and nerves and contribute to heart and blood vessel disease.

If your blood sugar falls too low (low blood sugar), it may be the result of taking too much diabetic medicine, eating very little or nothing at all, exercising for too long, or drinking alcohol without eating. Low blood sugar can make you shaky, tired, confused, hungry, or nervous.

While researchers feverishly search for a cure for diabetes, they are losing the battle because so many Americans are overweight and leading a sedentary lifestyle. Overweight and obesity contribute not only to diabetes, but also to high blood pressure, heart disease, and stroke.

Contributing to this potentially deadly game are high levels of cholesterol and triglycerides.

While most of the books on diabetes are devoted to menus, oral medications, insulin pumps, transplants, and the like, that is not the purview of this book. Although these aspects of the disease are important, I preferred to go in a different direction by showing through worldwide research how many of the important studies on vitamins, minerals, herbs, and other natural supplements are being virtually ignored.

I hope that much of this research will open the eyes of many researchers and patients alike. For example, diabetics who are not taking the mineral chromium are missing out on an opportunity to possibly control their disease. Type 2 diabetics can often be taken off insulin with a high-fiber diet. Other chapters in this book are equally enlightening. Your doctor can provide further information as well as suggesting a suitable menu for your particular case.

As Americans become fatter and fatter—especially children—diabetes will continue to be one of our most life-threatening disorders.

Writing in the October 9, 2002, issue of *The Journal of the American Medical Association,* Katherine M. Flegal, Ph.D., and colleagues at the National Center for Health Statistics, CDC, in Hyattsville, Maryland, said, "It likely will be difficult to reverse the increasing prevalence of overweight and obesity in the United States. Even as long ago as 1960, almost 50% of men and 40% of women were overweight, and 11% of men and 16% of women were obese." They added, "The potential health benefits from reduction in overweight and obesity are a matter of considerable public importance."

In a separate article in the same publication, Cynthia L. Ogden, Ph.D., et al., of the same affiliation, said that the prevalence of overweight among children in the U.S. is continuing to increase, especially among Mexican-Americans and non-Hispanic black adolescents.

Since many people have diabetes and don't know it, it is important to review the telltale signs and to seek medical advice as soon as possible, since the disease is life-threatening. For these patients and for those who already have Type 1 or Type 2 diabetes, I am hopeful that the worldwide research synthesized in this book will help them to control their disease.

Part One
Reducing Your Risk of Developing Diabetes

1 Diabetes: An Epidemic in the Making

Diabetes, the seventh leading cause of death in the United States, increased by about 6% in 1999, the latest year tabulated, and is headed for epidemic proportions. An estimated 800,000 new cases are recorded annually. Almost 16 million Americans have the disease, and the sharpest increase, about 70%, is found in those between the ages of 30 and 39. Treatment costs for the disease amount to about $100 billion annually. The rapid rise of the disease can be reversed with modest lifestyle changes and losing as little as 10 pounds. Major risk factors are obesity, lack of exercise, avoiding five or more daily servings of fruits and vegetables, smoking, and not getting enough of the antioxidant vitamins and minerals.

Diabetes, which is the leading cause of blindness, kidney failure, amputations, and is a major risk factor for heart attacks in the United States, increased by about 6% in 1999, the latest year tabulated, in what the government called an unfolding epidemic. It is the seventh leading cause of death in the U.S. An estimated 800,000 new cases are tabulated annually. The rise is attributed to obesity, which rose by 57% from 1991, according to the Centers for Disease Control and Prevention (CDC) in Atlanta, Georgia. A couch-potato mentality, computer-centered lifestyles, fast food, and limited spaces for exercising outdoors are blamed for the increase in overweight.[1]

The CDC reported that the incidence of adults diagnosed with Type 2 diabetes increased from about 6.5% in 1998 to 6.9% in 1999, amounting to almost 16 million Americans who have the disease. The sharpest increase–about 70%–was found in those between the ages of 30 and 39. In 1999, the largest increase was among African-Americans–above 10% in one year. Whites, Hispanics, and other ethnic groups also had higher rates in 1999, the CDC continued.

An increase in diabetes will get worse over the next several years, according to Robert Sherwin, M.D., president of the American Diabetes Association. "The American way of life tends to favor inactivity," he said. "We're going to need a major education program in the schools to reverse this trend."

A rapid rise in diabetes in the United States can be reversed with modest lifestyle changes—eating less fat, exercising two and a half hours a week, and losing a moderate amount of weight, according to the National Institutes of Health (NIH) in Bethesda, Maryland. This could cut the incidence of diabetes by more than half among those most at risk. The study focused on Type 2 diabetes, which is linked to risk factors such as overweight and lack of exercise.

The CDC statistics, published in more detail in the February 2001 issue of *Diabetes Care*, are based on a telephone survey of 150,000 Americans. By 2025, the number of diabetics in the U.S. is expected to reach 22 million.[2] "This disease used to come late in life," said Ali H. Mokdar, M.D., an epidemiologist at the CDC. "Now it's affecting people as young as the early 20s. That's alarming."

Commenting on the role of obesity in the development of diabetes, Mokdar said, "Over time, humans evolved the capacity to store food in their bodies when it wasn't easily available. Now, food is available all the time, everywhere. If we don't exercise, we'll never lose the weight and we'll increase our risk of diabetes."[3]

A rapid rise in diabetes in the United States can be reversed with modest lifestyle changes–eating less fat, exercising two and a half hours a week, and losing a moderate amount of weight, according to the National Institutes of Health (NIH) in Bethesda, Maryland. This could cut the incidence of diabetes by more than half among those most at risk. The study focused on Type 2 diabetes, which is linked to risk factors such as overweight and lack of exercise.[4]

The study involved 3,234 volunteers at twenty-seven medical centers, ranging in age from 25 to 85, and was the largest study in the U.S. to suggest that diet and exercise might prevent the disease. It was the first study to include large numbers of participants from minority groups at high risk for the disease. While risk factors such as age, race, and family history of the disease cannot be changed, those at risk can control two main factors—obesity and physical activity, reported the *New York Times*.

Smaller studies in Finland and China came to similar conclusions about diet and exercise, but it was not clear whether those findings would apply to the diverse racial and ethnic groups in the United States. Almost half of the participants in the U.S. study, which was sponsored by the National Institute of Diabetes and Digestive and Kidney Diseases, included African-Americans, Hispanics, Asian-Americans, and Native Americans, who are generally more prone than non-Hispanic whites to develop the disease. While metformin, a drug to treat diabetes, helps to prevent the disease, it does not work as well as diet, exercise, and weight loss, the researchers said. Treatment costs for the disease amount to approximately $100 billion annually.

The NIH added that, in addition to kidney failure, blindness, heart disease, and stroke, circulatory problems associated with diabetes are the leading cause of amputations of feet and legs. Type 2 diabetes accounts for 90 to 95% of the cases, while the remaining patients are Type 1 diabetics, which is not generally associated with obesity. Among volunteers who took metformin, 7.8% a year developed diabetes, a reduction of about one-third. But the drug has little effect in older people or those who are not overweight.

The NIH said that of the volunteers who changed their eating and exercise habits, only 4.8% a year developed diabetes, a reduction of more than half compared with the control group. In those who were 60 or older, the drop was even steeper, nearly three-quarters. In one-third of this group, blood glucose levels returned to normal during the 24-week study.

"We weren't asking the participants to train for a marathon," said David M. Nathan, M.D., of Massachusetts General Hospital in Boston, who headed the study. "They're a bunch of pretty normal people who are at high risk for diabetes. We didn't grow them in a test tube. What we asked them to do, in the end, was not overwhelming. I don't see this as out of reach for the 10 million people who are a high risk for diabetes."

Understanding Diabetes

Diabetes develops when there is too much glucose (sugar) in the blood. The cells require glucose for fuel, but when glucose builds up in the blood instead of going into the cells, the cells are starved for energy. High blood sugar levels can eventually harm your eyes, nerves, kidneys, and heart.

Type 1 diabetes mellitus was formerly called insulin-dependent diabetes or juvenile diabetes. Type 1 diabetes usually occurs in those under the age of 30; however, it can develop at any age. In those with Type 1 diabetes, the pancreas cannot produce enough insulin and they must take insulin injections to live.

Formerly called non-insulin-dependent diabetes or adult-onset diabetes, Type 2 diabetes mellitus usually occurs in those over 40. While these patients may often be treated with diet and exercise, they may require insulin or other oral medications.

Gestational diabetes mellitus occurs in up to 5% of nondiabetic women during the later stages of their pregnancy. The problem usually disappears after delivery, but they are sometimes candidates for Type 2 diabetes within five to ten years.

While all volunteers were advised to restrict their diet, exercise, and lose weight, only those who attended diet and exercise classes and received follow-up coaching achieved the greatest benefit from the study, the NIH said.

Commenting on the NIH study in *Time*, Christine Gorman reported that the greatest benefits were found among those who were physically active at least 30 minutes a day, five days a week, and who lost between 5 and 7% of their body weight or an average of 15 pounds. Walking was the preferred form of exercise. As for calories, the goal was to consume 25% of calories from fat—compared with 30 to 35% in the average American diet. For those who eat 1,500 calories daily, this translates to 42 grams of fat. To put this in perspective, a Big Mac and fries can register 14 grams over the limit.[5]

Many of the 6 million or so people in the U.S. who don't know they have diabetes are going untreated because they were tested at the wrong time of day, according to Maureen I. Harris, M.D., of the National Institute of Diabetes and Digestive and Kidney Diseases in Washington, D.C. She added that if patients were given blood tests in the afternoon instead of the morning, their possible diabetes may be overlooked. That is because blood glucose levels, used to determine if a person is diabetic, vary from morning to afternoon. Those tested in the morning were twice as likely (2.8%) as those tested in the afternoon to have a diagnosis of diabetes. The study analyzed blood-plasma tests for more than 12,000 people.[6]

"Typically, a patient being tested for diabetes is instructed to fast overnight and come in to the doctor's office in the morning," Harris said. "If the blood test shows a certain plasma glucose (sugar) or higher, it is considered evidence of diabetes. But many patients also come in for tests in the afternoon, when it is unclear how long they have been fasting."

At some point the economics of the diabetes epidemic will force the issue as our medical system runs out of money for the dialysis units, medications, and other treatments needed to sustain the new sick patients, wrote Ronald Halweil, M.D., in a letter to the *New York Times*, Aug. 28, 2000.[7]

Added another writer, Dick Smith, "One major cause of this epidemic has been the promotion for many years of low-fat diets. Reducing fat is not enough. So-called low-fat products are loaded with sugars of various sorts. So are the soft drinks and so many other delights that reportedly supply the average American with 20.5 teaspoons of added sugar a day (or 68.5 pounds per person each year).

People 30 years of age and older are certainly not immune from getting diabetes, reported Lauran Neergaard, a writer for the Associated

Risk Factors for Diabetes

Have you noticed increased thirst?	Yes	No
Has there been an increase in urination lately?	Yes	No
Have you experienced increased appetite?	Yes	No
Are you overweight?	Yes	No
Do you suffer with a dry or burning mouth?	Yes	No
Have you recently required a decided change in your prescription for eyeglasses?	Yes	No
Do you have tenderness of the gums?	Yes	No
Is there a history of diabetes in your family?	Yes	No
Have you lost considerable weight lately?	Yes	No
Have you ever been told that your blood sugar was suspiciously high?	Yes	No
Do you have periodontal disease?	Yes	No
Do you crave sweet foods and beverages?	Yes	No
For men, do you have a problem with impotency?	Yes	No
For women, do you suffer with vaginal itching or other signs of a possible infection?	Yes	No
For women, have you had a baby who weighed more than 9 pounds at birth?	Yes	No

Source: Emanuel Cheraskin, M.D., D.M.D., Ringsdorf, W. Marshall, Jr., M.S., D.M.D., and Sisley, Emily L., Ph.D. *The Vitamin C Connection*. New York: Harper & Row, 1983, pp. 104–105.

Press. In fact, cases of Type 2 diabetes are up 70% among 30-somethings during the past decade. Since the disease can fester for years, half of Type 2 diabetics have suffered serious damage to eyes, kidneys, nerves, and arteries by the time they learn they are affected, Neergaard said.[8]

The close association between diabetes and heart disease is well known, but a survey reported by the American Heart Association found that only one-third of diabetics realized that heart disease was among the "most serious" complications for which they are at risk. Almost twice that number would have a cardiovascular problem.[9] "Diabetes patients still tend to treat heart disease as a separate concern," stated Sidney C. Smith, Jr., M.D., the association's chief science advisor.

A survey of 532 people with Type 2 diabetes showed that many of them were not taking basic precautions. For example, only 53% said they were eating the recommended number of fruits and vegetables daily (five or more servings). One-third said they did not exercise regularly, and many did not monitor their weight.

The survey further found that there was widespread ignorance about insulin resistance, which plays an active role in both Type 2 diabetes and in cardiovascular problems. Those with insulin resistance are unable to effectively use their body's insulin. They are also prone to imbalances in blood lipids (fats), in which they have too much LDL-cholesterol (the bad kind), too little HDL-cholesterol (the good kind), and they are apt to have higher amounts of triglycerides, which put them at risk for hardening of the arteries.

Researchers at the Karolinska Institute in Stockholm, Sweden, have found that children of mothers who smoke are more likely to develop Type 2 diabetes and obesity later in life. The researchers used data from the British National Child Mortality Survey, which studied some 17,000 children born in 1958. Participants of mothers who had smoked ten or more cigarettes weekly during pregnancy were at least four times as likely to develop Type 2 diabetes as those whose mothers did not smoke. Further, teenagers who smoked had an independent, similarly increased risk of eventually developing diabetes.[10]

An estimated 300,000 Americans die annually from illnesses related to obesity, and the toll may soon overtake tobacco as the chief cause of preventable deaths, reported the *New York Times*. About 60% of American adults are overweight, as are nearly 13% of children, said David Satcher, M.D., the U.S. Surgeon General. Deaths due to obesity have been on the rise and threaten to wipe out progress in fighting heart disease and cancer, Satcher said.[11]

People are consuming more calories and shunning fruits and vegetables in favor of super-size junk foods. But losing 10 pounds can reduce the risk of getting diabetes and heart disease, as can walking 30 minutes a day, he added.

Keeping diabetes under control or reducing glucose intolerance can reduce blood glucose in the lens and protect the eyes, according to researchers at Virginia Polytechnic Institute and State University in Blacksburg, Virginia. In people younger than 65, diabetes can increase cataract prevalence three- to fourfold. And obesity is a major risk factor for Type 2 diabetes. The research team added that, in animal models at least, calorie restriction has enhanced aging and reduced cataracts, so that weight control is a prudent strategy to reduce diabetic risk. Avoiding smoking and exposing the eyes to high-energy radiation is also suggested.[12]

To protect the eyes, the researchers continued, people should increase their antioxidant intake, including copper, iron, manganese, zinc, selenium, and vitamin B_2. Also recommended is consuming free-radical scavengers such as vitamins C and E and beta-carotene. Antioxidants that help to absorb damaging ultraviolet light include beta-carotene, lutein, and zeaxanthin. Other measures to be taken include reducing vascular disease risk for the wet form of acute age-related macular degeneration by reducing fat intake to less than 25%, and reducing the risk of Type 2 diabetes by being less than 20% overweight, exercising, and cutting back on calories.

In a study, 522 Finnish adults at high risk of developing Type 2 diabetes reduced their risk of developing the disease by about 60% by losing as little as 10 pounds, increasing exercise, and making dietary changes, according to Jaakko Tuomilento, M.D., Ph.D., at the National Public Health Institute in Helsinki and other facilities in Finland. The volunteers, with a mean age of 55, were assigned to either an intervention group or a control group. Those in the intervention group were given individualized counseling to reduce weight, intake of saturated fat, and total intake of fat, and to increase their intake of fiber and physical exercise.[13]

Every year thousands of people experience the malaise and nagging thirst that are characteristic of untreated Type 1 diabetes, according to Nathan Seppa in *Science News*. The disease is caused by the death of beta cells in the pancreas. However, Japanese researchers have found that some patients have a kind of diabetes that doesn't fit this pattern. In most of these patients, their own immune cells destroy the beta cells. But instead of immune cells, an unknown agent—perhaps a virus or a chemical in the environment—apparently destroys the beta cells. Further, these patients become ill rather rapidly. David C. W. Lau, M.D., of the University of Calgary in Canada, commented that "the Japanese study establishes an important subtype of Type 1 diabetes that is different from the conventional diabetes that we associate with children."[14]

Patients with this type of diabetes showed signs that the whole pancreas, not just the beta cells, was affected. Ake Lernmark, M.D., an endocrinologist at the University of Washington at Seattle, added that damage to the pancreas might arise from an environmental factor, such as chemicals called nitrosamines, which are derived from nitrates found in smoked meats and other cured foods. In the past, nitrosamines have been weakly associated with diabetes.

A report from the Air Force, while highly criticized, suggested that Agent Orange might be linked to diabetes in Vietnam veterans, reported Gina Kolata in the *New York Times*. Beginning in 1962, about 19 million gallons of Agent Orange and other herbicides were sprayed over South Vietnam to destroy the camouflage the jungle provided Communist supply routes and base camps. Agent Orange is named after the orange-striped barrels in which the herbicide was transported.

The study compared the health of 859 veterans of Operation Ranch Hand, in which the defoliant Agent Orange was sprayed on foliage during the Vietnam war, to the health of 1,232 service personnel who did not use the chemical. It was found that 16.9% of the Ranch Hand personnel were diabetic, compared to 17% in the control group.[15]

"The diabetes effect only showed up when scientists looked at the levels of dioxin, the main chemical in Agent Orange, in the men's blood," Kolata reported. "After adjusting for factors like age and body fat levels, they concluded that the Ranch Hand participants with the lowest levels of dioxin in their blood had a 47% lower risk of diabetes than those with the highest levels of dioxin in their blood."

A major criticism of the Air Force study, said Joel E. Michalek, M.D., an Air Force statistician, was that it is hard to sort out a dioxin effect from an effect of simply being overweight.

Dioxin is stored in fat, so the fatter a person, the higher the dioxin levels are likely to be, Kolata said. But the fatter a person is, the more likely he is to develop diabetes. So is the effect due to dioxin or obesity?

A dissenting view came from Michael Gough, M.D., who was chairman of the federal advisory panel for the Ranch Hand study from 1990 to 1995: "The conclusion I've come to is that there is no evidence whatsoever between low-level dioxin exposure and any human disease." However, John Sommer, executive director of the Washington office of the American Legion, said, "Based on the evidence I have seen, the V.A. should make a decision that diabetes is presumed to be service-connected, based on Agent Orange exposure."

Even so, diabetes is not among the nine diseases, including Hodgkin's disease and respiratory cancers, that the Department of Veterans Affairs has listed as possibly linked to Agent Orange exposure, reported Philip Shenon in *The New York Times*. However, the government provides benefits to the children of Vietnam veterans who suffer from spina bifida, a congenital birth defect of the spine that is linked to the herbicide.[16]

References

1. "Diabetes as Looming Epidemic," *New York Times,* Jan. 30, 2001, p. F8.

2. McClam, Erin. "Obesity Fuels Diabetes Epidemic," Associated Press, Jan. 26, 2001.

3. Hoffman, Barbara. "Type 2 Diabetes Rising to Epidemic Proportions," *New York Post,* Jan. 30, 2001, p. 50.

4. Chang, Kenneth. "Diet and Exercise are Found to Cut Diabetes by Over Half," *New York Times,* Aug. 9, 2001, p. A16.

5. Gorman, Christine. "A Step or Two Against Diabetes," *Time,* Aug. 20, 2001, p. 73.

6. Nagourney, Eric. "When Diabetes Diagnoses Go Awry," *New York Times,* Jan. 2, 2001, p. F8.

7. "Act Now to Prevent Diabetes," *New York Times,* Aug. 28, 2000, p. A16.

8. Neergaard, Lauran. "Diabetes Strikes Adults in 30s," Associated Press, Aug. 27, 2001.

9. Nagourney, Eric. "Diabetics Reminded of Heart Risk," *New York Times,* May 22, 2001, p. F6.

10. Stephenson, Joan, Ph.D. "Maternal Smoking-Diabetes Link Is Described," *Journal of the American Medical Association* 287(6): 706, Feb. 13, 2002.

11. "U.S. Warning of Death Toll from Obesity," *New York Times,* Dec. 12, 2001, p. A26.

12. Bunce, G. E. "Nutrition and Eye Disease of the Elderly," *Journal of Nutritional Biochemistry* 5:66–77, Feb. 1994.

13. Tuomilehto, Jaakko, M.D., Ph.D. "Prevention of Type 2 Diabetes Mellitus by Changes in Lifestyle Among Subjects with Impaired Glucose Tolerance," *New England Journal of Medicine* 344: 1343–1350, 2001.

14. Seppa, Nathan. "Novel Diabetes Strain Has Rapid Onset," *Science News* 157(6): 86, Feb. 5, 2000.

15. Kolata, Gina. "Agent Orange and Diabetes: Diving Into Murky Depths," *New York Times,* March 30, 2000, p. A16.

16. Shenon, Philip. "Air Force Links Agent Orange to Diabetes," *New York Times,* March 29, 2000, p. A23.

2 What Is Diabetes?

Diabetes mellitus has plagued mankind since at least 1550 B.C. This is a disorder of metabolism in which our bodies use digested food for energy. After food is digested, glucose (sugar) passes into the bloodstream, where it is needed by cells for growth and energy. Before glucose can enter the cells, it must have insulin, a hormone produced by the pancreas. In Type 1 diabetes, the pancreas produces little or no insulin, so the patient must take insulin daily. In Type 2 diabetes, the body may produce enough insulin, but for some reason, the body cannot use the insulin effectively.

Symptoms of diabetes include increased thirst and urination, blurred vision, weight loss, fatigue, and other conditions. Out-of-control diabetes can lead to blindness, heart and blood vessel diseases, strokes, kidney failure, amputations, and nerve damage. Regular monitoring is essential.

As explained throughout this book, numerous vitamins, minerals, herbs, and other natural nutrients can help to prevent or control diabetes. If your doctor is not familiar with the literature, ask him/her to read the papers detailed in the endnotes. As for diet and recipes, I do not dwell on these subjects, leaving them to be answered by the patient's doctor or health care provider. My goal is to lead doctors and patients alike to the vast literature supporting a nutritional approach to diabetes.

Writings from the earliest civilizations in Asia Minor, China, Egypt, and India have documented the problems with diabetes mellitus, referring to patients with boils, infections, excessive thirst, loss of weight, and pass-

A Primer on Insulin

Insulin: A hormone that helps the body use glucose (sugar) for energy. The beta cells of the pancreas (in the islets of Langerhans) make the insulin. When the body cannot make enough insulin, a diabetic must inject insulin from other sources (beef, pork, human insulin—recombinant DNA origin—or human insulin—pork-derived, semisynthetic).

Insulin allergy: When a person's body has an allergic or bad reaction to taking insulin made from pork, beef, or bacteria, or because the insulin is not exactly the same as human insulin, or because it has impurities. A local allergy is indicated when the skin becomes red and itchy around the place where the insulin is injected. In a systemic allergy, a person's whole body can have a bad reaction—there can be hives or red patches all over the body, or changes in the heart rate and in the rate of breathing.

Insulin antagonist: Something that opposes the action of insulin. Insulin lowers the level of glucose in the blood, whereas glucagon raises it. Therefore, glucagon is an antagonist of insulin.

Insulin binding: This happens when insulin attaches itself to something else. When a cell needs energy, insulin can bind with the outer part of the cell. The cell then can bring glucose inside and use it for energy. With the help of insulin, the cell can do its work very well. However, sometimes the body acts against itself.

In this case, insulin binds with the proteins that are supposed to protect the body from outside substances (antibodies). If the insulin is an injected form and not made by the body, the body sees the insulin as an outside or foreign substance. When the injected insulin binds with the antibodies, it does not work as well as when it binds directly to the cell.

Insulin-dependent diabetes: Now called Type 1 diabetes.

Insulin reaction: Hypoglycemia.

Insulin receptors: Areas on the outer part of the cell that allow the cell to bind with insulin that is in the blood. When the cell and insulin bind together, the cell can take sugar from the blood and use it for energy.

Insulin resistance: Many people with Type 2 diabetes produce enough insulin, but their bodies do not respond to the action of insulin. This may happen if the person is overweight and has too many fat cells, which do not respond well to insulin. As people age, their body cells lose some of the ability to respond to insulin.

Insulin resistance is linked to high blood pressure and high levels of fat in the blood. Insulin resistance may happen in those who take insulin injections. They may have to take high doses of insulin daily (200 units or more) to bring their blood sugar down to the normal range. This is also called insulin insensitivity.

Insulin sensitivity: This is said to be the normal state in which the cells of the body are receptive to the action of insulin.

Insulin shock: This occurs when the level of blood sugar drops quickly. The signs are shaking, sweating, dizziness, double vision, convulsions, and collapse. Insulin shock may occur when an insulin reaction is not treated quickly enough. (Also see **hypoglycemia** and **insulin reaction**.)

Hyperinsulinism: Too high a level of insulin in the blood. This generally means that the body produces too much insulin. Researchers believe that this condition may play a role in the development of Type 2 diabetes and hypertension. (Also see **Syndrome X**.)

ing copious amounts of honeysweet urine, which often drew ants and flies, according to *Foods & Nutrition Encyclopedia*. The term "diabetes" is derived from the Greek work meaning siphon, or the passing through of water, and "mellitus" comes from the Latin word for honeysweet. The Papyrus Ebers, an Egyptian paper dated about 1550 B.C., recommended that those afflicted with the disease go on a diet of beer, fruits, grains, and honey, which was said to stifle the excessive urination. Indian writings from the period attributed diabetes to overindulgence in food and drink.[1]

"Accounts of the diets of the middle class in northern European countries during the 15th, 16th and 17th centuries described meals consisting of many courses of roast meats dripping in fat, rich and sugary pastries and plenty of butter and cream, but little coarse bread or green, leafy vegetables," the encyclopedia reports. "It is, therefore, not surprising that many cases of diabetes were reported during these times of abundance. It is noteworthy, too, that during this period doctors had to taste the urine of patients for sweetness in order to detect the disease."

Eventually, doctors centered on two schools of thought concerning diet. One school suggested dietary replacement of the sugar lost in the urine, while the other camp believed in restriction of carbohydrates in order to reduce the effects attributed to an excess of sugar. The first school was exemplified by Willis, a British physician who, in 1675, recommended a diet limited to milk, barley water, and bread. The diet was high in carbohydrates but low in calories.

The other school was promoted by Rollo, a British military surgeon who, in 1797, began the trend toward high-fat, high-protein, and low-carbohydrate diets by prescribing mainly meat and fat. Some of the patients apparently were helped by the diets, as evidenced by reductions in the amounts of sugar spilled in the urine. Caloric restriction appears to have been the most effective therapy, since the French physician Bouchardat found that the limited availability of food in Paris during the Franco-Prussian War of 1870–1871 brought marked reductions in the sugar spilled by his diabetic patients.

A major breakthrough in understanding the pathology of diabetes came in the latter part of the nineteenth century when Langerhans, a German physician, while examining a pancreas under a microscope, discovered tiny cells that were different from the rest of the pancreatic tissue; these were later named the islets of Langerhans. Many physicians attempted to cure diabetes

---

Pancreas Basics

Pancreas: An organ behind the lower part of the stomach that is about the size of a human hand. It makes insulin so that the body can use glucose for energy. It also makes enzymes that help the body digest food. Spread over the pancreas are areas called the islets of Langerhans. The cells in these areas have a special purpose. The alpha cells make glucagon, which raises the level of glucose in the blood. The beta cells make insulin. The delta cells make somatostatin. Little is known about PP and D cells.

Islets of Langerhans: Special group of cells in the pancreas. They make and secrete hormones that help the body break down and use food. Named after Paul Langerhans, the German scientist who discovered them in 1869, these cells sit in clusters in the pancreas. There are five types of cells in an islet: beta cells, which make insulin; alpha cells, which make glucagon; delta cells, which make somatostatin; and PP and D cells, about which little is known.

Delta cell: A cell in the pancreas in the islets of Langerhans. These cells make somatostatin, a hormone that is thought to control how the beta cells make and release insulin and how the alpha cells make and release glucagon.

with extracts of the pancreatic islets, but these attempts were unsuccessful. This was because the extracts were contaminated with digestive juices from the pancreas that destroyed the activity of insulin, which is a protein.

In 1921, Banting and Best, working at the University of Toronto in Canada, discovered that they could obtain biologically active insulin from dogs and that the insulin they obtained cured the diabetes of dogs who had had their pancreases removed. The insulin was later given to a male diabetic human, who experienced a remarkable recovery. The use of insulin brought a dramatic drop in deaths due to diabetic coma and greatly increased the years of survival following detection of the disease. However, the insulin initially used brought sharp drops in blood sugar levels (hypoglycemia), which resulted in distressing symptoms.

New forms of the hormone were developed by chemically modifying the substance so as to slow its action. One modification was developed in 1936 by Hagedorn, a Danish researcher, who added protamine, a protein-like substance. This and other modifications of insulin made it possible to use only one daily injection, instead of the three or four originally required.

While the nature of diabetes is still being investigated today, we know that the disease is a disorder of metabolism, that is, the way our bodies use digested food for energy, according to the U.S. Department of Health and Human Services (National Institutes of Health), Bethesda, Maryland. Most of the food we ingest is broken down into glucose, the form of sugar in the blood and the main source of fuel for the body.[2]

After food is digested, glucose passes into the bloodstream, where it is needed by cells for growth and energy. However, in order for glucose to enter the cells, it must have insulin, which is a hormone produced by the pancreas.

"When we eat, the pancreas is supposed to automatically produce the right amount of insulin to move glucose from blood into our cells," the NIH publication stated. "However, in people with diabetes, the pancreas either produces little or no insulin, or the cells do not respond appropriately to the insulin that is produced. Glucose builds up in the blood, overflows into the urine and passes out of the body. Therefore, the body loses its main source of fuel, even though the blood contains large amounts of glucose."

What Are the Types of Diabetes?

The three main types of diabetes are: Type 1 diabetes (formerly called juvenile diabetes); Type 2 diabetes (formerly called adult-onset diabetes); and gestational diabetes, which affects pregnant women.

Type 1 Diabetes: Type 1 diabetes is an autoimmune disease that results when the body's system for fighting infection—the immune system—turns against a part of the body. For diabetics, the immune system attacks the insulin-producing beta cells in the pancreas and destroys them. The pancreas then produces little or no insulin, which requires the diabetic to take insulin daily.

"At present, scientists do not know exactly what causes the body's immune system to attack the beta cells, but they believe that both genetic factors and environmental factors—possibly viruses—are involved," the NIH publication adds. "Type 1 diabetes accounts for about 5 to 10% of diagnosed diabetics in the United States."

Type 1 diabetes develops generally in children and young adults, but this disorder can appear at any age. Symptoms of the disease usually develop over a short period, although beta cell destruction can begin years earlier.

Symptoms of Type 1 diabetes include: 1) increased thirst and urination; 2) constant hunger; 3) weight loss; 4) blurred vision; and 5) extreme fatigue. If the disease is not diagnosed and treated with insulin, the patient can lapse into a life-threatening diabetic coma, also called diabetic ketoacidosis.

Type 2 Diabetes: This is the most common form of diabetes mellitus, affecting 90 to 95% of the people diagnosed with the disease. It usually develops in adults age 40 and older and is commonly found in adults over the age of 55. Roughly 80% of those with Type 2 diabetes are overweight. This disorder is usually part of a metabolic syndrome that includes obesity, elevated blood pressure, and high levels of blood fats. Unfortunately, as more children become overweight, Type 2 diabetes is becoming more common in young people.

"When Type 2 diabetes is diagnosed, the pancreas is usually producing enough insulin, but, for unknown reasons, the body cannot use the insulin effectively, a condition called insulin resistance," the NIH publication states. "After several years, insulin production decreases. The result is the same as for Type 1 diabetes—glucose builds up in the blood and the body cannot make efficient use of its main source of fuel."

Symptoms of Type 2 diabetes develop gradually. In fact, some people have no symptoms. Typical symptoms may include fatigue, nausea, frequent urination, unusual thirst, weight loss, blurred vision, frequent infections, and the slow healing of wounds and sores.

Gestational Diabetes: This type of diabetes develops only during pregnancy. Like Type 2 diabetes, it occurs most often in African-Americans, American Indians, Hispanic Americans, and those with a family history of diabetes. Although gestational diabetes usually disappears after delivery, the mother is at increased risk of getting Type 2 diabetes later in life.

What Tests Are Recommended?

The fasting plasma glucose test is the preferred test for diagnosing Type 1 and Type 2 diabetes. However, a diagnosis of diabetes is made for any one of three positive tests, with a second positive test on a different day:

- A random plasma glucose value (taken any time of day) of 200 mg/dl (milligrams per deciliter) or more, along with the presence of diabetes symptoms.

- A plasma glucose value of 126 mg/dl or more, after a person has fasted for 8 hours.

- An oral glucose tolerance test, plasma glucose value of 200 mg/dl or more in the blood sample, taken two hours after a person has consumed a drink containing 75 g of glucose dissolved in water. This test, taken in a lab or doctor's office, measures plasma glucose at timed intervals over a 3-hour period.

However, there are other tests for assessing glucose metabolism, such as:

- Impaired fasting glucose. A person has impaired fasting glucose when fasting plasma glucose is 110 to 125 mg/dl. This is higher than normal but less than the level indicating diabetes. Approximately 13.4 million people in the United States—or about 7% of the population—have impaired fasting glucose.

Diabetes Facts

Diabetes is widely recognized as one of the leading causes of death and disability in the United States. According to death certificates, diabetes contributed to the deaths of more than 193,140 people in 1996. In 1997, diabetes cost the United States $98 billion. But indirect costs, including disability payments, time lost from work, and premature death, totaled $54 billion. Direct medical costs for diabetes care, including hospitalizations, medical care, and treatment supplies, totaled $44 billion.

"Diabetes is associated with long-term complications that affect almost every part of the body," according to the NIH. "The disease often leads to blindness, heart and blood vessel disease, strokes, kidney failure, amputations and nerve damage. Uncontrolled diabetes can complicate pregnancy, and birth defects are more common in babies born to women with diabetes."

In American males, diabetes is the seventh leading cause of death. Other causes of death related to diabetes in the Top 10 causes are: Heart disease (1st); stroke (3rd); kidney disease (9th); and liver disease and cirrhosis (10th).[3]

All About Glucose

Blood glucose: The main sugar that the body makes from proteins, fats, and carbohydrates, mostly from carbohydrates. Glucose is the major source of energy for living cells and is carried to the cells via the bloodstream. Cells cannot use glucose without the help of insulin.

Blood glucose monitoring: A way of testing how much glucose is in the blood. A drop of blood, usually taken from the fingertip, is placed on the end of a specially coated strip, called a testing strip, which has a chemical on it that makes it change color according to how much glucose (sugar) is in the blood.

Telling whether the level of glucose is low, high, or normal can be determined by comparing the color on the end of the strip to a color chart that is printed on the side of the test strip container, or by inserting the strip into a small machine, called a meter, which reads the strip and shows the level of blood glucose in a digital window display.

Blood testing is more accurate than urine testing in monitoring blood glucose levels, since it shows what the current level of glucose is, rather than what the level was an hour or so previously.

Fasting blood glucose test: A method for finding out how much glucose (sugar) is in the blood. The test can show if a person has diabetes. A blood sample is taken in the lab or doctor's office. The test is usually done in the morning before a person has eaten.

The normal, nondiabetic range for blood glucose is from 70 to 100 mg/dl, depending on the type of blood being tested. If the level is over 140 mg/dl it usually means the person has diabetes, except for newborns and some pregnant women.

Glucagon: A hormone that raises the level of glucose (sugar) in the blood. The alpha cells of the pancreas (in the islets of Langerhans) make glucagon when the body needs to put more sugar into the blood. An injectable form is often used to treat insulin shock. (Also see **alpha cell**.)

Glucose: A simple sugar found in the blood. Also known as dextrose, it is the body's main source of energy.

Glucose tolerance test: A test to see if a person has diabetes. The test is given in a lab or doctor's office in the morning before the patient has eaten. A first sample of blood is taken, then the person drinks a liquid that has sugar in it. After one hour, a second blood sample is drawn, and after another hour, a third sample is taken. The idea is to see how well the body deals with the glucose in the blood over time.

Glycemic response: The effect of different foods on blood glucose levels over time. Researchers have discovered that some kinds of foods may raise blood glucose levels more quickly than other foods containing the same amount of carbohydrates.

Glycogen: A substance made up of sugars. It is stored in the liver and muscles and releases glucose into the blood when needed by the cells. Glycogen is the chief source of stored fuel in the body.

Hyperglycemia: Too high a level of glucose in the blood. It's a sign that diabetes is out of control. It occurs when the body does not have enough insulin or cannot use the insulin it does have to turn glucose into sugar. Signs of hyperglycemia are a great thirst, dry mouth, and a need to urinate often. For those with Type 1 diabetes, this may lead to diabetic ketoacidosis.

Hypoglycemia: Too low a level of sugar in the blood. This occurs when a person with diabetes has injected too much insulin, eaten too little food, or has exercised without extra food. The person may feel nervous, shaky, weak, or sweaty and have a headache, blurred vision, and hunger. Taking small amounts of sugar, sweet juice, or food with sugar, cheese, et cetera, will usually help the person feel better within 10 to 15 minutes. Also called low blood sugar. (Also see **insulin shock**.)

Impaired glucose tolerance: Blood glucose levels higher than normal but not high enough to be called diabetes. Those with IGT may or may not develop diabetes. Names for IGT no longer used include borderline, subclinical, chemical, or latent diabetes.

• Impaired glucose tolerance (IGT). This means that blood glucose during the oral glucose tolerance test is higher than normal but not high enough for a diagnosis of diabetes. IGT is diagnosed when the glucose level is 141 to 199 mg/dl two hours after a person is given a drink containing 75 g of glucose.

Who Should Be Tested?

In patients with impaired glucose tolerance that was documented by a baseline glucose tolerance test, there was a greater chance that they would develop diabetes. The researchers said that only 6% of those with normal glucose tolerance tests developed diabetes, compared with 25% of those with impaired glucose tolerance. The researchers also found that a weight loss of 4.5 kg reduced the risk of diabetes in both those with normal and abnormal glucose tolerance tests at the beginning of the study. They added that making the behavioral changes when beginning a weight loss program is easier than maintaining the behavioral changes to keep the weight off.[4]

People with diabetes should see a doctor who helps them learn to manage their diabetes and monitors their diabetes control, according to the U.S. Department of Health and Human Services (National Institutes of Health). An endocrinologist is one type of doctor who may specialize in diabetes care. Also, those with diabetes often see ophthalmologists for eye examinations, podiatrists for routine foot care, and dietitians and diabetes educators to help teach the skills of day-to-day diabetes management.[5]

Other Complications of Diabetes

A number of researchers have implicated viruses as instigators of beta-cell damage in Type 1 diabetics, especially enteroviruses, which are a group of viruses (such as poliomyelitis virus) that hang out in the gastrointestinal tract but may also be associated with respiratory ailments, meningitis, and neurological disorders. Other viruses related to diabetes include mumps, measles, cytomegalo- and retroviruses.

Several studies have implicated cow's milk with Type 1 diabetes. In animal studies at least, wheat gluten has been associated with Type 1 diabetes. A more common association with diabetes is celiac disease, which is characterized by defective digestion and utilization of fats. Other possible causes of juvenile diabetes include excessive weight gain during the mother's pregnancy, older maternal age, and amniocentesis, in which a surgical needle is used to determine fetal sex or chromosome abnormalities.[6]

Researchers at the University of Chicago in Illinois report that the body's reaction to the loss of sleep resembles insulin resistance, the condition in which cells fail to effectively use this sugar-processing hormone. As reported earlier, insulin resistance produces high blood glucose concentrations that can lead to Type 2 diabetes. A hundred years ago, Americans averaged nine hours of sleep a night, compared to an average of less than seven hours today.[7]

A research team, headed by Bryce A. Mander, Ph.D., brought together 13 people who were chronically short of sleep, averaging less than 6.5 hours nightly, and 14 volunteers who typically slept more than 7.5 hours a night. For 8 days, the recruits wore a wrist device that monitored nighttime movement and sleep patterns. On the last night, the volunteers left a saliva sample, slept through the night, and then skipped breakfast.

Before eating, the volunteers were given an intravenous dose of glucose to determine how each processed the sugar. Those who slept less during the preceding week needed to produce 50% more insulin to metabolize the glucose. In addition, insulin sensitivity—the measure of how well cells take up the hormone and use it to process sugars—was only about 60% as efficient in those getting less sleep as in the more-rested individuals. Additional tests showed that the saliva of short-sleepers contained excess cortisol, a stress hormone, Mander said.

Sleep-disordered breathing is prevalent in the general population, and this has been linked to chronically elevated blood pressure, according to a research team at the University of Wisconsin Medical School at Madison. As previously stated, elevated blood pressure is a risk factor for Type 2 diabetes. Since sleep-disordered breathing is highly prevalent, affecting as many as 9% of women and 24% of men in the United States, a casual association could be responsible for a substantial number of cases of hypertension, including cardiovascular and cerebrovascular morbidity and mortality. The data involved sleep habits of 709 volunteers at the Wisconsin Sleep Cohort Study.[8]

Screening studies in the United States, Europe, and Australia have shown that a substantial proportion of the adult population has mild-to-moderate sleep-disordered breathing, a condition characterized by repeated episodes of apnea (interrupted breathing patterns) and hypopnea (shallower or slower than normal breathing) during sleep, the researchers said. These conditions cause temporary elevation in blood pressure and may cause elevated blood pressure during the daytime and, eventually, sustained high blood pressure.

As reported in the *American Journal of Clinical Nutrition*, the thickness of the carotid artery's intima-media, which is a layer of cells in the blood vessel wall, suggests a person's risk of developing cardiovascular disease, one of the complications of diabetes. A thicker intima-media is more of a risk factor than a thinner one.[9]

A research team evaluated the antioxidant content of blood vessels, along with the intima-media thickness of the carotid artery and the degree of narrowing of blood vessels in 468 elderly volunteers. It was found that men with high blood levels of beta-carotene (provitamin A) and vitamin C had a relatively thin intima-media. And men with low blood levels of vitamin E were two and one-half times more likely to have a narrowing of blood vessels. Women did not exhibit any significant effects with the antioxidants.

The researchers suggested that high levels of antioxidants may help to prevent heart disease in men. Therefore, they recommended that additional studies are needed to evaluate the role of vitamin E, vitamin C, and beta-carotene on the earliest stages of cardiovascular disease.

An estimated 11 million Americans suffer strokes each year that are never detected since there are no obvious symptoms. About 750,000 more people have classic stroke symptoms, such as slurred speech, dizziness, and numbness on one side, according to papers read at the American Stroke Association meeting in Fort Lauderdale, Florida, February 16, 2001.[10]

Megan C. Leary, M.D., of the UCLA Medical Center in California, and her colleagues, released data from two surveys involving brain scans on about 5,500 Americans. They found that strokes are rare before the age of 30, but by the time people reach their 70s, one in three has a silent stroke every year. "Silent strokes are epidemic in this country," Leary said. "They do not cause symptoms right away, but their effects accumulate over the years." The meeting was told that strokes can be prevented by keeping blood pressure under control, lowering cholesterol, treating diabetes, and stopping smoking. Added Sarah E. Vermeer, M.D., of Erasmus Medical Center in Rotterdam, the Netherlands, "Up until now, we have not told people about silent strokes because we didn't know what they mean. Now we have evidence that silent strokes do count."

Elderly people with Type 2 diabetes have an 8.8% increased risk of developing dementia, including Alzheimer's disease, according to Alewjin

Ott, M.D., and colleagues at Erasmus University Medical School in the Netherlands. The study involved 6,370 volunteers, 55 and older, who had not been diagnosed with dementia. Of the study patients, 692 were found to have Type 2 diabetes, and those at highest risk were diabetics who needed insulin.[11]

"Type 2 diabetes is notorious for vascular complications," the Dutch research team said. "It is a well known risk factor for strokes, which, if they accumulate or strike vital brain segments, may cause dementia. An increase in vascular dementia by diabetes is to be expected."

"Type 2 diabetes is notorious for vascular complications," the Dutch research team said. "It is a well known risk factor for strokes, which, if they accumulate or strike vital brain segments, may cause dementia. An increase in vascular dementia by diabetes is to be expected."

As to why there is an association between diabetes and Alzheimer's disease, the researchers said that this was found in patients who were initially treated with insulin. They added that patients on insulin may have more severe diabetes, or a longer history of diabetes, and are thus longer exposed to diabetes-related risk factors. The detailed study was published in the December 10, 1999, issue of *Neurology*.

In the same issue of *Neurology*, Simon Lovestone, Ph.D., of the Institute of Psychiatry in London, England, said, "The demonstration that insulin resistance is associated with risk is important as it might suggest that it is not the long-term aftereffect of diabetes, but something to do with the action of insulin or the regulation of glucose metabolism."

In evaluating serum IgA (immunoglobulin antibody) concentrations in 1,251 Type 1 and 2,224 Type 2 diabetics, researchers in Spain found that IgA levels were significantly higher in the diabetics compared to controls. For example, elevated IgA concentrations were reported in 23.1% of all diabetics. High IgA levels were much greater in males than in females among Type 1 patients. Increased IgA levels are a generalized phenomenon among diabetics, and high levels are a nonspecific sign for the development of diabetic complications.[12] Immunoglobulins, such as IgA, IgD, etc., are antibodies or special proteins that the body produces as a defense against invading substances—antigens.

A study by researchers at the Regional Hospital in Wilton, Cork, Ireland, evaluated 122 Type 1 diabetics for dietary intakes. Daily protein intake was 18% of the calories and significantly higher than the general population. Dietary fat was 37% of the caloric intake, which was also higher than the usual recommendation. Saturated fat was higher than recommended, and polyunsaturated fat intake was low. The average carbohydrate intake was 42% of total calories, which was much lower than recommended and similar to the general population. Sugar intake was lower, and starch intake was higher than in the general population. Fiber intake was found to be lower than recommended but higher than in the general population.[13]

The goal of diabetes management is to keep blood glucose levels as close to the normal range as safely possible, the NIH says. A recent major study—the Diabetes Control and Complications Trial, sponsored by the National Institute of Diabetes and Digestive and Kidney Diseases—showed that keeping blood glucose levels as close to normal as possible reduces the risk of developing major complications of Type 1 diabetes.

The 10-year study, which was completed in 1993, included 1,441 people with Type 1 diabetes. The study compared the effect of two treatment approaches—intensive management and standard management—on the development and progression of eye, kidney, and nerve complications of diabetes. The study found that intensive treatment aimed at keeping hemoglobin A1C as close to normal as possible (6%) was recommended.

Hemoglobin A1C reflects average blood sugar over a 2- to 3-month period. Study participants who maintained lower levels of blood glucose through intensive management had significantly lower rates of these complications. A follow-up study showed that the ability of intensive control to lower the complications of diabetes persists up to four years after the trial ended.

A 1998 European study—the United Kingdom Prospective Diabetes Study—found that intensive control of blood glucose and blood pressure reduced the risk of blindness, kidney disease, stroke, and heart attack in those with Type 2 diabetes.

A variety of supplements may contribute to sugar control and prevention or management of diabetic complications, reported Michael Janson, M.D., in *Dr. Janson's New Vitamin Revolution*. He noted that diabetes mellitus (commonly called sugar diabetes) results from either the reduced function of the pancreas, which produces insulin, or more commonly from the inability of the cells to respond to insulin (i.e., insulin resistance).[14]

His supplement recommendations include: bilberry (100 mg), twice daily; bioflavonoid mix (1,000 mg), twice daily; chromium (200 mcg), twice in the morning and twice in the afternoon; coenzyme Q10 (200 mg), once daily; Ginkgo biloba (60 mg extract), once in the morning and once in the afternoon; gamma linolenic acid from borage oil (240 mg), once daily; alpha-lipoic acid (333 mg), once in the morning and twice in the afternoon; magnesium aspartate (200 mg), once in the morning and once in the afternoon.

References

1. Ensminger, A., et al. *Foods and Nutrition Encyclopedia.* Clovis, Calif.: Pegus Press, 1983, pp. 555ff.

2. "Diabetes Overview," U.S. Department of Health and Human Services, National Institutes of Health, Washington, D.C., Nov. 2000.

3. "Health and Medicine, Quarterly Guide," *U.S. News & World Report,* March 11, 2002, p. 67.

4. Wylie-Rosett, Judith, E.D.D, R.D. "Efficacy of Diet and Exercise in Reducing Body Weight and Conversion to Overt Diabetes," *Diabetes Care* 21(3): 334–335, March 1998.

5. "Diabetes Overview."

6. Vaarala, O., et al. "Environmental Factors in the Aetiology of Childhood Diabetes," *Diab. Nutr. Metab.* 12(2): 75–85, 1999.

7. Seppa, Nathan. "Does Lack of Sleep Lead to Diabetes?" *Science News* 160(2): 31, July 14, 2001.

8. Peppard, Paul E., Ph.D., et al. "Prospective Study of the Association Between Sleep-Disordered Breathing and Hypertension," *New England Journal of Medicine* 342: 1378–1384, May 11, 2000.

9. Gale, C. R., et al. "Antioxidant Vitamin Status and Carotid Atherosclerosis in the Elderly," *American Journal of Clinical Nutrition* 74: 402–408, 2001.

10. Haney, Daniel Q. "Study: Millions Suffer Silent Strokes," Associated Press, Feb. 16, 2001. Also, "'Silent Strokes' Affect 11 Million, Study Finds," *New York Times,* Feb. 17, 2001, p. A11.

11. Colchamiro, Russ. "Type 2 Diabetes Increases Risk of Dementia," *Medical Tribune* 41(1): 5, Jan. 2000.

12. Rodriguez-Segade, Santiago, et al. "High Serum IgA Concentrations in Patients with Diabetes Mellitus: Agewise Distribution and Relation to Chronic Complications," *Clinical Chemistry* 42(7): 1064–1067, 1996.

13. Humphreys, M., et al. "Are Nutritional Recommendations for Insulin-Dependent Diabetic Patients Being Achieved?" *Diabetic Medicine* 11:79–84, 1994.

14. Janson, Michael, M.D. *Dr. Janson's New Vitamin Revolution.* New York: Avery/Penguin/Putnam, 2000, pp. 134–135.

3 Beware of High Blood Pressure

High blood pressure (hypertension) is reported more often in Type 1 and Type 2 diabetics than in the general population. A lower blood pressure goes a long way in preventing heart disease and stroke. In determining a blood pressure reading, physicians evaluate the systolic pressure (when the heart is beating) and diastolic pressure (when the heart rests between beats). Both systolic and diastolic pressures are measured in millimeters of mercury (mmHg). Blood pressure increases with age, and it is more prominent among African-Americans than other racial groups. A reading of 140/90 is considered mild hypertension.

There are numerous ways of lowering blood pressure naturally without the use of drugs. These include vitamin C, vitamin E, coenzyme Q10, fiber, fish oil, magnesium, potassium, calcium, garlic, flavonoids, and others. Caffeine, alcohol, and licorice can elevate blood pressure in susceptible people.

Almost 50 million Americans (25% of the adult population) have blood pressure of 140/90 mmHg or more or take antihypertensive medications, according to *Medical and Health Annual, 1994.* Hypertension (high blood pressure) increases with age and is more prevalent among African-Americans than in whites.[1]

To understand high blood pressure as a diabetes risk factor, let's first look at the basics of the heart. The heart is the center of the circulatory system, which supplies tissues and organs with blood, thus delivering vital nutrients and removing the products of metabolism, the publication said.

The heart's pumping action brings a flow of blood through a series of tubes (arteries) that have an ability to expand or contract. The arteries, which carry blood from the heart to the tissues, divert into vessels of progressively smaller diameter as they distance themselves from the heart, finally dividing into millions of tiny aristoles that cannot be seen by the naked eye. Pulsatile high-pressure flow is converted to the continuous low-pressure flow that is needed for the exchange of material between capillaries—the smallest blood vessels in the body—and the cells. Finally, blood is returned to the heart through the veins.

A person's heartbeat changes the pressure inside the arteries, with the maximum pressure, reached during the heart's contraction (systole), being called systolic or beating blood pressure. The minimum pressure, which occurs when the heart relaxes during beats (diastole), is diastolic blood pressure. Both systolic (the first number in a blood pressure readout) and diastolic (the second number) pressures are measured in millimeters of mercury (mmHg).

"Sometimes kidney disease or impaired circulation to one or both kidneys due to a narrowing of the kidney artery is the culprit in hypertension," the publication continued. "However, congenital narrowing of the aorta or an adrenal gland tumor is implicated. This cause of high blood pressure is documented in fewer than 10% of patients. When no cause is identified, hypertension is called 'essential' or primary. . . . Levels of various hormones produced and secreted by the adrenal glands are elevated in some cases but not in others. Renin (not to be confused with rennin, an enzyme that coagulates milk), an enzyme released by the kidneys, may be present in high, normal or low amounts."

The publication added that even those with well-controlled hypertension have an increased risk of cardiovascular and kidney complications compared with those with normal blood pressure (120/80 mmHg). The relative risk of coronary heart disease rises progressively at every level of systolic blood pressure, from 100 to 129 mmHg upward. A large clinical study estimated that 49% of the coronary heart disease deaths that occurred in more than 360,000 men aged 35 to 57 years of age were attributable to systolic blood pressure above the optimal level. Interestingly, about one-fifth of the deaths were in those with systolic blood pressures of 130 to 139 mmHg, which is considered "high-normal" blood pressure. A number of studies have documented a similar increased risk in women, the publication said.

High blood pressure, as we know, is a major risk factor for coronary heart disease. In one instance, prevalence of hypertension in adults over

18 years of age was 24%. In 1994, for example, 32.1% of all deaths were attributed to heart disease and 6.8% to stroke.[2]

High blood pressure is reported with greater frequency in Type 1 and Type 2 diabetics than in the general population, according to Seymour L. Alterman, M.D., and Donald A. Kullman, M.D. Uncontrolled diabetes contributes to the accelerated buildup of fatty deposits in the arteries (atherosclerosis), and it plays a prominent role in the development of high blood pressure.

It also has been suggested that hypertension may be related to insulin resistance that is found in diabetes and in obesity, they said.[3] With insulin resistance, many Type 2 diabetics produce enough insulin, but their bodies do not respond well to the hormone. This can be due to a person being overweight or having too many fat cells which do not react to insulin. In addition, as people age, their body cells lose some of their ability to handle insulin.

Irving S. Cutter, M.D., of Northwestern University Medical School in Chicago, Illinois, has stated that a relationship between insulin and high blood pressure has been shown by epidemiologic studies since the mid-1980s. The relationship is most prominent in obese, hypertensive patients, as well as in lean hypertensives. Insulin is a vasodilator (it expands blood vessels) and it also stimulates the sympathetic nervous system and promotes the absorption of sodium in the kidneys, he said.[4]

At the Saitama Medical School in Japan, in evaluating 470 men without a history of gastrectomy (removal of part or all of the stomach), it was found that those with a blood pressure exceeding 150 and/or 90 mmHg had a significantly higher frequency of diabetes associated with excess cholesterol in the blood and mild obesity.[5]

When evaluating the men for too much insulin in the blood after a 75 g glucose load, those with hyperinsulinemia (high levels of insulin in the blood) showed a higher blood pressure. Those with too much insulin had a greater incidence of glucose intolerance, abnormal amounts of triglycerides in the blood, low HDL-cholesterol (the beneficial kind), elevated cholesterol levels and obesity. These individuals may be at a greater risk for cardiovascular episodes, the researchers said.

At the National Institutes of Health, National Heart, Lung and Blood Institute, Bethesda, Maryland, Claude Lenfant, M.D., reported that the following lifestyle modifications can benefit people with high blood pressure: 1) lose weight if overweight; 2) limit alcohol intake to no more than 1 oz. (30 ml) of ethanol (alcohol) per day for men, which is equal to 24 oz. of beer, 10 oz. of wine, or 2 oz. of 100-proof whiskey, and 0.5 oz. of ethanol per day for women and lighter-weight people; 3) increase physical activity to 30 to 45 minutes most days of the week; 4) reduce sodium intake to no more than 2.4 g of sodium or 6 g of sodium chloride (table salt) per day; 5) maintain an adequate intake of dietary potassium from fruits and vegetables; 6) maintain an adequate amount of dietary calcium and magnesium; 7) stop smoking; and 8) reduce dietary saturated fat and cholesterol. Caffeine may increase blood pressure acutely, but there is a tendency for the body to tolerate caffeine, a tendency which develops rapidly, he said.[6]

Let's look now at how foods and nutrients can affect blood pressure.

Dietary Foods: At the Kaiser Permanente Center for Health Research in Portland, Oregon, William M. Vollmer, Ph.D., and colleagues reported that a diet rich in fruits and vegetables and low-fat dairy foods, along with reduced saturated and total fat, can significantly reduce blood pressure.[7]

The study evaluated 459 adults with systolic pressures of less than 160 mmHg and diastolic pressures of 80 to 95 mmHg. They were fed a control diet low in fruits, vegetables, and dairy products, with a fat content similar to the average American diet for 3 weeks. The volunteers then ate a control diet that was rich in fruits and vegetables, or a combination diet rich in fruits, vegetables, and low-fat dairy products, along with reduced saturated and total fat for 8 weeks.

The research team reported that the combination diet reduced systolic and diastolic blood pressure by 5.5 and 3 mmHg, respectively, when compared to the control diet. The fruit and vegetable diet lowered systolic blood pressure by 2.8 mmHg more and diastolic pressure by 1.1 mmHg more than the control diet. In 133 volunteers with high blood pressure who ate the combination diet, systolic and diastolic pressures were reduced by 11.4 and 5.5 mmHg, respectively, more than the control diet. Among 326 participants without high blood pressure, the corresponding reductions were 3.5 and 2.1 mmHg.

Studies have demonstrated that consumption of fruits, vegetables, wine, and tea may protect against stroke, which is a potential consequence of high blood pressure. Flavonoids—flavonols, flavones, and isoflavones—have been shown to be inversely associated with mortality from coronary heart disease and stroke. Therefore, increasing flavonoid intake may reduce the risk of high blood pressure.[8] Flavonoids, which were formerly collectively called vitamin F, are found in citrus fruits, berries, wine, green tea, black tea, onions, grapes, kale, cherries, red cabbage, broccoli, beets, radishes, apples, tomatoes, leeks, endive, green beans, and others.[9]

Researchers at the Harvard School of Public Health in Boston, Massachusetts, studied 208 volunteers with high blood pressure (47 years of age, 59% females), who were on the Dietary Approaches to Stop Hypertension (DASH) diet, compared with 204 people (49 years of age, 54% females) on the control diet. The research team found that reducing salt intake from high to intermediate levels reduced systolic blood pressure by 2.1 mmHg during the control diet and by 1.3 mmHg on the DASH diet.[10]

Salt Intake: Reducing salt intake from the intermediate level to the low level brought additional reductions of 4.6 mmHg during the control diet and 1.7 mmHg during the DASH diet. When compared to the control diet with a high sodium intake, the DASH diet with a low salt level led to a mean systolic blood pressure reduction that was 7.1 mmHg lower compared with control diet patients without high blood pressure, and 11.5 mmHg lower in those with hypertension.

The DASH diet proved that a diet emphasizing fruits, vegetables, and low-fat dairy products and which included whole grains, poultry, fish, and nuts, and only small amounts of red meat, sweets, and sugar-containing beverages, with lower amounts of total and saturated fat and cholesterol, can lower blood pressure in those with and without hypertension.

In evaluating forty-six studies on the relationship between blood pressure and diet in children and adolescents, it was found that in thirty-seven trials higher sodium intake is related to higher blood pressure. In fifteen studies, potassium did not give a clear picture of a relationship with hypertension. Nine studies were inconclusive with regard to calcium and high blood pressure. And in five observational trials, magnesium was useful in lowering blood pressure.[11]

Potassium: In a study involving 8 patients over 68 years of age, they were given potassium supplements for 5 months. This reduced their systolic blood pressure by an average of 15 points. The mineral can be found in cantaloupe, potatoes, avocados, bananas, broccoli, milk, and citrus fruits. However, in patients with poor kidney function, excessive potassium may be of concern.[12] The Food and Drug Administration has agreed to allow health claims for potassium in reducing the risk of high blood pressure and stroke. It was found that more than 80% of Americans do not get the recommended dietary allowance for the mineral, which is 400 mg/day. An 8-oz. glass of orange juice contains about 450 mg of potassium.[13]

Garlic: A research team at the University of South Australia in Adelaide evaluated eight trials using dried garlic powder in 415 volunteers to determine the herb's effect on blood pressure. The dose range was between 600 and 900 mg/day, which was equivalent to 1.8 to 2.7 g of fresh garlic daily. The median duration of the trials was 12 weeks.[14]

Of the seven studies that compared the effect of garlic with placebo, three showed a significant reduction in systolic blood pressure, and four found lower diastolic blood pressure. The researchers suggested that garlic preparations may be beneficial for patients with mild hypertension.

Coffee: At Johns Hopkins Medical Institutions in Baltimore, Maryland, a research team evaluated thirty-six studies, eleven of which met the inclusion for evaluating the effect of coffee consumption on blood pressure in 522 people. The median duration of the studies was 56 days and the median dose of coffee was 5 cups/day. It was reported that systolic and diastolic blood pressures increased 2.4 mmHg and 1.2 mmHg, respectively, with coffee consumption, compared to those who did not drink coffee. The researchers added that there was an independent, positive relationship between cups of coffee consumed and subsequent changes in systolic pressure. The effect of coffee on blood pressure was more pronounced in younger people.[15]

At Royal Perth Hospital in Western Australia, researchers evaluated 22 normotensive and 26 hypertensive, nonsmoking men and women (mean age of 72.1 years), following 2 weeks of a caffeine-free diet. (Normotensive means the volunteers had average blood pressures for their age group.) Participants were then randomized to continue with a coffee-free diet as well as abstaining from caffeine-containing drinks or to drink instead 5 cups/day of coffee (equal to 300 mg of caffeine daily), in addition to a caffeine-free diet for an additional 2 weeks.[16]

In the group with high blood pressure, the rise in mean 24-hour systolic blood pressure was greater by 4.8 mmHg, and an increase in mean 24-hour diastolic pressure was higher by 3 mmHg in the coffee drinkers, when compared to abstainers. The researchers suggested that coffee intake restriction may be of benefit to older people with high blood pressure.

In 11 patients with orthostatic hypotension (abnormally low blood pressure while standing), the average systolic blood pressure was 120 mmHg while seated and 80 mmHg while standing. The volunteers were told to drink 16 oz. of tap water, and 30 minutes later the average blood pressure was 145 mmHg while seated and 110 mmHg while standing. The water brought positive effects within 5 minutes of drinking, and peaked about 25 minutes later. The water enhanced the effects of a 14-mg dose of phenylpropanolamine, a drug used to treat hypotension (low blood pressure). In a healthy individual, a 16-oz. glass will generally raise blood pressure by about 11 mmHg.[17]

Vitamin C: At the Boston Medical Center in Massachusetts, 20 volunteers given a placebo were compared with 19 participants (average age of 49 and 48, respectively) who were given 2 g/day of vitamin C, followed by 30 days of 500 mg/day of the vitamin. One month following supplementation, there was a reduction in systolic blood pressure from a mean of 155 to 142 mmHg. There was no effect among the placebo takers. After 1 month, vitamin C reduced diastolic blood pressure; however, this response was not significantly different from that obtained by placebo.[18]

A Western-Electric Study evaluated blood pressure changes over an 8-year period in more than 1,800 white, middle-aged men. It was found that over time, changes in systolic blood pressure were inversely related to the intake of vitamin C and beta-carotene (provitamin A). In other words, those with the highest intakes of vitamin C and beta-carotene would be expected to have a less than 2 mmHg rise in blood pressure over 10 years. Diastolic pressure was similarly affected, although the association was weaker than with systolic pressure. The researchers believe that dietary antioxidants (vitamin C, vitamin E, etc.) may help to protect against blood pressure changes often seen in aging Americans.[19]

At the General Hospital of Athens in Greece, researchers recommended that smokers should have a much higher intake of vitamin C in order to avoid high blood pressure. In fact, smokers need 100 mg/day more of vitamin C than nonsmokers.[20]

Tobacco Use: The study involved 38 habitual smokers who smoked 25 to 40 cigarettes a day. Twenty were normotensive and 18 had essential hypertension. Initially, cigarette smoke produced a significant increase in blood pressure and heart rate in a few minutes in both groups. Pretreatment with vitamin C led to a smaller blood pressure increase, while the heart rate remained unchanged. It has been estimated that the content of human plasma is depleted on average by 50% after exposure to one puff of cigarette smoke, and each puff causes oxidation of about 0.09 mg of vitamin C. Therefore, the risk of cardiovascular disease increases, the researchers said.

Magnesium: At the Norrlands University Hospital in Sweden, researchers conducted a randomized crossover study with magnesium or placebo in 39 patients, ranging in age from 26 to 69. Magnesium was given at 365 mg three times daily for 8 weeks. The researchers reported that 365 mg/day of the mineral given to mild to moderate hypertensive patients treated with beta-blockers could bring a significant decrease in resting and standing blood pressure.[21]

At the Center of Hope Medical Center in Duarte, California, Jerry Nadler, M.D., gave 260 mg/day of magnesium, twice daily for 6 weeks, to 7 Type 2 diabetics with high blood pressure and low magnesium levels in their blood. The controls were 7 patients without diabetes or high blood pressure. The mineral brought a fall in blood pressure from an average of 157/96 mmHg to 128/77 mmHg. The magnesium therapy controlled the blood pressure in these patients. In addition, platelets became less sticky and thromboxane was decreased. Those with abnormal kidney function need to be monitored if using magnesium therapy. The effect on Type 1 diabetes was not reported.[22]

Calcium: In nine studies involving people with normal blood pressure for their age group, calcium supplements resulted in lower blood pressure, while ten other studies found that calcium did not help. In those with high blood pressure, twelve studies found an inverse association with calcium supplements and twelve did not. Reasons for these inconsistencies are not known. Possible reasons are: 1) single nutrient supplementation; 2) high calcium levels in the blood when the study began; 3) small sample size; 4) short follow-up periods; 5) inconsistent screening of participants for other factors (salt intake, salt sensitivity, and calcium imbalance); 6) inadequate doses of calcium; 7) variable blood pressure readings; 8) calcium absorption variables; and others.

However, the researchers said that it is evident from epidemiologic literature that dietary calcium plays an important part in the maintenance of normal blood pressure, and that an adequate intake of the mineral may help to reduce the risk of hypertension. They added that it is also necessary to evaluate the mineral's interaction with potassium, magnesium, and sodium.

At the University of Mississippi, 30 normotensive and 20 hypertensive pregnant women, between the ages of 18 and 28, were randomly assigned to either a control or supplemental group of 1,000 mg/day of calcium for 20 weeks. The researchers reported that there was a significant inverse relationship between dietary calcium intake and blood pressure. The women were taking a familiar over-the-counter calcium supplement.[23]

In another study at the University of Mississippi, researchers evaluated 75 adults, between the ages of 19 and 25, who either were in a control group, or received 1,000 mg/day of calcium, in two 500 mg doses, or were given 24 fluid oz. of milk (skimmed, 2% or whole) daily while following their normal diets. All systolic blood pressures, regardless of the treatment group, declined during a 6-week period. Diastolic pressures went down only in the two calcium-supplemented groups. When total calcium intakes through diet and supplements were studied, the treatment group intakes were above the Recommended Daily Allowance for this age group.[24]

Coenzyme Q10: Ten patients (5 men and 5 women), with a mean age of 61, with essential arterial high blood pressure, were treated at the University of Firenze Medical School in Italy. Each was given 50 mg of coenzyme Q10 twice daily for 10 weeks. Following treatment, systolic blood pressure decreased from 161.5 mmHg on average to 142.2 mmHg. Diastolic pressure went down from 98.5 mmHg to 83.1 mmHg. During this time, total serum cholesterol dropped from 227 to 203, and serum HDL-cholesterol, the beneficial kind, went up from 42 mg/dl to 45.9 mg/dl.[25]

At another study at the University of Firenze, 18 volunteers with essential hypertension were taken off all blood pressure medications for 2 weeks and then given either 100 g/day of coenzyme Q10 or a placebo for 10 weeks. There was a washout period for 2 weeks in which no supplements were given, and then the groups were crossed over to the other treatment for an additional 10 weeks. Following 10 weeks of CoQ10 therapy, the systolic blood pressure went down about 10 points, while diastolic pressure dropped 7 points on average.[26]

Fish Oils: At the University of Iowa Hospitals and Clinics in Iowa City, researchers found that a high dose of 15 g/day, but not a low dose of 3 g/day, of omega-3 fatty acids (fish oils) brought a significant decline in systolic and diastolic blood pressure. These data were confirmed in a large population-based trial in Norway, in which patients with high blood pressure who did not habitually eat fish had a reduction in blood pressure with a 6 g/day of eicosapenataenoic acid but not with a similar amount of corn oil.[27] At Memorial Hospital of Rhode Island in Pawtucket, researchers conducted a randomized, double-blind study of 16 patients, 8 of whom were given 50 g of vegetable oil while the others received 50 g of marine oil. It was found that diastolic blood pressure went down significantly in the fish oil group; however, systolic blood pressure did not change. Triglycerides dropped 30% in the fish oil group.[28]

Fiber: In a 4-year study at Harvard University in Boston, it was found that 30,000 men who ate more than 24 g/day or 1 oz. of fiber daily were less likely to develop high blood pressure compared to those who ate less than 12 g/day of fiber. Fiber from fruit was the most protective.[29]

The men who ate more than 24 g/day of fiber reduced their risk of developing hypertension by 57%, compared with an intake of less than 12 g/day. In addition, those who consumed more than 3.6 g/day of potassium reduced their risk of high blood pressure by 54%, compared to a minimal intake of less than 2.4 g/day. Further, men with intakes of 0.4 g/day of magnesium had a 49% reduction in high blood pressure, compared to those getting less than 0.25 g/day. This study found no significant relationship between sodium and calcium and hypertension.

Vitamin E: High amounts of vitamin E may relieve high blood pressure during pregnancy and lower the risk of preeclampsia. A research team found low levels of the vitamin and high levels of lipid peroxides in women with severe gestational hypertension or preeclampsia. Lipid peroxides are fats that are damaged by free radicals, which increase the risk of preeclampsia. Preeclampsia, which affects about 7% of pregnancies, is a serious disorder in which high blood pressure, fluid retention, and protein in the urine develop during the second half of a woman's pregnancy. It is a common problem for diabetics. Preeclampsia can lead to eclampsia, which brings seizures and may lead to the death of the woman or her fetus.[30]

The men who ate more than 24 g/day of fiber reduced their risk of developing hypertension by 57%, compared with an intake of less than 12 g/day. In addition, those who consumed more than 3.6 g/day of potassium reduced their risk of high blood pressure by 54%, compared to a minimal intake of less than 2.4 g/day.

Exercise: Researchers at the University of Auckland, New Zealand, studied 181 volunteers who followed a sedentary lifestyle and who were on drug therapy for high blood pressure. They were asked to walk briskly for 40 minutes, three times weekly, with or without reducing salt in their diet. It was found that there was significant reduction of up to 7 mmHg in systolic blood pressure for three months for brisk walking alone and salt restriction alone, but not for the combined intervention. There are no changes reported in diastolic blood pressure. The researchers concluded that it is possible to lower blood pressure for short periods, when hypertensive patients increase physical activity and reduce salt intake.[31]

General Recommendations: Researchers at the University of Helsinki in Finland reported that dietary sodium is positively associated with blood pressure, and a reduction in salt intake can reduce blood pressure in some patients. Potassium, calcium, and magnesium can be protective electrolytes in some individuals. They added that omega-3 polyunsaturated fatty acids (fish oils) may help to lower blood pressure. Coffee, alcohol, and habitual licorice consumption may also increase blood pressure, they said. A daily intake of more than 100 g of licorice (equivalent to 300 mg of glycyrrhetinic acid) is usually required to raise blood pressure markedly.[32]

References

1. Roccella, Edward J., Ph.D., M.P.H., et al. "Hypertension," *Medical and Health Annual.* Chicago: Encyclopaedia Britannica, 1994, pp. 333ff.

2. Osborne, Carl G., D.V.M., et al. "Evidence for the Relationship of Calcium to Blood Pressure," *Nutrition Reviews* 54(12): 365–381, Dec. 1996.

3. Alterman, Seymour L., M.D., and Donald A. Kullman, M.D. *How to Prevent, Control and Cure Diabetes.* Hollywood, Fla.: Frederick Fell Publishers, 2000, p. 207.

4. Landsberg, Lewis. "Insulin and Hypertension: Introduction," *Experimental Biology and Medicine,* 1995, pp. 315–316.

5. Maruno, Yoshiko, M.D., et al. "Hyperinsulinemia in Relation to Hypertension and Other Coronary Risk Factors in Japanese Men," *Japanese Heart Journal* 38(5): 685–696, Sept. 1997.

6. Lenfant, Claude, M.D. "The Sixth Report of the Joint National Committee on Prevention, Detection, Evaluation and Treatment of High Blood Pressure," *Archives of Internal Medicine* 157: 2413–2446, Nov. 1997.

7. Appel, Lawrence J., M.D., et al. "A Clinical Trial of the Effects of Dietary Patterns on Blood Pressure," *New England Journal of Medicine* 336: 1117–1124, April 17, 1997.

8. Moline, J., et al. "Dietary Flavonoids and Hypertension: Is There a Link?" *Medical Hypothesis* 55(4): 306–309, 2000.

9. Ronzio, Robert A., Ph.D. *The Encyclopedia of Nutrition and Good Health.* New York: Facts on File, Inc., 1997, pp. 180–181.

10. Sacks, F. M., et al. "Effects on Blood Pressure of Reduced Dietary Sodium and the Dietary Approaches to Stop Hypertension (DASH) Diet," *New England Journal of Medicine* 344(1): 3–10, Jan. 3, 2001.

11. Simons, Morton, Denise G. and Eva Obarznek. "Diet and Blood Pressure in Children and Adolescents," *Pediatric Nephrology* 11:244–249, 1997.

12. "Blood Pressure and Potassium," *International Journal of Clinical Practice* 51: 219–222, 1997.

13. "Blood Pressure and Potassium," *Nutrition Week* 30(42): 7, Nov. 3, 2000.

14. Silagy, Christopher A., and Andrew W. Neil. "A Meta-Analysis of the Effect of Garlic on Blood Pressure," *Journal of Hypertension* 12: 463–468, 1994.

15. Jee, S. H., et al. "The Effect of Chronic Coffee Drinking on Blood Pressure: A Meta-Analysis of Controlled Clinical Trials," *Hypertension* 33: 647–652, Feb. 1999.

16. Rakie, V., et al. "Effects of Coffee on Ambulatory Blood Pressure in Older Men and Women," *Hypertension* 33: 869–873, Feb. 1999.

17. Zoler, M. L. "Water Consumption Can Boost Low Blood Pressure," *Family Practice News,* Feb. 1, 2001, p. 11.

18. Duffy, S. J., et al. "Treatment of Hypertension with Ascorbic Acid," *Lancet* 354: 2048–2049, Dec. 11, 1999.

19. Stampler, J., et al. "Antioxidants Protective Against Rising Blood Pressure," *Circulation* 89(2): 932, 1994.

20. Efstratopoulos, Aris D., and Sofia M. Voyaki. "Effects of Antioxidants on Acute Blood Pressure Response to Smoking in Normotensive and Hypertensives," *Journal of Hypertension* 11 (Suppl. 5): S112–S113, 1993.

21. Wirell, M. P., et al. "Nutritional Dose of Magnesium in Hypertensive Patients on

Beta Blockers Lowers Systolic Blood Pressure: A Double-Blind Cross-Over Study," *Journal of Internal Medicine* 236: 189–195, 1994.

22. Nadler, Jerry, M.D. "Magnesium Lowers Blood Pressure in Type 2 Diabetics," *Practical Cardiology* 16(10): 4, Oct. 1990.

23. Knight, Kathy B., and Robert E. Keith. "Calcium Supplementation on Normo-tensive and Hypertensive Pregnant Women," *American Journal of Clinical Nutrition* 55: 891–895, 1992.

24. Knight, Kathy B., and Robert E. Keith. "Effects of Oral Calcium Supplementation Via Calcium Carbonate Versus Diet on Blood Pressure and Serum Calcium in Young, Normotensive Adults," *Journal of Optimal Nutrition* 3(4): 152–158, 1994.

25. Digiesi, V., et al. "Mechanism of Action of Coenzyme Q10 in Essential Hypertension," *Current Therapeutic Research* 51(5): 668–672, May 1992.

26. Digiesi, V., et al. "Effect of Coenzyme Q10 on Essential Arterial Hypertension," *Current Therapeutic Research* 47(5): 841–845, May 1990.

27. Knapp, Howard R., M.D. "Fatty Acids and Hypertension," *World Review of Nutrition and Diet* 76: 9–14, 1994.

28. Levinson, Paul D., et al. "Effect of N-3 Fatty Acids in Essential Hypertension," *American Journal of Public Health* 13: 754–760, 1990.

29. Faivelson, Saralie. "Fiber and Fruit Protects Against Hypertension," *Medical Tribune* 33(22): 1, Nov. 26, 1992.

30. "Pregnancy, Hypertension and Vitamin E," *Nutrition Week* 28(36): 7, Sept. 18, 1998.

31. Arroll, Bruce, MB, et al. "Salt Restriction and Physical Activity in Treated Hyper-tensives," *New Zealand Medical Journal,* July 14, 1995, pp. 266–268.

32. Nurminen, M. L., et al. "Dietary Factors in the Pathogenesis and Treatment of Hypertension," *Annals of Medicine* 30: 143–150, 1998.

4 The Complications of Cardiovascular Disease

About three-fourths of the deaths among diabetics are caused by cardiovascular complications, including heart attacks, strokes, high blood pressure,and impaired circulation in both large and small blood vessels. Hardening of the arteries and fatty deposits in arteries appear at an earlier age and advance more quickly in diabetics. High blood glucose levels may play a role in the development of hardening of the arteries. Strict glucose control can have long-term benefits by helping diabetics to avoid heart disease.

Nutrition plays a significant role in preventing diabetes, cardiovascular disease, hardening of the arteries, and other complications. Also related to diabetes and heart disease is the refining of our grains and sugar cane, which removes vast amounts of essential nutrients for controlling these diseases: vitamin E, chromium, magnesium, zinc, and others.

Another reason for an increase in heart disease since the beginning of the twentieth century has been the increasingly large amounts of sugar that Americans eat. This contributes to low blood sugar, a major cause of heart attacks. A diet to avoid low blood sugar is given here. Dosages for important vitamins and minerals to avoid diabetes and cardiovascular diseases are included here and in various chapters throughout this book.

About three-fourths of the deaths among diabetics are caused by cardiovascular complications, according to the Columbia University College of Physicians and Surgeons Complete Home Medical Guide. In fact, those with diabetes have a much higher rate of heart disease and circulatory problems than the general population. These problems range from an increased risk of heart attacks, strokes, and high blood pressure to impaired circulation in both large and small blood vessels. In addition, hardening of the arteries (arteriosclerosis) and a buildup of fatty deposits in the arteries (atherosclerosis), which affect many in the general population, appear at an earlier age and advance more rapidly in diabetics.[1]

"High levels of blood cholesterol and triglycerides are common among both men and women with diabetes," the publication said. "Women, who ordinarily have lower blood lipid levels and a lower incidence of heart disease than men, often have very high levels of blood lipids (fats) when they have diabetes. High blood pressure, which increases the risk of strokes and heart attacks, also is very common among diabetic patients."

It is unclear how diabetes promotes cardiovascular and circulatory abnormalities, but a number of researchers believe the answer lies in the abnormally high blood glucose levels in diabetics. High blood glucose affects a number of blood components, especially red blood cells and platelets (which affect clotting), and these abnormalities may play a role in the development of hardening of the arteries.

Insulin seems to increase lipid synthesis in the artery walls, which may promote the buildup of fatty deposits. Since many Type 2 diabetics have high levels of insulin, even though their bodies do not correctly utilize it, a number of researchers think that this may be a factor in the high degree of fatty deposits among these patients. For Type 1 diabetes, insulin therapy inhibits the atherosclerotic process by normalizing blood sugar, the publication said.

Diabetes also damages capillaries, or the microcirculation, which nourish body cells. However, with diabetes there is a thickening of the "basement" membranes, the substances that separate the epithelial cells lining the various body surfaces and the underlying structures. When the capillary membranes become thickened, the vessels are sometimes unable to carry sufficient blood to the tissues they serve, which causes poor circulation, the publication continued.

"The limbs are particularly vulnerable to these circulatory problems, partly explaining why diabetic patients have a high incidence of leg and foot problems," the publication added. "Poor circulation to the lower limbs is particularly common in diabetes, resulting in chronic skin ulcers; leg cramps or pain, especially when walking or climbing stairs; and, in some cases, gangrene and amputation can be prevented by early treatment of infections or other problems."

Glucose Control: Insulin collects in the blood when cells fail to respond to the hormone's signal to take up glucose, as in the case of Type 2 diabetes, said James B. Meigs, M.D., of the Massachusetts General Hospital and Harvard Medical School in Boston. This increases a diabetic's risk of developing heart disease, and it goes beyond the dangers attributed to high blood pressure and elevated cholesterol. It is theorized that the insulin buildup inhibits the patient's ability to break down blood clots efficiently.[2]

The research involved 2,962 healthy volunteers, with an average age of 53, who fasted overnight and then were tested for their metabolism of glucose. It was found that 80% of the volunteers processed the simple sugar normally, while 15% were glucose intolerant, a condition that often precedes Type 2 diabetes. The remaining 5% had diabetes but did not know it.

"Our data strongly suggest that insulin resistance is linked to arterial clotting, but it's still unclear whether physicians could determine patients' risk of heart disease by measuring insulin or other substances that influence clotting," Meigs said.

A relatively new study headed by David M. Nathan, M.D., at the Harvard Medical School in Boston, suggests that strict glucose control can have long-term benefits by helping diabetics to avoid heart disease. Between 1983 and 1993, the researchers tracked 1,441 Type 1 diabetics. The team had chosen half of the volunteers to receive insulin and standard counseling for their disease, while the remaining ones had followed a program of checking blood glucose more frequently and taking insulin injections as needed.[3]

All of the participants were placed on a strict glucose program. After 6 more years, the research team utilized ultrasound to measure the thickness of each patient's carotid arteries, which supply the brain with blood. Thickness of the vessel wall is an indicator of the beginning stages of hardening of the arteries.

Nathan reported that those who had been intensively monitored and treated for 10 years had only 76% as much artery thickening as did those originally on standard treatment. The study reinforces previous studies which show that strict glucose control reduces eye, nerve and kidney complications stemming from Type 1 diabetes.

Chronic Inflammation: Signs of chronic, low-grade inflammation precede the development of Type 2 diabetes, according to Paul M. Ridker, M.D., of Brigham and Women's Hospital in Boston. He said that various studies have shown that inflammation is the underlying factor that links obesity, heart disease, and diabetes. However, other researchers suggest that inflammation may not cause the disease but are merely signals of early stages of the disorders.[4]

The researchers analyzed data from a subset of women in an ongoing study of heart disease, which was reported in depth in the July 18, 2001, issue of the *Journal of the American Medical Association*. During the first 4 years of the study, 188 women in the subset developed diabetes. The women's medical records were compared to those of 362 participants of similar ages who were not diabetics.

The research team found that blood samples taken from both groups at the beginning of the study showed that those who had had higher concentrations of two biochemical markers of inflammation were more likely to develop Type 2 diabetes. Other risk factors for the disease, such as obesity and high blood pressure, were factored in.

It was reported that the quarter of women whose blood had the highest concentrations of C-reactive protein, or CRP, were 4.2 times as likely to develop diabetes after 4 years as were the quarter of the women with the lowest concentrations. The quarter of women with the highest amounts of Interleukin-6 were 2.3 times as likely to have developed the disease. CRP is a protein in blood serum involved in inflammation. IL-6 is involved in the body's immune system.

The Role of Nutrition: Nutrition can play a role in the prevention of diabetes, cardiovascular disease, dental caries, hardening of the arteries, osteoporosis, and other disabling diseases. Nutrition is the keystone of preventive health care, and the knowledge of nutrition as prevention is the responsibility not only of the physician, but also of the general public. All health professionals should be exposed to educational programs in nutrition, but alas, it is well known that physicians and nurses have little training in nutrition, he said. The prevention of disease could result in enormous cost savings to both physicians and hospitals, he continued.[5]

Carbohydrates: In a 6-year study involving more than 65,000 women, those who ate diets high in carbohydrates from white bread, potatoes, white rice, and pasta had two-and-one-half times the risk for Type 2 diabetes than those who ate a diet rich in high-fiber foods such as whole wheat bread and whole grain pasta, according to Walter Willett, M.D., professor of epidemiology and nutrition at the Harvard School of Public Health in Boston. He suggested that white bread and potatoes should be moved to the sweets category on the Food Pyramid, since metabolically they are basically the same.[6]

"What's important in the diet is not just the total amount of carbohydrates but the type of carbohydrate, and the Food Pyramid is remiss in not pointing that out," Willett said.

Low-fiber carbohydrates such as pasta behave like white sugar during digestion, and fiber helps to reduce the rate of carbohydrate absorption. A number of studies have shown that whole grains lower the risk of coronary heart disease and other disorders, Willett said.

Refined Grains: Refining splits the whole grain into bran, germ, and endosperm, and it also removes all but the endosperm, which is the kernel's starchy center, Willett added. Ground fine, the endosperm is converted into flour that makes light and airy white bread, while the bran and germ are segregated to use in bran muffins and mixed into heavier breads that most Americans avoid.

Enriched white flour is nutritionally stripped so that, of the 15 key nutrients in white flour, including vitamin E, only five of them equal or surpass levels found in whole wheat flour. In addition, unground whole wheat is better than ground whole wheat. In studying blood glucose levels in 16 patients with diabetes who had eaten breads made with varying ratios of whole grains and milled flours, it was found that the higher proportion of whole grains, that is, unmilled grains, the lower the blood glucose, Willett said.

Vitamin E: In a study at University Hospital, Queen's Medical Centre, Nottingham, England, researchers reported that fatty deposits in the arteries account for 70% of the deaths in patients with diabetes, and a two- to fourfold excess mortality in those with impaired glucose tolerance. Vitamin E is lipophilic (it likes fats), and when it is incorporated into LDL-cholesterol, this inhibits oxidation. Dosages between 100 IU/day and 800 IU/day have been shown to reduce hardening of the arteries. The vitamin also improves insulin sensitivity, the researchers said.[7] Vitamin E, vitamin C, and other antioxidants fight off unstable free radicals that damage tissues and contribute to heart disease, cancer, arthritis, and other disorders.

Magnesium: A magnesium deficiency is prevalent in diabetes, and this may result in increased risk for cardiac arrhythmias, high blood pressure, myocardial infarction (heart attack), and altered glucose metabolism, reported Robert K. Rude, M.D., of the University of California School of Medicine at Los Angeles.

Actually, the association between low magnesium levels and diabetes has been documented since 1946. Insulin may enhance magnesium transport into the cells, and therefore, insulin resistance may result in intracellular magnesium deficit, he said. In Type 2 diabetes, insulin resistance results when the diabetics produce enough insulin, but their bodies do not know how to handle it. Insulin resistance is also linked to high blood pressure and high levels of fats in the blood.[8]

Rude went on to say that magnesium supplements, either intravenously or by mouth, may prevent complications in those at risk for magnesium deficiency, such as diabetics and those using diuretics (water pills). Initial oral doses of 300 mg/day may be given, but doses gradually increased up to 600 mg/day may be needed to achieve maximum therapeutic effect, he added. Divided doses are recommended in order to prevent diarrhea. However, caution should be taken for those with impaired kidney function.

Chromium: Thirty-five years of research suggests that chromium plays a considerable role in the progression of glucose intolerance and the increased risk of developing diabetes and cardiovascular disease, even though this suggestion has been generally ignored, reported Walter Mertz, Ph.D. Thirteen out of fifteen studies evaluating the mineral's effect on glucose tolerance show benefit by maintaining glucose levels with lower insulin output. In one study, chromium supplements reduced elevated cholesterol, LDL-cholesterol, and increased HDL-cholesterol. A chromium deficiency results in insulin resistance, which can improve when chromium supplements are recommended.[9]

Insulin resistance is a significant risk factor for cardiovascular disease, Mertz said, and it may be more significant in the cause of cardiovascular disease than LDL-cholesterol, the so-called bad kind. Also, he said, it may be more important in the cause of cardiovascular disease than blood LDL-cholesterol levels. Since there is not a good way of diagnosing a chromium deficiency, many physicians ignore the potential benefits of chromium supplementation, he added. (For suggested dosages, refer to the chapter on chromium.)

Physical Exercise: In studying 31,432 person-years from 5,125 female nurses with diabetes in the Nurses' Health Study, over a 14-year follow-up period, there were 323 new cases of cardiovascular disease, of which 225 were coronary heart disease and 98 were strokes. It was found that physical activity was inversely associated with coronary heart disease and ischemic stroke. A faster walking pace was independently associated with a lower risk of cardiovascular disease.[10]

Red Wine: In a study reported in the *European Journal of Clinical Investigation*, 20 Type 2 diabetics (12 men and 8 women), with an average

age of 55.1 years, who had diabetes for an average of 9.2 years, were studied during fasting consumption of 300 ml of red wine, or during a meal including or not including wine. The researchers found that red wine consumption during a meal significantly preserved plasma antioxidant defenses and reduced LDL-cholesterol oxidation and thrombotic activation. Therefore, a moderate amount of red wine during meals may help prevent cardiovascular disease in diabetics.[11]

Sugar Consumption: As Ruth Adams and I reported in *Improving Your Health with Zinc*, numerous scientists have pointed out that the refining of our grains and sugar cane has contributed to all kinds of ill-health, especially heart disease. For example, in the refining of grains to make white flour, 40% of the chromium is removed, along with 86% of the manganese, 76% of the iron, 89% of the cobalt, 68% of the copper, 78% of the zinc, and 48% of the molybdenum, according to Henry Schroeder, M.D., an expert on minerals at Dartmouth College. Only some of the iron is restored in the so-called enrichment program, along with some of the B_1, B_2, and B_3.[12]

When sugar cane is refined into white sugar, he said, 93% of the chromium is removed, along with 89% of the manganese, 98% of the cobalt, 83% of the copper, 98% of the zinc, and 98% of the magnesium.

Carl C. Pfeiffer, Ph.D., M.D., reported that chromium is essential in regulating blood sugar levels, yet much of it is removed during the refining of grains. He wondered whether or not this is one reason that statistics on diabetes are soaring. Chromium and zinc are essential for the health of the eyes, and the removal of these minerals from grains may play a role in the increasing rates of glaucoma, cataract, and other problems.

He added that zinc is essential for the proper activity of the pancreas, which is disordered in diabetics. Yet few doctors prescribe zinc. Manganese is also related to blood sugar regulation, he said.

Writing in *Is Low Blood Sugar Making You a Nutritional Cripple?*, Ruth Adams and I reported that, as long ago as 1933, Dr. J. H. P. Paton, a British researcher, wrote in the British journal *Lancet* that the great increase in the intake of refined sugar may be the cause of the great increase in coronary heart disease and heart attack. He added that there are a number of diseases—obesity, hardening of the arteries, and diabetes—that have long been associated clinically with the excessive carbohydrate intake, which is largely, if not entirely, due to the prodigious increase in the use of sugar.[13]

Speaking at a meeting of the Institute of Food Technologists in May 1974, Fred A. Kummerow, M.D., said that evidence seemed to show that dietary fat cannot be the only cause or even the chief cause of heart and artery conditions. He reported that he had fed an artificial, cholesterol-free egg mixture to laboratory rats, and that all of their offspring fed the new product died within weeks of weaning.

Added David Kritchevsky, Ph.D., of the Wistar Institute, fibrous diets decrease the threat of cholesterol by sweeping the waxy substance out of the digestive tract before it can enter the bloodstream. Other studies reported at the meeting showed that cholesterol in meals had almost no relationship to blood cholesterol. In fact, in one study, animals fed a low-cholesterol diet developed gallstones.

In an article in the *American Journal of Clinical Nutrition* in April 1974, Richard A. Ahrens, Ph.D., said that smoking, obesity, sedentary lifestyle, and stress have been implicated as possible causes of heart attacks, but that "the most striking dietary change (in the past 100 years or so) has been a sevenfold increase in the consumption of sucrose (sugar)."

He went on to say that "it is relevant to observe that the pandemic of arteriosclerotic heart disease continues to increase on a worldwide scale in rough proportion to the increase in sucrose consumption, but not in proportion with saturated fat consumption."

For many years, Benjamin Sandler, M.D., a North Carolina physician, wrote and spoke about how low blood sugar is related to heart attacks. In his landmark book, *How to Prevent Heart Attacks* (now out of print), he outlined his theories on how low blood sugar produces the conditions that lead to heart fatalities. In the book, he discussed a paper written in 1954 by Paul Dudley White, M.D., who was President Eisenhower's physician, and colleagues, who explained that heart attacks were almost never seen before the beginning of the twentieth century.

The authors (in 1954) said, "To realize that the first cause of death in the United States is a disease little known 50 years ago comes as something of a surprise to physicians and public alike. . . . No disease has ever come so quickly from obscurity to the place coronary heart disease now occupies, to maintain itself there with a permanence presumably to endure in this country for years to come."

The answer, according to Sandler, is the suddenness with which sugar became available very inexpensively. He added that our individual consumption of sugar rose from 44 pounds a year per person to well over 100 pounds annually within 50 to 75 years. Today, he said, we are eating vast amounts of the white stuff and the heart attack figures continue to climb.

What foods would Sandler remove from supermarket shelves if everyone in the country were to go on a diet to prevent low blood sugar: practically all of the packaged and processed foods. The only foods the person with hypoglycemia can eat are fresh foods—meat, fish, poultry, eggs, dairy products, fresh vegetables and fruits, nuts, and seeds. White sugar and refined carbohydrates are no-nos. Commercial cereals, loaded with sugar, are also forbidden.

The diet Sandler recommends to prevent heart attacks is very simple and easy to follow. You eliminate from your meals all foods that contain the quickly absorbed carbohydrates (sugar and refined starches mostly), and you eat considerable amounts of protein and moderate amounts of fat. You should eat often during the day so that you do not become hungry and fatigued. Snacks must be high-protein foods such as chicken, cheese, and nuts.

Since they contain considerable carbohydrates, the following foods should be eaten in moderation: baked beans, pasta, rolls, bread, corn, split peas, sweet and white potatoes, lentils, rice, noodles, and all cereals. Because of their sugar content, fruits should be eaten in limited quantities.

References

1. Tapley, Donald F., M.D., et al. *The Columbia University College of Physicians and Surgeons Complete Home Medical Guide.* New York: Crown, 1985, p. 481.

2. Seppa, Nathan. "Poor Glucose Metabolism Risks Clots," *Science News* 157(5): 77, Jan. 29, 2000.

3. Seppa, Nathan. "Glucose Control Spares Arteries in Diabetes," *Science News* 159(26): 406, June 30, 2001.

4. Christensen, Damaris. "Inflammation Linked to Diabetes," *Science News* 160(6): 89, Aug. 11, 2001.

5. Kretchmer, Norman. "Nutrition Is the Keystone of Prevention," *American Journal of Clinical Nutrition* 60:1, 1994.

6. Folz-Gray, Dorothy. "Against the Grain?" *Hippocrates,* Nov. 1997, pp. 54–61.

7. Gazis, Anastasios, et al. "Vitamin E and Cardiovascular Protection in Diabetes: Antioxidants May Offer Particular Advantage in This High Risk Group," *British Medical Journal* 314: 1845–1846, June 28, 1997.

8. Rude, Robert K., M.D. "Magnesium Deficiency and Diabetes Mellitus: Causes and Effects," *Postgraduate Medicine* 92(5): 217–223, Oct. 1992.

9. Mertz, Walter. "Chromium in Human Nutrition: A Review," *Journal of Nutrition* 123: 626–633, 1993.

10. Hu, F. B., et al. "Physical Activity and Risk for Cardiovascular Events in Diabetic Women," *Annals of Internal Medicine* 134(2): 96–105, Jan. 16, 2001.

11. Ceriello, A., et al. "Red Wine Protects Diabetic Patients from Meal-Induced Oxidative Stress and Thrombosis Activation: A Pleasant Approach to the Prevention of Cardiovascular Disease in Diabetes," *European Journal of Investigation* 31(4): 322–328, 2001.

12. Adams, Ruth, and Frank Murray. *Improving Your Health with Zinc.* New York: Larchmont Books, 1978, pp. 108-109, 114–115.

13. Adams, Ruth, and Frank Murray. *Is Low Blood Sugar Making You a Nutritional Cripple?* New York: Larchmont Books, 1975, pp. 18ff.

5 Obesity: A Continuing Problem for Diabetics

Obesity and weight gain are associated with an increased risk of diabetes. In the U.S. each year, an estimated 300,000 adults die as a result of being overweight, and many of them are diabetics. In 1997 alone, the health care costs associated with diabetes amounted to an estimated $98 billion. Because of the complexity of obesity and diabetes, it is necessary for each diabetic to have a diet and exercise regimen tailored to their specific needs. The bottom line is that many of the research studies outlined in this book, if practiced by physicians, might go a long way in reducing the astronomical health care costs related to obesity and diabetes.

Evidence from several studies indicates that obesity and weight gain are associated with an increased risk of diabetes, according to Ali M. Mokdad, Ph.D., and colleagues at the National Center for Chronic Disease Prevention and Health Promotion and other facilities in Atlanta, Georgia. Each year, he continued, an estimated 300,000 U.S. adults die of causes related to obesity. Overall, the direct costs of obesity and physical inactivity account for about 9.4% of U.S. health care expenditures. The direct and indirect costs of health care associated with diabetes in 1997 were an estimated $98 billion, Mokdad reported in the September 21, 2001, issue of the *Journal of the American Medical Association.*[1]

Mokdad went on to say that, in 2000, the prevalence of obesity was 19.8%; of diabetes, 7.3%; and the prevalence of both combined was 2.9%.

Mississippi had the highest rates of obesity at 24.3% and of diabetes at 8.8%. Colorado had the lowest rate of obesity at 13.8%, while Alaska had the lowest rate of diabetes at 4.4%.

It was reported that 27% of U.S. adults did not engage in any physical activity and another 28.2% were not regularly active. Also, only 24.4% of American adults consumed fruits and vegetables five or more times daily. Of obese patients who had had a routine checkup during the previous year, 42.8% had been advised to lose weight. Among those trying to lose or maintain weight, 17.5% were told to eat fewer calories and increase physical activity to more than 150 minutes/week.

"In the past 25 years," the authors concluded, "several promising approaches have been identified as targets for clinical and public health action. To control these dual epidemics, now is the time for implementing multicomponent interventions for weight control, healthy eating and physical activity."

A research team from the Netherlands, Canada, and the United States, headed by Jacob C. Seidell, M.D., stated in the *American Journal of Clinical Nutrition* that a large waist and hip circumference in men and women were associated significantly with low HDL-cholesterol concentrations and high fasting triglycerol, insulin, and glucose concentrations. In women alone, they said, a large waist circumference was also associated with high LDL-cholesterol concentrations and blood pressure.

Conversely, a narrow hip circumference was associated with low LDL-cholesterol (the bad kind) and high glucose concentrations in men, and high triglycerol and insulin concentrations in men and women. They added that hip girths showed different relations to body fat, fat-free mass, and visceral fat accumulation.[2]

The researchers pointed out that other studies have shown that the wasting of leg muscle or low leg muscle mass may be associated with an increased risk of cardiovascular disease and diabetes. "An increased waist circumference is most likely associated with elevated risk factors because of its relation with visceral (internal organs) fat accumulation, and the mechanism may involve excess exposure of the liver to fatty acids, although this issue is a matter of debate," the Netherlands team reported.

They went on to say that the reason relatively narrow hip circumferences are related to unfavorable concentrations of insulin, HDL-cholesterol, and triglycerides is not known. However, there are several theories. For example, narrow hips may reflect peripheral muscle wasting or low muscle mass, which may contribute to both a low insulin clearance from the muscle and low muscle lipoprotein lipase mass and activity with a concomitant reduction in the capacity of muscle to use fatty acids.

The study also showed that the total amount of fat in legs and hips was negatively associated with risk of cardiovascular diseases. They suggested that increased leg fat may reflect underlying hormonal factors (e.g., estrogens) that regulate preferential deposition of fat in the hip and thigh area. In addition, the protective effect of a large hip circumference may, alternatively, be due to the high lipoprotein lipase activity and low fatty acid turnover of gluteofemoral (buttocks and thigh) adipose tissue. The cross-sectional study involved 313 men and 382 women living in Quebec City, Canada.

A research team from Madrid, Spain, found that 54 obese patients were able to lose weight induced by caloric restriction and consuming a Mediterranean-type diet consisting of 35% energy from carbohydrate and 43% from fat. This improved insulin sensitivity and most of the typical cardiovascular risk factors.[3]

Researchers in the United States and Japan have reported that a hormone produced by fat cells may be a link between obesity and insulin resistance that is typically found in Type 2 diabetics, according to Joan Stephenson, Ph.D., in the September 12, 2001, issue of the *Journal of the American Medical Association*. A protein known as adiponectin, or Acpr30, is reduced in laboratory mice and humans, suggesting a role in regulating energy balance. A deficiency in the protein may be involved in the obesity-dependent development of diabetes.[4]

Researchers in the United States and Japan have reported that a hormone produced by fat cells may be a link between obesity and insulin resistance that is typically found in Type 2 diabetics. A protein known as adiponectin, or Acpr30, is reduced in laboratory mice and humans, suggesting a role in regulating energy balance. A deficiency in the protein may be involved in the obesity-dependent development of diabetes.

In two models with Type 2 diabetes, researchers at the University of Tokyo reported that treating the mice with physiological doses of the protein decreased insulin resistance. Insulin resistance was partially reversed in one group of animals by giving them adiponectin or leptin, which is another protein secreted by fat cells. At the Albert Einstein College of Medicine, Bronx, New York, researchers found that giving other strains of obese and diabetic mice injections of adiponectin lowered their blood glucose levels.

While diet and obesity are obviously related to diabetes, this complicated subject is not dealt with to any extent in this book. There are many books now available that go into great detail about diet, menus, and so on. Since each diabetic is an individual, one's diet recommendations need to be reviewed by his/her physician. It is impossible to outline a one-size-fits-all dietary approach to this complicated disease.

References

1. Mokdad, Ali H., Ph.D., et al. "The Continuing Epidemics of Obesity and Diabetes in the United States," *Journal of the American Medical Association* 286(10): 1195–1200, Sept. 12, 2001.

2. Seidell, Jacob C., et al. "Waist and Hip Circumference Have Independent and Opposite Effects on Cardiovascular Disease Risk Factors: The Quebec Family Study," *American Journal of Clinical Nutrition* 74: 315–321, 2001.

3. Calle-Pascual, A. L., et al. "Changes in Nutritional Pattern, Insulin Sensitivity and Glucose Tolerance During Weight Loss in Obese Patients from a Mediterranean Area," *Hormone Metabolism Research* 27: 499–502, 1995.

4. Stephenson, Joan, Ph.D. "Obesity-Diabetes Link," *Journal of the American Medical Association* 286(10): 1167, Sept. 12, 2001.

6 Why a Healthful Diet Is Important

Since diabetes is such a complex disease, nutritionists don't always agree on the best dietary solutions. They do agree that obesity, lack of exercise, and coffee and alcohol consumption are major risk factors for diabetes. A vegetarian, monounsaturated-fat diet is useful for some diabetics. This helps to lower blood pressure, the risk of stroke and heart disease, and other complications that befall diabetics. A number of foods contribute to helping diabetics keep fit, such as soy, nuts, mushrooms, blueberries, olive oil, and others. It's always best for diabetics to have their physician/nutritionist tailor a nutritional program for their specific needs, since some patients have a variety of risk factors and others do not.

A research team at the Harvard School of Public Health, Boston, Massachusetts, headed by Frank B. Hu, M.D., tracked the eating habits of more than 42,000 men over a 12-year period, and found proof that the typical Western diet increases the chances of developing diabetes. Further, they said that a diet high in red meat, processed meat, high-fat dairy products, refined grains, and sweets increases the risk of developing Type 2 diabetes. The risk is worse for those with a sedentary lifestyle.[1]

The researchers, whose complete study appeared in the February 2002 issue of *Annals of Internal Medicine*, divided the volunteers into two groups based on their eating habits: 1) those who followed a Western-type diet; and 2) those who followed a "prudent" diet, characterized by a high consumption of fruit, vegetables, whole grains, fish, and poultry. During the study, 1,321 new cases of Type 2 diabetes were diagnosed. Men with the so-called worst diets were said to be 16% more likely to develop diabetes than were men with the best diets. The health professionals involved in the study ranged in age from 40 to 75.

At the University of Vermont at Burlington, Nancy F. Sheard, Sc.D., R.D., said that the dietary formula most frequently prescribed for diabetics is 15 to 20% calories from protein, less than 30% from fat, and 50 to 60% from carbohydrates. However, she said, recent studies had shown that such a diet may increase triglycerides, the major class of fats in the diet, which is often associated with Type 2 diabetes, lower HDL-cholesterol (the beneficial kind), increased hypoglycemia, and increased insulin levels in some people.[2]

She added that Type 2 diabetics often have lower amounts of fats, glucose, and insulin when following an increased monounsaturated fatty acid diet when compared to the traditional high-carbohydrate, low-fat diet. Vegetable oils such as olive and canola are typical monounsaturated fats. She found that her data support the hypothesis that substituting monounsaturated fat for carbohydrates improves blood glucose, triglyceride, and insulin concentrations while not adversely affecting the LDL– and HDL-cholesterol.

After analyzing a meta-analysis (a complication of many studies) comparing the low-saturated-fat, high-carbohydrate diet or the high-monounsaturated-fat diet for diabetics, researchers at the University of Texas Southwestern Medical Center at Dallas reported that a diet rich in monounsaturated fat may be beneficial for both Type 1 and Type 2 diabetics who are trying to maintain or lose weight. Further, a high-monounsaturated-fat diet helped to control blood sugar levels. As an example, a high-monounsaturated-fat diet reduced triglycerides and VLDL-cholesterol (very-low-density cholesterol) by 19 and 22.6%, respectively.[3]

At the Kerala Agricultural University in India, researchers evaluated the effect of a food on blood sugar levels of 20 Type 2 diabetics, who consumed meals containing 60% carbohydrate, 20% protein, and 20% fat. It was found that the wheat-based meals showed the lowest glycemic response, followed by ragi, a type of millet cultivated in India. The researchers said that the low glycemic response to wheat may be attributed to the high amylose content, which is 27%. Amylose is a component of starch.[4]

As reported in *Metabolism*, 12 patients with Type 2 diabetes had serum total cholesterol levels of 235 mg/dl and triglycerides of 180 mg/dl. The volunteers were given home-prepared meals in which olive oil was the main edible fat, accounting for 8 to 25% of daily energy expenditures in the low- and high-fat diets, respectively. The researchers said that a diet high in total and monounsaturated fat is a good alternative diet to the traditional low-fat diet that has been used for patients with Type 2 diabetes.[5]

In this study at least, the traditional low-fat, high-carbohydrate diabetic diet and a diet enriched with monounsaturated fatty acids, given for 6 weeks, had similar effects on body weight, glucose metabolism, and fasting and after-eating lipids in diabetic volunteers who had fair glycemic control and no significant dyslipidemia (abnormal levels of fats in the blood) at the beginning of the study. High blood pressure and dyslipidemia are associated with abnormalities in insulin metabolism that are independent of overweight and body weight.

In a study reported in the *American Journal of Clinical Nutrition*, 91 Type 2 diabetics were given either about 10% of their energy from a low-glycemic-index breakfast cereal (see chapter 20 on the glycemic index), a high-glycemic-index cereal or oil or margarine containing monounsaturated fatty acids (MUFAs) for 6 months. Seventy-two volunteers completed the study. Those given the cereals consumed about 10% more energy from carbohydrates than did those in the MUFA group.[6]

It was stated that HDL-cholesterol, the good kind, increased about 10% in the MUFA group when compared with those who were given either the high- or low-glycemic-index cereals. Also, the ratio of total HDL-cholesterol was higher in the volunteers who consumed the high-glycemic-index cereal than in the MUFA group when measured at 3 months, but not after 6 months.

The researchers added that a 10% increase in carbohydrate intake associated with breakfast cereal consumption had no adverse effects on glycemic control (control of blood sugar levels) or blood fats during 6 months in Type 2 diabetics. The increase in plasma insulin and the reduction of free fatty acids associated with higher carbohydrate intake may reduce the rate of progression of diabetes, the researchers said.

While evaluating 9,665 volunteers for about 20 years, researchers found that 1,018 had developed diabetes. The participants ranged in age from 25 to 74. It was found that the mean daily intake of fruits and vegetables, and the percentage of those consuming five or more fruits and vegetables daily, was lower among those who developed diabetes when compared to those who did not get the disease. After adjusting for variables, the ratio of those who consumed five or more servings of fruits and vegetables daily compared to those who did not eat any was 0.75 for all volunteers—0.54 for women and 1.09 for men.[7]

A study chronicled the relationship between diet and the risk of Type 2 diabetes. It involved more than 84,360 women in the United States. During the 6 years of follow-up, 702 women were diagnosed with diabetes. The researchers found that body mass index (a formula involving height and weight) was a powerful risk factor for determining overweight and for getting the disease. After allowing for body mass index, previous weight change and alcohol intake, the researchers found no association between intakes of energy, protein, sucrose, carbohydrate, or fiber and the risk of developing diabetes. The researchers concluded that the prevention of obesity is more likely to reduce the incidence of Type 2 diabetes than any modification of intake of specific nutrients.[8]

In a study involving 7 patients with Type 2 diabetes who were vegans, they were compared with 4 diabetics on a low-fat diet. The researchers found that blood glucose levels went down an average of 28% in the vegan group, but only 12% in the low-fat controls. The vegans lost more weight (an average of 16 pounds) than the low-fat group, which lost about 8 pounds. One of the vegans was able to wean himself off hypoglycemic drugs, and 3 others were able to reduce their dosages.[9]

At the Weimar Institute in California, Milton O. Crane, M.D., and colleagues studied 21 patients with Type 2 diabetes and systemic distal polyneuropathy (a nerve disorder). Average age of the participants was 64. The volunteers were placed on a low-fat (10 to 15% fat), a high-fiber total vegetarian diet of unrefined foods, and a planned exercise program in a 25-day, in-residence study. This brought a complete resolution of systemic distal polyneuropathy pain in 17 of 21 patients, in 4 to 16 days. Weight loss averaged 4.9 kg during the study, and fasting blood glucose levels were 35% lower on average in 11 patients. Five patients no longer needed hypoglycemic drugs.[10]

The researchers added that serum triglycerides and total cholesterol had gone down 25 and 13.6, respectively, within 2 weeks. In a follow-up of 17 of 21 patients for 1 to 4 years, it was found that 71% remained on the diet and exercise program. The research team added that a total vegetarian diet is simple and economical and can benefit some patients with Type 2 diabetes.

A high-monounsaturated-fat/low-carbohydrate diet has clinical and metabolic benefits for Type 2 diabetics, according to researchers at the University of Naples in Italy.

In their study, 10 Type 2 diabetics, with a mean age of 52, randomly received either a high-monounsaturated-fat/low-carbohydrate diet (carbohydrates 4.0%, fat 40%, protein 20%, fiber 24 g) or a low-monounsaturated-fat/high-carbohydrate diet (carbohydrates 60%, fat 20%, protein 20%, fiber 24 g) for 15 days. The participants were then switched to the alternate diet.[11]

The research team found that with the high-monounsaturated-fat/low-carbohydrate diet, there was a decrease in glucose and blood insulin levels following a meal, along with lower triglyceride levels.

Researchers in Denmark studied 12 Type 2 diabetics, who were given 300 mg of mashed potato in combination with 40 g of olive oil, 80 g of olive oil, 50 g of butter, or 100 g of butter. The research team found that blood glucose levels after potatoes with 100 g of butter were significantly lower than that after the other four meals. Insulin levels increased with 50 and 100 g of butter, but the addition of 40 to 80 g of olive oil had no effect.[12]

The researchers also reported that the triacylglycerol (triglyceride) levels went up with the fat content of the meals, regardless of the type of fat. However, it was found that butter increases insulin levels more than olive oil, and that large amounts of butter increase fatty acid and triacylglycerol concentrations.

Coffee Consumption: Countries with the highest coffee consumption per capita had the highest incidence of Type 1 diabetes, according to researchers at the National Public Health Institute in Helsinki, Finland. The country has the highest incidence of Type 1 diabetes in the world, and incidence has increased during recent years as has the consumption of coffee, the researchers said.[13]

According to the Diabetes Epidemiologic Research International Study Group, caffeine, the most widely used psychotropic agent, could be a risk factor in utero (in the womb) for Type 1 diabetes. Its half-life is prolonged in pregnancy and is known to cross the placenta into the fetus. The report added that pregnant women who consume large amounts of coffee have an increased risk of spontaneous abortions, premature deliveries, and giving birth to infants with low birth weights. The study added that these results can only generate a hypothesis and must be interpreted with caution.

Blueberries: Anthocyanins, which are natural components found in blueberries and European bilberries, give the berries their color. They also have a high antioxidant capacity. Of the 40 different fruits and vegetables researchers tested, blueberries contained the highest antioxidant capacity. The berries are said to reduce eye strain, control diabetes, and improve circulation.[14]

Nuts: A research team from Pennsylvania State University at University Park has found that, in a review of 11 existing published epidemiological studies, people who consume 1 oz. of tree nuts or peanuts more than five times a week can have a 25 to 39% reduction in coronary heart disease risk. An ounce of nuts equates to about 4 to 5 tablespoons. Among the nuts consumed in the studies were almonds, Brazil nuts (a rich source of selenium), cashews, hazelnuts, macadamia nuts, pecans, pistachios, walnuts, and peanuts.[15]

Nuts are a valuable source of unsaturated fatty acids, the good fats, and they are low in saturated fats, the bad fats. They are also a good source of plant protein, dietary fiber, antioxidant vitamins, minerals, and other bioactive substances. And, of course, they contain no cholesterol.

"However, you can't simply add nuts, nut butters or nut oils to your usual diet without making some adjustments," explained Penny Kris-Etherton, Ph.D., a professor of nutrition at Penn State. "You have to replace some of the calories you usually consume with nuts and substitute the unsaturated fat in nuts for some of the saturated fat in your diet."

Vegetable Fat: The Center for Nutrition Information, Washington, D.C., reported that there is considerable evidence that vegetable fat may enhance the risk of chronic disease when it is converted by hydrogenation to harmful trans fatty acids. A good example is margarine. Diseases that may be affected by these fats are diabetes, coronary artery disease, cancer, as well as reproduction.[16]

Researchers in Japan gave 1 g/day of maitake mushroom *(Grifola frondosa)* to genetically diabetic mice. The mushroom therapy brought reduction in blood glucose, insulin, and triglycerides in the mushroom-treated animals.[17]

Soy Protein: Studies have shown that soy protein, rich in antioxidant isoflavones, can lower low-density lipoprotein cholesterol (LDL) by about 13%, and triglycerides by some 10%. Two studies revealed that soy can lower blood pressure in both men and women. Animal studies have found that isoflavones help to prevent blood clots, which are related to strokes and cardiovascular disease, and another study involving primates reported that soy can improve blood level function, a marker for cardiovascular disease.[18]

In a study involving 24 volunteers, they were asked to eat diets with high-isoflavone and low-isoflavone soy foods for two and a half weeks. The researchers evaluated levels of isoprostanes, which are markers of free radicals—dangerous chemicals inside the body—and free radical oxidation of low-density lipoprotein cholesterol. Those eating a high-isoflavone diet (found in soy) had about one-fourth reductions of isoprostane levels, compared to those eating the low-isoflavone regimen. Also the high-isoflavone diet increased the oxidation of LDL-cholesterol, which would reduce the risk of developing heart disease.[19]

It is known that when soy protein replaces animal protein, it can reduce cholesterol levels in those with elevated blood fats. In one study, 13 healthy premenopausal women, ranging in age from 18 to 35, ate different amounts of soy protein isolate, an isoflavone-rich extract, daily for three menstrual cycles. The women did not have elevated cholesterol levels. Following ingestion of the soy flavones, the women had reductions in their LDL from 7.6 to 10%, suggesting a reduced risk of coronary artery disease. Also, the ratios of total cholesterol to HDL, the beneficial kind, improved by almost 14%.

The study suggested that soy isoflavones can improve the blood-fat profile in women with normal cholesterol levels and that the effect goes beyond helping only those with elevated cholesterol levels, an obvious risk factor for heart disease and stroke in diabetics and others.[20]

References

1. Nagourney, Eric. "New Findings on Diabetes and Diet," *New York Times,* Feb. 12, 2002, p. F7.

2. Sheard, Nancy F., Sc.D., R.D. "The Diabetic Diet: Evidence for a New Approach," *Nutrition Reviews* 53(1): 16–18, 1995.

3. Garg, Abhimanyu. "High Monounsaturated Fat Diets for Patients with Diabetes Mellitus," *American Journal of Clinical Nutrition* 67 (Suppl.): 577S–582S, 1998.

4. Kavita, M. S., et al. "Glycemic Response to Selected Cereal-Based South Indian Meals in Non-Insulin Dependent Diabetics," *Journal of Nutritional and Environmental Medicine* 7:287–294, 1997.

5. Rodriguez-Villar, C., et al. "High-Monounsaturated Fat, Olive Oil-Rich Diet Has Effects Similar to a High-Carbohydrate Diet on Fasting and Postprandial State and Metabolic Profiles of Patients with Type 2 Diabetes," *Metabolism* 49(12): 1511–1517, Dec. 2000.

6. Tsihlias, E. B., et al. "Comparison of High- and Low-Glycemic-Index Breakfast Cereals with Monounsaturated Fat in the Long-Term Dietary Management of Type 2 Diabetes," *American Journal of Clinical Nutrition* 72: 439–449, 2000.

7. Ford, E. S., et al. "Fruit and Vegetable Consumption and Diabetes Mellitus Incidence Among U.S. Adults," *Preventive Medicine* 32: 33–39, 2001.

8. Colditz, Graham A., et al. "Diet and the Risk of Clinical Diabetes in Women," *American Journal of Clinical Nutrition* 55: 1018–1023, 1992.

9. "Diabetes Mellitus and Vegan Diet," *Nutrition Week* 29(35): 7, Sept. 17, 1999.

10. Crane, Milton G., M.D., and Clyde Sample, R.D. "Regression of Diabetic Neuropathy with Total Vegetarian (Vegan) Diet," *Journal of Nutritional Medicine* 4: 431–436, 1994.

11. Parillo, M., et al. "A High-Monounsaturated Fat/Low Carbohydrate Diet Improves Peripheral Insulin Sensitivity in Non-Insulin Dependent Diabetes Patients," *Metabolism* 41(12): 1373–1378, Dec. 1992.

12. Rasmussen, Ole, et al. "Differential Effects of Saturated and Monounsaturated Fat on Blood Glucose and Insulin Response in Subjects with Non-Insulin Dependent Diabetes Mellitus," *American Journal of Clinical Nutrition* 63: 249–253, 1996.

13. Tuomilehto, J., et al. "Coffee Consumption as a Trigger for Insulin Dependent Diabetes Mellitus in Childhood," *British Medical Journal* 300: 642–643, March 10, 1990.

14. "Anthocyanins and Blueberries," *Nutrition Week* 27(38): 7, Oct. 3, 1997.

15. Hale, Barbara. "Nuts Cut Coronary Heart Disease Risk," *Penn State News,* May 8, 2001.

16. McCullum, Christine, M.S., R.D. "How to 'Unmarket' Trans Fatty Acids Out of the Food Supply," *Nutrition Week* 26(7): 4–5, Feb. 16, 1996.

17. "Anti-Diabetic Activity Present in the Fruit Body of Grifola Frondosa (Maitake)," *Biological Pharmacology Bulletin* 17(8): 1106–1110, 1994.

18. Anthony, M. S. "Soy and Cardiovascular Disease: Cholesterol Lowering and Beyond," *Journal of Nutrition* 130: 662S–663S, 2000.

19. Wiseman, H., et al. "Isoflavone Phytoestrogens Consumed in Soy Decrease F2-Isoprostane Concentrations and Increase Resistance of Low-Density Lipoprotein to Oxidation in Humans," *American Journal of Clinical Nutrition* 72: 395–400, 2000.

20. Merz-Demlow, B. E., et al. "Soy Isoflavones Improve Plasma Lipids in Normocholesterolemic, Premenopausal Women," *American Journal of Clinical Nutrition* 71: 1462–469, 2000.

7 Diabetes and African-Americans

A study at the University of Alabama at Birmingham concluded that African-American children showed a greater disease risk than did the white children, even after body composition, social class background, and dietary patterns were adjusted for. In a USDA study, 28% of African-Americans had a poor diet compared with 16% for whites and 14% of other racial groups.

Insulin sensitivity has been reported to be nearly 50% lower, and insulin secretion higher, in African-American children than in whites, especially in girls. African-Americans are often deficient in vitamin C, magnesium, and other nutrients.

African-Americans generally have higher rates of Type 2 diabetes than do whites, presumably because of diet and lifestyle. Inner-city-dwelling African-Americans are at a high nutritional risk, due to tooth and mouth problems, lack of money for food, eating alone, inability to shop, cook, or eat on their own, and other problems.

The disparity in the prevalence of cardiovascular disease and Type 2 diabetes between African-Americans and whites has been well established, and ethnic differences in several risk factors for the disease are evident in childhood, according to Christine H. Lindquist and colleagues at the University of Alabama at Birmingham. They concluded that African-American children showed a greater disease risk than did the white children, even after body composition, social class background, and dietary patterns were adjusted for.[1]

The study involved 95 African-American and white children with a mean age of 10. Cardiovascular disease and Type 2 diabetes risk were determined on the basis of total cholesterol, triglyceride, and insulin sensitivity in which cells remain responsive to insulin's action. The researchers added that insulin sensitivity has been reported to be nearly 50% lower, and insulin secretion higher, in African-American children than in whites, especially in girls.

A study by the U.S. Department of Agriculture in Washington, D.C., found that on the Healthy Eating Index (HEI), computed on a regular basis by the USDA, the mean HEI score for African-Americans was 59, compared to 64 for whites and 65 for other racial groups, including Asian/Pacific Islander Americans, American Indians, and Alaskan Natives. Only 5% of African-Americans, when compared with 11% of whites, had a good diet.[2]

Overall, 28% of African-Americans had a poor diet compared with 16% of whites and 14% of other racial groups. African-Americans are especially prone to less-than-ideal diets, the USDA said.

A study reported in the *Journal of the American Geriatric Society* evaluated older inner-city black Americans to see if they were at nutritional risk. Four hundred people over 69 years of age in north St. Louis, Missouri, and a community-based sample of 115 residents aged 50 and older living in public housing in East St. Louis, Illinois, were compared to a 90% white group from New England.[3]

When compared with the mostly white population in New England, both of the African-American groups showed a particularly high prevalence for limited intake of fruits, vegetables, and milk. Tooth and mouth problems, lack of money for food, eating alone, inability to shop, cook, or eat on their own were some of the significant problems. The researchers said that these data suggest that inner-city-dwelling older African-Americans are at high nutritional risk. Improvement in the nutrient content of the diet, oral health, depressive symptoms, and general health could improve the status of these individuals. Group meals and assistance with shopping and cooking would be beneficial.

In a study of 120 nonpregnant patients, 18 years of age or older, it was found that there was a 20% prevalence of low magnesium levels among the predominantly female, African-American population. Low magnesium stores were most pronounced in those with a history of alcoholism, and among those having one or more of the following medical conditions: diabetes, high blood pressure, kidney disease, asthma, and elevated cholesterol and triglyceride levels.[4]

At Johns Hopkins Medical Institutions, Baltimore, Maryland, a study evaluated 87 healthy African-Americans, 27 to 65 years of age, with slightly elevated blood pressure. A 21-day intervention with a low-potassium diet, followed by a potassium supplement or a placebo, showed that the supplement reduced blood pressure substantially in the African-Americans consuming a low-potassium diet.[5]

A research team at the Veterans Affairs Medical Center in Washington, D.C., evaluated 46 men, ranging in age from 35 to 76, who were assigned to an exercise program plus a high blood pressure medication, or an antihypertensive drug alone. It was found that regular exercise reduced blood pressure and enlargement of the left ventricle (in the heart) in African-Americans who had elevated high blood pressure. The exercise programs lasted 16 to 32 weeks and involved working out on a stationary bike 3 times weekly for a median time of 44 minutes.[6]

At Colorado State University at Fort Collins, researchers studied 172 African-American volunteers (mean age 48) whose vitamin C levels were inversely related to malondialdehyde levels; their systolic and diastolic blood pressure, serum cholesterol, and HDL-cholesterol (the good kind) were positively correlated with the amount of vitamin C in their blood. Malondialdehyde is a marker for fatty acid oxidation.[7]

Researchers at the Centers for Disease Control and Prevention in Atlanta, Georgia, found that, overall, about 27% of Americans had low levels of vitamin E, but that 41% of African-Americans had low levels of the vitamin; 28% of Hispanics; and 32% of other racial groups. The conclusions came after analyzing blood levels of 16,000 people nationwide. They added that high intakes of vitamin E or supplementation may reduce the risk of chronic diseases.[8]

African-Americans, Asian-Americans, Latinos, and Native Americans have higher rates of Type 2 diabetes than do Caucasians: it's about 60% higher in African-Americans and about 110 to 120% higher among Latinos, according to Maria Thomas in *The Unofficial Guide to Living with Diabetes*. However, Native Americans have the highest incidence of Type 2 diabetes in the world.

For example, in some Native American groups, such as the Pima Indians, rates among adults are as high as 50%. It is suggested that, as Native Americans become assimilated into modern American culture, the transition from their traditional foods to a diet rich in processed foods, their metabolism is unable to cope with the change. Latino groups such as Mexican Americans, who share genes with Native American groups, have higher rates of Type 2 diabetes than do Latino people who do not share these genes, such as Cuban Americans, Thomas said.[9]

References

1. Lindquist, Christine H., et al. "Role of Dietary Factors in Ethnic Differences in Early Risk of Cardiovascular Disease and Type 2 Diabetes," *American Journal of Clinical Nutrition* 71: 725–732, 2000.

2. "Report Card on the Diet Quality of African-Americans," Center for Nutrition Policy and Promotion, USDA, Washington, D.C., *Nutrition Week* 28(28): 4–5, July 24, 1998.

3. Miller, Douglas L., et al. "Nutritional Risk in Inner-City-Dwelling Older Black Americans," *Journal of the American Geriatric Society* 44: 959–962, 1996.

4. Fox, C. H., et al. "An Investigation of Hypomagnesemia Among Ambulatory, Urban, African-Americans," *Journal of Family Practice* 48(8): 636-639, Aug. 1999.

5. Brancati, Frederick L., M.D., et al. "Effect of Potassium Supplementation on Blood Pressure in African-Americans on a Low-Potassium Diet," *Archives of Internal Medicine* 156: 61–67, Jan. 8, 1996.

6. Kokkinos, Peter F., Ph.D., et al. "Effects of Regular Exercise on Blood Pressure and Left Ventricular Hypertrophy in African-American Men with Severe Hypertension," *New England Journal of Medicine* 333(22): 1462–1467, Nov. 30, 1995.

7. Toohey, Lynn, et al. "Plasma Ascorbic Acid Concentrations Are Related to Cardiovascular Risk Factors in African-Americans," *Journal of Nutrition* 126: 121–128, 1996.

8. Ford, E. S., and A. Sowell. "Serum Alpha-Tocopherol Status in the United States Population: Findings from the Third National Health and Nutrition Examination Survey," *American Journal of Epidemiology* 150: 290–300, 1999.

9. Thomas, Maria, and Loren W. Greene, M.D. *The Unofficial Guide to Living with Diabetes*. New York: Macmillan, 1999, p. 43.

8 Diabetes and Women

Obesity, weight gain, cigarette smoking, a low-fiber diet, a diet with foods high on the glycemic index, and a sedentary lifestyle are some of the risk factors for diabetes in women. According to an article from the British Journal of Nutrition, *omega-3 fatty acids from fish oils inhibit the formation of thromboxane A2, which promotes blood thickness and may lead to blood clots in women with preeclampsia, a potentially dangerous condition during pregnancy. Free radicals, which are dangerous roving molecules that can cause cataracts, heart disease, aging, and other problems, can be inactivated with vitamins E and C, and other antioxidants.*

Women with gestational diabetes are often deficient in vitamin B_1, even though they may be getting a multivitamin supplement. The incidence of Type 2 diabetes in women could be reduced if they would switch from hydrogenated vegetable oils (margarine, etc.) to unhydrogenated polyunsaturated fatty acids (corn oil, safflower oil, etc.). A chromium deficiency may be related to gestational diabetes. Also, cod liver oil, rich in omega-3 fatty acids and vitamin D, may offer infants a protective effect against Type 1 diabetes.

Pregnant women with diabetes are often deficient in some vitamins and minerals due to losses from frequent urination. Magnesium, potassium, chromium, and vitamin B_6 are especially lacking, and supplements may be warranted.

Several lifestyle factors affect the incidence of Type 2 diabetes, especially in women, according to Frank B. Hu, M.D., and colleagues at the Harvard School of Public Health and other facilities in Boston,

Massachusetts. Obesity and weight gain dramatically increase the risk, and physical inactivity further elevates the risk, independently of obesity. They added that cigarette smoking is associated with a small increase, and moderate alcohol consumption with a decrease in the risk of diabetes. Also, a low-fiber diet with a high glycemic index has been associated with an increased risk of diabetes, and specific dietary fatty acids may differentially affect insulin resistance and the risk of diabetes.[1]

Several lifestyle factors affect the incidence of Type 2 diabetes, especially in women. Obesity and weight gain dramatically increase the risk, and physical inactivity further elevates the risk, independently of obesity. Cigarette smoking is associated with a small increase, and moderate alcohol consumption with a decrease in the risk of diabetes.

In the study, the researchers followed 84,941 female nurses from 1980 to 1996. The volunteers were free of diagnosed cardiovascular disease, diabetes, and cancer as the study began. A low-risk group was defined according to various variables: a body-mass index (the weight in kilograms divided by the square of the height in meters) of less than 25; a diet that was high in cereal fiber and polyunsaturated fat and low in trans fat and glycemic load (which reflects the effect of diet on blood glucose levels); amount of moderate-to-vigorous physical activity for at least half an hour per day; no smoking; and the consumption of an average of at least half a drink of an alcoholic beverage daily.

"During 16 years of follow-up," the researchers reported, "we documented 3,300 new cases of Type 2 diabetes. Overweight or obesity was the single most important predictor of diabetes. Lack of exercise, a poor diet, current smoking, and abstinence from alcohol use were all associated with a significant increased risk of diabetes, even after adjustment for body-mass index."

The researchers concluded by saying that the majority of cases of Type 2 diabetes could be prevented by weight loss, regular exercise, modification of diet, abstinence from smoking, and limited amounts of alcohol, with weight control being of the greatest benefit.

A research team at Sansum Medical Research Foundation in Santa Barbara, California, reported that dietary intervention to minimize glucose changes and decrease insulin secretion, using low-carbohydrate diets, might result in decreasing the prevalence of diabetes in women who had previously been diagnosed with gestational diabetes, which develops during a women's pregnancy. In the study, calories consisted of nutritional supplement bars, except for the evening meal, which consisted of one-third of caloric needs. The 12-week trial involved 23 obese women, 13 of whom had had gestational diabetes.[2]

Each volunteer was allocated to a treatment regimen for 6 weeks, then crossed over to the alternate plan for another 6 weeks. The women with previous gestational diabetes were similar to the obese women without gestational diabetes, except that those with gestational diabetes had higher levels of glucose on a glucose tolerance test, and higher fasting insulin levels that were consistent with greater insulin resistance. Weight loss was similar in both groups for the first 6 weeks, but was reduced in all groups during the final 6 weeks, regardless of diabetic history or treatment group.

The participants with or without a history of gestational diabetes had higher triglycerides while on a 55% carbohydrate diet than while on a 40% carbohydrate diet. The researchers pointed out that a weight loss regimen that consists of 40% carbohydrates results in lower triglyceride levels than those attained with a 55% carbohydrate diet in obese women. Further, the hypoglycemic diet with the higher fat content brought the more favorable amounts of fat to all of the obese women. Those who switched to a 55% carbohydrate diet from 40% showed an increase in serum triglycerides, whereas those who switched to 40% from 55% showed a decrease.

At the Center for Child Diabetes in Denver, Colorado, researchers determined that the use of oral contraceptives by young women with Type 1 diabetes does not pose an additional risk for diabetic retinopathy and/or nephropathy (eye or kidney problems). The study involved 43 diabetic women who had used the pill for an average of 3.4 years, compared with 43 diabetic women who had not used contraceptives. Mean age and duration of diabetes was 22.7 and 13.8 years. The researchers reported that hemoglobin A1C levels, mean albumin excretion rates, and mean eye grades were not significantly different between the two groups. Eye and kidney problems are difficult to control in some diabetics.[3]

A study at the Department of Obstetrics and Gynecology in Leuven, Belgium, evaluated the excretion of urinary thromboxane A2 metabolites in 24 Type 1 pregnant diabetics, and 20 women with normal pregnancies between 28 and 32 weeks of gestation. The amount of the two metabolites measured was significantly higher in the diabetic women. These findings imply a role for thromboxane in the development of preeclampsia, especially in diabetics. Preeclampsia is the development of high blood pressure during pregnancy, which is sometimes life-threatening. Thromboxanes are any of several substances which can promote blood clots, among other things.[4]

According to an article in the *British Journal of Nutrition,* omega-3 fatty acids from fish oils inhibit the formation of thromboxane A2, which promotes the clumping of platelets and leads to clotting. Fish oils may have a greater effect than aspirin because they increase the production of prostacyclin 13, which is useful in lowering blood pressure, increasing blood viscosity and other variables which prevent preeclampsia.[5]

In studying 43,500 women in the Nurses' Health Study, it was found that body-mass index, the waist-hip ratio, and waist circumference were powerful independent predictors for Type 2 diabetes in American women.[6]

Writing in the *American Journal of Epidemiology,* researchers stated that free radicals play key roles in aging and the development of degenerative diseases. Free radicals, which often contain oxygen, are unstable molecules produced by external sources and in-body metabolism, which can damage cells and lead to high blood pressure, hardening of the arteries, cataracts, aging, and other problems.[7]

The researchers evaluated more than 60,000 middle-aged nurses who have participated in the long-term study on the relationship between diet, lifestyle, and disease. Their focus was on the relationship between cataract, diabetes, and heart disease.

It was found that the risk of cataract was higher among those women with diabetes than without the disease. The finding is significant because both diseases are associated with raised levels of free radicals. Also, cataracts were strongly associated with eventual death from heart disease, which is also related to high levels of free radicals. The researchers added that antioxidants—vitamins E and C—may serve as a beneficial intervention.

Thiamine, B_1: In evaluating 77 mothers and newborns at birth, 19% of the pregnancies were found to be deficient in thiamine (B_1), in spite of vitamin supplementation and treatment for gestational diabetes. The newborn's blood had significantly higher levels of vitamin B_1 than did the pregnant women. Cord blood from newborns born to mothers who were treated with insulin for gestational diabetes had significantly higher vitamin B_1 concentrations than other newborns. Low levels of B_1 are frequently found in pregnant women in spite of vitamin supplementation, suggesting that the fetus is getting first dibs on the vitamin.[8]

Physical Exercise: In the Nurses' Health Study, researchers at Harvard University in Boston, Massachusetts, evaluated 31,432 person-years from 5,125 female nurses with diabetes during a 14-year follow-up. During that time, 323 cases of cardiovascular disease were recorded, including 225 with coronary heart disease and 98 with strokes. Levels of exercise were inversely associated with coronary heart disease and ischemic stroke. Also, a faster walking pace was independently associated with a lower risk for cardiovascular disease.[9]

Fats: Excess body fat because of an imbalance between energy intake and physical activity is a major risk factor for Type 2 diabetes, according to Jorge Salmeron and colleagues at the Harvard School of Public Health and other facilities in Boston, Massachusetts. Their study suggests that total and saturated fat and monounsaturated fatty acid intakes are not associated with risk of Type 2 diabetes in women, but that trans fatty acids increase, and polyunsaturated fatty acids reduce, risk of developing the disease. Substituting nonhydrogenated polyunsaturated fatty acids for trans fatty acids would likely reduce the risk of Type 2 diabetes substantially, they additionally reported in the *American Journal of Clinical Nutrition.*[10]

Their study, based on a 14-year follow-up in the Nurses' Health Study, estimated that replacing 5% of energy from saturated fatty acids with energy from polyunsaturated fatty acids was associated with a 35% lower risk, and that replacing 2% of energy from trans fatty acids with polyunsaturated fatty acids was associated with a 40% lower risk of developing Type 2 diabetes.

"Because the average intake of trans fatty acids from partially hydrogenated vegetable oils (margarine, etc.) is less than 3% of energy in the United States, our data suggest that the incidence of Type 2 diabetes could be reduced by about 40% if these oils were consumed in their original unhydrogenated form (corn oil, safflower oil, sunflower oil, etc.)."

Chromium: A deficiency in chromium might be related to gestational diabetes in pregnant women, according to a study at the Israel Institute of Technology in Haifa, Israel. The results were determined after analyzing hair samples from normal and pregnant diabetic women.[11]

Fish Oils: In a study of 85 diabetic volunteers compared to 1,071 controls, the offspring of mothers who took cod liver oil during their pregnancy had a lower risk of diabetes, with an odds ratio of 0.30. Mothers given multivitamin supplements during their pregnancy, and infants given cod liver oil as well as other vitamin D supplements during the first year of life, were not significantly associated with diabetes. It is believed that either vitamin D or the omega-3 fatty acids EPA (eicosapentaenoic acid) and DHA (docosahexaenoic acid) that are found in cod liver oil, or a combination of the two, have a protective effect against Type 1 diabetes.[12]

Vitamins C and E: Preeclampsia, which generates toxic compounds in pregnant women, raises blood pressure and endangers the lives of both mother and fetus, often resulting in premature delivery. Researchers in England gave women either 400 IU/day of natural vitamin E (d-alpha tocopherol) and 1,000 mg/day of vitamin C, or placebos, to 160 women at risk for preeclampsia. Supplements were begun at 16 and 22 weeks of gestation.

Women given the two supplements had a 76% lower risk of developing preeclampsia when compared to those in the control group getting look-alike supplements. The researchers concluded that the supplements are a safe and inexpensive way of preventing preeclampsia.[13]

Calcium: Calcium supplementation lowers diastolic blood pressure (when the heart is resting between beats) in women with pregnancy-induced high blood pressure, but not in normotensive women, that is, those with normal blood pressure, according to a research team at Auburn University in Alabama. The study involved 20 pregnant women with high blood pressure and 30 pregnant women without the problem. The women ranged in age from 18 to 28. During the 20-week study, the women received 1,000 mg/day of calcium. The volunteers entered the study at 12 weeks of gestation and were evaluated until they delivered.[14]

Supplementation: At the Samsun Medical Research Foundation in Santa Barbara, California, Lois Jovanovic-Peterson, M.D., stated that pregnant women with diabetes need extra vitamins and minerals because of increased nutrient losses in the urine because of frequent urination. For example, deficiencies are often found in magnesium, potassium, chromium, and vitamin B6. Vitamin and mineral supplements may help to prevent pregnancy-related glucose intolerance, especially when the above-mentioned nutrients are prescribed.[15]

Estrogen: Physicians often prescribe estrogen-based drugs to reduce the risk of coronary artery disease in women. Unfortunately, these drugs often increase the risk of side effects, according to an article in *Circulation.*[16]

The researchers studied the effects of genistein, the predominant antioxidant isoflavone in soybeans. Genistein is a weak estrogenic compound that has about 1/100th the potency of the hormone estrogen. It is thought that some of the beneficial effects of soy include the lowering of cholesterol levels in the blood, the result of this subtle estrogen-like effect.

In the study, the researchers inoculated genistein, one of four main isoflavones in soy, into the forearms of healthy men, ranging in age from 20 to 51, and healthy premenopausal women, ages 29 to 33. The research team also measured the effects of daidzein, another soy isoflavone, as well as actual estrogen.

It was reported that genistein increased forearm vasodilation (expansion of blood vessels) by two to three times, with the effect being about the same as with estrogen. There was no benefit from daidzein. Improved vasodilation is a sign of healthy blood vessels.

References

1. Hu, Frank B., M.D., et al. "Diet, Lifestyle and the Risk of Type 2 Diabetes in Women," *New England Journal of Medicine* 345(11): 790–797, Sept. 13, 2001.

2. Peterson, Charles M., M.D., and Lois Jovanovic-Peterson, M.D. "Randomized Crossover Study of 40% Versus 55% Carbohydrate Weight Loss Strategies in Women with Previous Gestational Diabetes Mellitus and Non-Diabetic Women of 130-200% Ideal Body Weight," *Journal of the American College of Nutrition* 14(4): 369–375, 1995.

3. Garg, Satish K., M.D., et al. "Oral Contraceptives and Renal and Retinal Complication in Young Women with Insulin-Dependent Diabetes Mellitus," *Journal of the American Medical Association* 271(14): 1099–1102, April 13, 1994.

4. Van Assche, F. Andre, M.D., et al. "Increased Thromboxane Formation in Diabetic Pregnancy as a Possible Contributor to Preeclampsia," *American Journal of Obstetrics and Gynecology* 168(1): 84–87, Jan. 1993.

5. Olsen, Sjurdur F., and Niels J. Secher. "A Possible Preventive Effect of Low-Dose Fish Oil on Early Delivery and Preeclampsia: Indications from a 50-Year-Old Controlled Trial," *British Journal of Nutrition* 64: 599–609, 1990.

6. Carey, Vincent J., et al. "Body Fat Distribution and Risk of Non-Insulin Dependent Diabetes Mellitus in Women: The Nurses' Health Study," *American Journal of Epidemiology* 145(7): 614–619, 1997.

7. Hu, F. B., et al. "Prospective Study of Cataract Extraction and Risk of Coronary Heart Disease in Women," *American Journal of Epidemiology* 153: 875–881, 2001.

8. Baker, H., et al. "Thiamin Status of Gravidas Treated for Gestational Diabetes Mellitus Compared to Their Neonates At Parturition," *Internal Journal of Vitamin and Nutrition Research* 70(6): 317–320, 2000.

9. Hu, F. B., et al. "Physical Activity and Risk for Cardiovascular Events in Diabetic Women," *Annals of Internal Medicine* 134(2): 96–105, Jan. 16, 2001.

10. Salmeron, Jorge, et al. "Dietary Fat Intake and Risk of Type 2 Diabetes in Women," *American Journal of Clinical Nutrition* 73: 1019–1026, 2001.

11. Aharoni, A., et al. "Hair Chromium Content of Women with Gestational Diabetes Compared with Nondiabetic Pregnant Women," *American Journal of Clinical Nutrition* 55: 104–107, 1992.

12. Stene, L. C., et al. "Use of Cod Liver Oil During Pregnancy Associated with Lower Risk of Type 1 Diabetes in the Offspring," *Diabetologia* 43: 1093–1098, 2000.

13. Chappell, L. C., et al. "Effect of Antioxidants on the Occurrence of Preeclampsia in Women at Increased Risk: A Randomized Trial," *Lancet* 354: 810–816, 1999.

14. Knight, K., et al. "Calcium Supplementation on Normotensive and Hypertensive Pregnant Women," *American Journal of Clinical Nutrition* 55: 891–895, 1992.

15. Jovanovic-Peterson, Lois, M.D. "Vitamin and Mineral Deficiencies Which May Predispose to Glucose Intolerance of Pregnancy," *Journal of the American College of Nutrition* 15(1): 14–20, 1996.

16. Walker, H. A., et al. "The Phytoestrogen Genistein Produces Acute Nitric Oxide-Dependent Dilation of Human Forearm Vasculature with Similar Potency to 17 Beta-Estradiol," *Circulation* 103: 258–262, 2001.

9 Diabetes and Children

Recent estimates suggest that Type 2 diabetes may now account for as many as half of all new cases of diabetes in certain pediatric groups. Prior to this, children were thought to have juvenile-onset, or Type 1, diabetes.

Risk factors for Type 2 diabetes in children–previously a form that only affected adults–include obesity, ethnicity, age, sex, sedentary lifestyle, family history, and perinatal influences. Type 2 diabetes is more common in American Indian, African-American, and Hispanic children than in the general population. This epidemic raises the possibility of coronary heart disease becoming a disease of young adulthood.

Some diabetic children have a beta-cell autoimmunity, in which the immune system produces antibodies that attack the beta cells of the pancreas, which make and release insulin. This destruction may be inhibited by antioxidants, such as vitamin E, which destroy harmful free radicals.

Diabetic children should be screened for celiac disease, a disorder in which they cannot digest the gluten in certain grains, especially wheat, rye, oats, and barley. At least one study has shown that breast-feeding during the first two months of life protects individuals against Type 2 diabetes. Too much coffee or tea can increase the chances of children developing Type 1 diabetes.

Diabetes mellitus has always been classified as either juvenile-onset (Type 1) or adult-onset (Type 2), due to distinct differences in the usual age of presentation of the two conditions, explains David S. Ludwig, M.D.,

Ph.D., and Cara B. Ebbeling, Ph.D., of Children's Hospital in Boston, Massachusetts. However, with the increasing prevalence of Type 2 diabetes in children, these terms are now inaccurate.[1]

"Recent estimates suggest that Type 2 diabetes mellitus may now account for as many as half of all new cases of diabetes in certain pediatric populations," the authors reported in the *Journal of the American Medical Association.* "This apparent epidemic, attributable to the increased rates of obesity in children, carries enormous long-term public health implications."

Currently there are no nationwide epidemiological data focusing on Type 2 diabetes in children, but prevalence has been estimated at between 2 and 50 per 1,000 in various populations, the authors said. These rates have increased as much as tenfold in the last two decades. In two studies reported in the 1990s of people aged 10 to 19 years of age, Type 2 diabetes accounted for 33 to 46% of all diabetes in those age groups.

In addition to obesity, risk factors for Type 2 diabetes in children include ethnicity, age, sex, sedentary lifestyle, family history, and perinatal influences. Also, Type 2 diabetes is more common in American Indian, African-American, and Hispanic children than in the general population. For example, in a study in a Midwestern metropolitan area, 69% of the children with Type 2 diabetes were African-Americans, although blacks represented only 9.7% of patients with Type 1 diabetes, and 14.5% of the local population.

"The peak age of diagnosis of Type 2 diabetes in youth is between 12 and 16 years of age, corresponding to the midpubertal period," the authors added. "Sedentary lifestyle is associated with significantly increased risk of Type 2 diabetes in adults, and this association is likely to exist among children as well. Family history constitutes another important risk factor. In one study, 80% of Mexican-American children with Type 2 diabetes had at least one affected first-degree relative."

The authors went on to say that risk appears to increase with either low or high birth weight, perhaps because undernutrition or overnutrition in utero (in the womb) may cause permanent metabolic and hormonal changes that promote obesity, insulin resistance, and beta-cell dysfunction later in life. (Beta cells make and release insulin, which controls the level of glucose or sugar in the blood.)

As a result of this epidemic, the authors continued, we face the prospect of coronary heart disease becoming a disease of young adulthood. This calls for a public health campaign to identify novel treatments for obesity and insulin resistance, public schools to promote physical activity and fitness, the commercial food industry to market healthful foods to children, and parents to model and support healthful lifestyle choices, among other things, the authors concluded.

In a study involving 165 children, with an average age of 3 years, who had a parent or sibling with Type 1 diabetes, 18 were found to have beta-cell autoimmunity. Autoimmune disease is a disorder of the immune system in which the immune system mistakenly destroys body tissue that it considers to be foreign. Type 1 diabetes is an example, in that the immune system produces antibodies that attack insulin-producing beta cells of the pancreas that release insulin.[2]

Two of the 18 children had been given vitamin supplements during their first year of life. By comparison, 47 of the remaining 147 children who did not have beta-cell autoimmunity had been given vitamin supplements during their first year of life. After controlling for various variables, the protective benefit of vitamin supplements remained. This prompted Jill Harris, Ph.D., of the University of Colorado Health Sciences Center at Denver, to say that vitamin supplementation helps to prevent beta-cell autoimmunity rather than eliminate it. She believes that it is probably the antioxidants, specifically vitamin E, that help protect the beta cells from free-radical damage.

A research team at the Department of Child and Youth Psychiatry in Lund, Sweden, studied 67 Type 1 diabetics between the ages of newborn and 14 years, and 61 healthy matched controls. They found that stress early in life increased the risk of Type 1 diabetes, due to an autoimmune response. Negative events during the first two years of life were more prevalent in the diabetics than in the controls.[3]

There is no doubt that sugar causes dental caries, according to Iain C. Mackie, Ph.D., of the Turner Dental School in Manchester, England. Sugar-containing medications (cough syrups, etc.) usually contain sucrose, the most cariogenic sugar. Therefore, having a spoonful of sugar-containing medicine is like taking a spoonful of sugar. There is also concern about sugar in medicines in uncontrolled diabetes; these patients should have sugar-free medications.[4]

At Children's Hospital in Valencia, Spain, a research team reported that all diabetic children should be routinely screened for celiac disease. This disorder, also called nontropical sprue and gluten-induced enteropathy, is a severe allergy to the proteins in certain grains, specifically wheat, rye, oats, and barley. Gluten-free flours are quinoa, amaranth, corn, rice, and potato. Millet and spelt can often be tolerated.[5]

In the study, 141 Type 1 diabetics were screened for serum immuno-globin IgA antigliadin antibodies. Twelve volunteers with positive IgA antigliadin antibodies in their blood on two or more consecutive meas-urements underwent a small intestinal biopsy, and 4 of them were diag-nosed with celiac disease. Children who have diabetes and celiac disease have an onset of Type 1 diabetes at a younger age than nonceliac patients, the researchers said. The prevalence of celiac disease in these Type 1 dia-betics is 2.85%, greater than in the general population, which is one in 2,500 live births.

A study was conducted of 720 Pima Indians, ranging in age from 10 to 39, of whom 325 were exclusively bottle-fed. They had significantly higher age-adjusted and sex-adjusted mean relative weights than 144 who were exclusively breast-fed or 251 who were partially breast-fed. However, those who were breast-fed had significantly lower rates of Type 2 diabetes when compared to those who were bottle-fed in all age groups.[6] The researcher at the National Institute of Diabetes and Digestive and Kidney Diseases in Phoenix, Arizona, reported that those breast-fed exclusively for the first two months experienced a significantly lower rate of Type 2 diabetes.

In a study of 600 newly diagnosed diabetic children, and 536 controls, researchers at the University of Helsinki in Finland evaluated the relation-ship of coffee and tea consumption in the children and their parents and the risk of diabetes.[7] The research team found that the risk of Type 1 dia-betes was increased in children who drank at least two cups of coffee a day or those who consumed one or two cups of tea daily. Coffee consumption by the mother during pregnancy was not a factor.

References

1. Ludwig, David S., M.D., Ph.D., and Cara B. Ebbeling, Ph.D. "Type 2 Diabetes Mellitus in Children," *Journal of the American Medical Association* 286(12): 1427–1430, Sept. 26, 2001.

2. Baker, Barbara. "Infant Vitamins May Protect Against Diabetes," *Family Practice News,* July 15, 1996, p. 4.

3. Thernlund, Gunilla, M.D., et al. "Psychological Stress and the Onset of Insulin-Dependent Diabetes Mellitus in Children," *Diabetes Care* 18(10): 1323–1329, Oct. 1995.

4. Hamilton, Kirk. "Dental Caries and Sugar-Free Medication," *The Experts Speak*. Sacramento, Calif.: I.T. Services, 1997, p. 61. Also, Mackie, Iain C., Ph.D. "Promoting Sugar-Free Pediatric Medicines to Parents," *Health Visitor* 68(8): 327–338, Aug. 1995.

5. Calero, P., et al. "IgA Antigliadin Antibodies as a Screening Method for Nonovert Celiac Disease in Children with Insulin-Dependent Diabetes Mellitus," *Journal of Pediatric Gastroenterology and Nutrition* 23: 29–33, 1996.

6. Pettit, David J. "Breastfeeding and Incidence of Non-Insulin-Dependent Diabetes Mellitus in Pima Indians," *Lancet* 350: 166–168, July 19, 1997.

7. Virtanen, S. M., et al. "Is Children's or Parents' Coffee or Tea Consumption Associated with the Risk of Type 1 Diabetes Mellitus in Children," *European Journal of Clinical Nutrition* 48: 279–285, 1994.

10 Does Cow's Milk
Cause Diabetes?

Researchers cannot agree on whether or not cow's milk proteins cause Type 1 diabetes. Some say they do, some say they don't, depending on how much milk a child drinks. The more conservative researchers suggest that it is premature to remove cow's milk from the diet of growing children, and that more research is needed.

Canadian researchers suggest that Type 1 diabetes is very likely caused by diabetes-causing foods, such as wheat and soy, and to a lesser degree, cow's milk. The development of Type 1 diabetes may be related to genetic disposition and environmental factors, such as viruses, dietary factors, toxins, and so on, which can damage beta cells, which make and release insulin, the hormone that controls the amount of glucose (sugar) in the blood.

The jury is still out as to whether or not cow's milk proteins are involved in Type 1 diabetes. The issue becomes more clouded when pro-vegetarian groups, such as the Physician's Committee for Responsible Medicine, enter the picture. It's best to take what they say with a grain of salt. Their main guru was the late Benjamin Spock, M.D., who did not recommend milk for children under the age of 1 year.

Meanwhile, researchers at the University of Florida at Gainesville suggest that diabetes may be induced by something in the environment. Evidence indicates that there is only one in every three pairs of identical twins affected by Type 1 diabetes, and that the incidence of childhood diabetes is increasing.[1]

The Florida researchers refer to research that supports the long-held suspicion that proteins in cow's milk could be the key environmental factor in the disease. They added that breast-feeding may provide a protective influence against the risk of Type 1 diabetes later in life, and that increased frequencies of antibodies to cow's milk proteins in children with newly diagnosed Type 1 diabetes have been reported. The frequency of Type 1 diabetes parallels the frequency with which cow's milk is consumed around the world; however, the Florida researchers suggest that it is premature to eliminate cow's milk from the diets of growing children considered to be at risk for Type 1 diabetes.

In his study at the Hospital for Sick Children in Toronto, Canada, Jukka Karjalainen, M.D., said that previous research had implicated cow's milk as a possible trigger of an autoimmune response, which destroyed the beta cells in the pancreas in genetically susceptible people, causing diabetes.

At the University of Colorado School of Medicine at Denver, researchers studied 253 children, ranging in age from 9 months to 7 years, from 171 families of those with Type 1 diabetes, who were screened for beta-cell autoimmunity.[2]

Beta cells are a type of cell in the islets of Langerhans that make and release insulin. As we know, insulin is a hormone that controls the level of glucose (sugar) in the blood. Autoimmune disease is a disorder of the body's immune system in which the immune system destroys body tissue that it mistakenly considers foreign. For example, insulin-dependent diabetes is an autoimmune disease since the immune system destroys the insulin-producing beta cells.

In the Colorado study, 18 cases of beta-cell autoimmunity were found. As controls, the research team used 153 unrelated autoantibody-negative children.

It was reported that there was no difference between the proportion of cases and controls who were exposed to cow's milk or foods containing cow's milk or to cereal, fruit and vegetable, or meat protein by 3 months or

The Florida researchers refer to research that supports the long-held suspicion that proteins in cow's milk could be the key environmental factor in the disease. They added that breast-feeding may provide a protective influence against the risk of Type 1 diabetes later in life, and that increased frequencies of antibodies to cow's milk proteins in children with newly diagnosed Type 1 diabetes have been reported.

6 months of age. Children with beta-cell autoimmunity were breast-fed for a slightly longer time than the controls. It was concluded that beta-cell autoimmunity is not associated with cow's milk or other dietary protein. Therefore, they added, avoiding cow's milk as a preventive measure for Type 1 diabetes is questionable.

Type 1 diabetes is very likely to be initiated by food-containing diabetogens, substances that cause diabetes, such as wheat, soy, and to a lesser degree, cow's milk given early in life, according to Canadian researchers. Type 1 diabetes may be prevented or delayed by avoiding these foods until weaning or even as late as adolescence.[3]

In diabetic rodent models, wheat and soy are the major diabetogens in plant-based rodent diets. However, in diabetes-prone animals, cow's milk is a weaker diabetogen. Most diabetics require long-term food exposure to diabetogens after infancy, with the time around puberty being of special significance. The research team added that the probability of preventing diabetes by avoiding only one dietary diabetogen in the first six months of life is small. Diet is thought to have a major effect on both target cells and attacking leukocytes (white blood cells).

In an opposing view, researchers at the University of Helsinki in Finland reported that avoidance of cow's milk protein in early infancy could prevent Type 1 diabetes in genetically susceptible infants. The development of Type 1 diabetes may be related to genetic predisposition and the interaction of environmental factors, such as viruses, dietary factors, toxins, and others, which result in autoimmunity to the beta cells, their destruction, and subsequent development of the disease. The researchers added that the indirect evidence from animal models and observations in human beings are sufficient to justify intervention trials to determine whether or not cow's milk protein is associated with Type 1 diabetes.[4]

Viruses have been implicated as potential inducers of beta-cell damage. Viruses that have been associated with Type 1 diabetes include the enteroviruses, mumps, measles, cytomegalo- and retroviruses. Cow's milk proteins have been suggested as a cause of Type 1 diabetes in various countries, and wheat gluten exposure has been linked to the disease in animal studies.[5]

Researchers have also linked celiac disease and Type 1 diabetes. Also, a lack of vitamin D may contribute to the risk of developing the disease. Other causes may be incompatibility with the mother's blood group, older maternal age, and amniocentesis (a surgical procedure into the uterus to determine the sex of a child or to uncover chromosomal abnormalities).

Celiac disease, a malabsorption syndrome, is characterized by swelling (edema), malnutrition, skeletal disorders, anemia, abnormal stools, and nerve damage. Abnormalities in the intestinal lining of the stomach require a gluten-free diet.

A research team at McMaster University Department of Medicine in Hamilton, Ontario, Canada, reported that there is a relationship between early cow's milk exposure and the development of Type 1 diabetes. This exposure to cow's milk protein could result in beta-cell-directed autoimmunity and subsequent Type 1 diabetes. However, the data are insufficient at present to conclude that these observations are causal or to alter recommendations for infant feeding. International randomized trials are recommended, the researchers added.[6]

At the University of Helsinki in Finland, a research team evaluated milk consumption with levels of cow's milk protein antibodies in 697 newly diagnosed diabetic children, 415 sibling-control children, and 86 birth-date- and sex-matched population-based controls. It was found that there were inverse correlations between the duration of breast-feeding or age when dairy products and antibodies were introduced, and positive correlations between milk consumption and antibodies in the three populations studied.[7]

The researchers reported that high IgA antibody levels to cow's milk formula were associated with a greater risk of Type 1 diabetes in both diabetic-population-control and diabetic-sibling-control pairs. The results indicated that young age introduction of dairy products and high milk consumption during childhood can increase the level of cow's milk antibodies. In addition, high IgA antibodies to cow's milk are associated with an increased risk of Type 1 diabetes in susceptible children.

At the University of Tampere in Finland, the same researchers as in the previous study reported that when adjusted for variables, high milk consumption in childhood (more than 3 glasses/day) was associated with more frequent emergence of Type 1 diabetes-associated autoantibodies than low consumption (less than 3 glasses/day). There was a nonsignificant association between high milk consumption and the progression of Type 1 diabetes, the researchers said.[8]

Two studies show the benefits of breast-feeding and confirm the theory that infants fed cow's milk–based formula in the first three months of life have an increased risk of developing Type 1 diabetes, *Medical Tribune* reported. One study involved 90% of the infants who developed diabetes in New South Wales, Australia, over an 18-month period when compared to healthy controls. Infants fed exclusively breast milk for the first three months of life had a 34% lower risk of developing diabetes than those not breast-fed. Children fed cow's milk–based formula during the first three months of life were 52% more likely to develop diabetes than those not given cow's milk formula.[9]

A previous study found that bovine serum albumin, a protein in cow's milk, somewhat resembles a molecule on the surface of beta cells in the pancreas. This resemblance results in an autoimmune attack that causes beta-cell destruction. In nine regions of Italy, it was reported that there was an 88% correlation between the amount of milk that children drank and their risk of developing diabetes. It was also stated that Nutramigen, an infant formula developed by Mead Johnson for children with allergies, protects against the risk of developing diabetes.

References

1. MacLaren, Noel, M.D., and Mark Atkinson, Ph.D. "Is Insulin-Dependent Diabetes Mellitus Environmentally Induced?" *New England Journal of Medicine* 327(5): 348–349, July 30, 1992.

2. Norris, Jill M., Ph.D., et al. "Lack of Association Between Early Exposure to Cow's Milk Protein and Beta-Cell Autoimmunity," *Journal of the American Medical Association* 276(8): 609–619, Aug. 28, 1996.

3. Scott, Fraser W., and Hubert Kolb. "Cow's Milk and Insulin-Dependent Diabetes Mellitus," *Lancet* 348: 613, Aug. 31, 1996.

4. Akerblom, Hans K., et al. "Cow's Milk Protein and Insulin-Dependent Diabetes Mellitus," *Scandinavian Journal of Nutrition* 40: 98–103, 1996.

5. Vaarala, O., et al. "Environmental Factors in the Aetiology of Childhood Diabetes," *Diab. Nutr. Metab.* 12(2): 75–85, 1999.

6. Gerstein, H. C., and J. VanderMeulen. "The Relationship Between Cow's Milk Exposure in Type 1 Diabetes," *Diabetic Medicine* 13: 23–29, 1996.

7. Virtanen, S. M., et al. "Diet, Cow's Milk and the Risk of IDDM in Finnish Children," *Diabetologia* 37: 381–387, 1994.

8. Virtanen, S. M., et al. "Cow's Milk Consumption, Disease-Associated Autoantibodies and Type 1 Diabetes Mellitus: A Follow-Up Study in Siblings of Diabetic Children," *Diabetic Medicine* 15: 730–738, 1998.

9. Hurley, Dan. "Studies Confirm Diabetes Risk from Cow's Milk in Infants," *Medical Tribune,* Feb. 2, 1995, p. 11.

11 Take Care of Your Eyes

The most serious eye problems faced by diabetics are cataracts, glaucoma, diabetic retinopathy, and macular degeneration, some of which can lead to blindness. It is essential that diabetics have their eyes checked regularly by a doctor, and any condition—blurry vision, pressure, floating spots, red eyes—requires immediate attention. It is also important to regulate glucose levels and high blood pressure and to stop smoking.

As reported here, numerous studies show that nutritional supplements are helpful in preventing and treating eye problems. The list is rather long and includes vitamin C, vitamin E, vitamin A, the carotenoids (beta-carotene, lutein, zeaxanthin), zinc, B-complex vitamins, essential fatty acids, selenium, alpha-lipoic acid, and others. Many of these nutrients act as antioxidants to inactivate the harmful free-radicals, which can damage the eyes as well as other parts of the body. With many of these supplements, diabetics can enjoy a much fuller life.

Diabetics are prone to eye problems, which can lead to blindness, according to the American Diabetes Association. To understand how eye problems develop, we need to know something about the eye's structure.

The eye is a ball covered with a tough outer membrane and the covering is crystal clear. The curved area is the cornea, which focuses light while protecting the eye. After light passes through the cornea, it travels through the anterior chamber (which is filled with a protective fluid called the aqueous humor); through the pupil (which is a hole in the iris, the covered part of the eye); and then through the lens for more focusing. Finally, light passes through another fluid-filled chamber in the center of the eye (the vitreous); then it strikes the retina, the back of the eye.

Similar to the film in a camera, the retina records the images focused on it, but unlike film, the retina also converts these images into electrical signals, which the brain receives and decodes. A part of the retina (the macula) is specialized for seeing fine print or other detail. The retina is nourished by small vessels, the capillaries.[1]

The most serious eye problems for diabetics are glaucoma, cataracts, and retinopathy. Macular degeneration is also a harmful eye condition.

Glaucoma: Diabetics are 40% more likely than others to develop glaucoma. The longer one has had diabetes, the more likely one is to develop glaucoma, in which pressure builds up in the eye. Generally, drainage of the aqueous humor slows down and fluid builds up in the anterior chamber. Pressure pinches the blood vessels taking blood to the retina and optic nerve, and vision gradually diminishes as the retina and nerves are damaged.

Cataracts: While everyone is subject to cataracts, diabetics are 60% more likely to develop this eye condition, the American Diabetes Association reported. Diabetics are likely to develop cataracts at a younger age and to have them progress faster. When cataracts develop, the eye's clear lens clouds and blocks light from entering. If any light does pass through, it may be distorted. For mild cases of cataracts, diabetics may need to wear sunglasses or have glare-control lenses put in the glasses.

Retinopathy: Diabetic retinopathy refers to all disorders of the retina caused by diabetes. Non-proliferative retinopathy is the common, milder form, and it is also known as background retinopathy. While this form has no effect on vision and needs no treatment, it is important that diabetics have their eyes checked at least once a year to ensure that it is not progressing.

In non-proliferative retinopathy, capillaries balloon to form pouches. While the disorder does not usually cause a loss of vision at this stage, the capillary walls may lose their ability to control the passage of substances between the blood and the retina. However, the retina may become swollen and fatty deposits form. If the swelling affects the center of the retina, the problem is called macular edema, and it may cause the loss of vision.

Retinopathy may eventually progress to proliferative retinopathy, which is a more serious disorder. This is when the blood vessels are so damaged that they close off. Although new blood vessels may start growing in the retina, they are weak and can leak blood. This blocks vision and results in vitreous hemorrhage. The new blood vessels may generate scar tissue. If the scar tissue shrinks, it can distort the retina or pull out of place, resulting in retinal detachment.

Unfortunately, the retina can be damaged before a diabetic notices any vision changes. That is why patients should have their eyes examined by an eye doctor regularly, even though there may be no symptoms of eye damage.

A number of factors determine whether or not a diabetic will develop retinopathy. Type 1 diabetics will suffer various complications, such as blood glucose control, blood pressure levels, how long they have had diabetes, and their genes. Almost everyone with Type 1 diabetes will develop retinopathy, but fortunately, proliferative retinopathy is far less common. Those with blood glucose levels near normal are less likely to have retinopathy. However, retinopathy is more common in Mexican Americans with Type 2 diabetes than others. Women are more likely to lose their eyesight than men.

To avoid eye problems, keep your blood glucose levels under tight control. In the Diabetes Control and Complications Trial, those on standard diabetes treatment got retinopathy four times as often as people who kept their blood glucose levels close to normal. In diabetics who had retinopathy, the condition progressed in the tight-control group only half as often. High glucose levels may cause vision to become temporarily blurry. It is important to bring high blood pressure under control and stop smoking.

Finally, see an eye doctor regularly, since a special exam can locate early stages of retinopathy. During this exam, the doctor will dilate (expand) your pupils with drops and check the retina. Only optometrists and ophthalmologists can detect retinopathy, and only ophthalmologists can treat retinopathy.

According to the American Diabetes Association, diabetics should see an eye doctor if:

• your vision becomes blurry
• you have trouble reading signs or books
• you see double
• your eyes hurt
• you feel pressure in your eye
• your eye gets red and remains that way

- you see floating spots or flashing lights
- straight lines do not look straight
- you can't see things at the side the way you used to

Macular Degeneration: As explained earlier, the macula is the part of the retina with the sharpest sight. In many Americans, mostly older people, the surface of the macula degenerates enough to cause legal blindness. The problem may be due to poor blood flow to the retina or it can be an inherited condition. In its early stages, magnifying glasses may enable the diabetic to read.[2] While macular degeneration might rightfully be covered under diabetic retinopathy, I have decided to give it a special section, since a great deal of research deals with this condition specifically.

How to Deal with Glaucoma

A research team in Italy suggested that polyunsaturated fatty acids are beneficial supportive therapy for the prevention and treatment of glaucoma. These substances have a vasodilating effect, perhaps because of increased nitric oxide levels.[3] Nitric oxide, a potentially toxic compound of oxygen and nitrogen, is produced by endothelial cells that line blood vessels, where it relaxes blood vessels, as well as helping to maintain blood pressure.

The study involved 25 males and 15 females, with a mean age of 48.9 years, and a mean increase in ocular pressure of 22.4 mmHg. In the double-blind trial, the volunteers were divided into two groups, in which one group was given 240 mg of DHA (docosahexaenoic acid), along with 340 mg of EPA (eicosapentaenoic acid), twice daily, for 3 months. The other group was given a look-alike pill. After 3 months of therapy, there were significant improvements in various parameters involving glaucoma.

In a study involving 49 sets of eyes, of which 39 people suffered from various types of glaucoma, and 9 were normotensive (having blood pressure typical of the group that one belongs to), the volunteers received a single oral dose of vitamin C (0.5 g/kg body weight), which brought a significant fall in intraocular pressure. In patients with hemorrhagic glaucoma or secondary glaucoma, the tension-lowering effect of the vitamin was less significant.[4]

Alpha-lipoic acid, when given to glaucoma patients, normalized the metabolism of the amino acid tyrosine, along with their cofactors of vitamin B_6, vitamin C, and iron. This therapy improved the pressure in the eyeball of the patients. Therefore, the researchers suggest alpha-lipoic acid, vitamin B_1, vitamin B_2, pantothenic acid, vitamin B_6, and vitamin C for glaucoma patients.[5]

Nine volunteers with glaucoma were exposed to normal daylight, and then given either a placebo or 0.5 mg of melatonin at 6 P.M. This brought a reduction by 30% of pressure in the eyeball, whereas the pressure in the control group went down 13%.[6] Melatonin, a hormone of the pineal gland, is also a major antioxidant to route free radicals. This over-the-counter supplement is being prescribed for insomnia, jet lag, and heart disease, among other things. A deficiency is known to increase blood levels of cholesterol and triglycerides.

In a study involving 25 volunteers, with an average age of 63, with moderate pressure in their eyes, 0.5 g of vitamin C four times daily for 6 days brought a significant decrease in intraocular pressure of 1.10 mmHg, but there was no significant change in the facility of outflow. In 19 patients, average age of 63, a 10% solution of vitamin C was given topically in one eye, three times daily for 3 days, while the other eye served as a control. The research team found that pressure in the test eye was significantly lower than in the control eye.[7]

How to Deal with Cataracts

Cataracts affect about 50% of people over 73, and they are the largest reimbursable item within the Medicaid budget, according to Allen Taylor, M.D., of Tufts University in Boston, Massachusetts. Epidemiologic data suggest that better nutrition (especially with vitamins C and E and the carotenoids) and fruit and vegetable consumption are the least costly and most practical measures to delay cataract formation. He added that two studies have shown that the consumption of vitamin C supplements for more than 10 years decreased the risk of cataracts.[8]

It has long been suspected that free-radical damage might influence the formation of cataracts. Thus began a study at the Harvard School of Public Health in Boston, which concluded that dietary intake of carotenoids and long-term supplementation with vitamin C might delay the development of cataracts, and prevent the condition from reaching a severe stage requiring extraction. The study involved dietary analysis of more than 50,800 nurses, ranging in age from 45 to 67, in 11 states.[9]

The researchers found that women in the upper fifth for total vitamin A intake, excluding supplements, had a 39% lower risk of developing cataracts in relation to the women in the lowest fifth. Although dietary intakes of vitamin B$_2$, vitamin E, multivitamins, or vitamin C were not associated with cataract risk, the researchers did find that women who had taken vitamin C supplements for 10 years or more had a 45% lower risk of developing cataracts than unsupplemented women. In a surprise development, carrots, a rich source of beta-carotene (provitamin A), did not necessarily protect against cataracts, suggesting that other carotenoids might be more beneficial in providing protection. There are more than 500 carotenoids that are synthesized from plants, such as beta-carotene, lutein, lycopene, zeaxanthin, and others.

Cataracts may be associated with inadequate levels of antioxidants in the eye, according to an article in *Diabetologia*. Several studies have suggested that alpha-lipoic acid, an antioxidant, may reduce the risk of diabetes-associated cataract.[10]

In the study, researchers induced diabetes in laboratory rats, noting that diabetes interferes with the way lens cells burn glucose. After feeding some of the animals with alpha-lipoic acid, the researchers noted that the animals getting the supplement were more resistant to glucose-related changes to the lenses of the eye, when compared to the animals not getting the supplement.

As we know, diabetes damages the eyes and increases the risk of cataracts and glaucoma. A number of studies have shown a strong association between abnormal levels of lutein and macular degeneration. Studies have also revealed that low levels of this carotenoid also increase the risk of cataracts.[11]

In a study of 36,000 male physicians, which lasted more than 8 years, it was found that men who consumed the greatest quantities of the carotenes lutein and zeaxanthin were 19% less likely to develop cataracts when compared to those who consumed little or none of the nutrients. Broccoli and spinach, both rich in lutein, were also associated with a lower risk of the disorder.

A number of studies have suggested that lutein and zeaxanthin may help to maintain normal visual acuity and reduce the risk of cataracts and macular degeneration. In a review appearing in *Archives of Biochemistry and Biophysics*, a research team discussed evidence supporting prevailing theories of how these two substances function in the eye. One view is that the macular pigment (containing lutein and zeaxanthin) acts like polarizing glasses, filtering out stray light and improving visual acuity. The contrasting view is that the macular pigment functions to keep eye tissues healthy by screening out harmful light, thereby acting as an antioxidant.[12]

It has long been known that vitamin A is essential for normal eyesight, and that the body converts some beta-carotene, or provitamin A, to vitamin A. As we have seen, lutein and zeaxanthin also play major roles in eye health, specifically by reducing the risk of cataracts and macular degeneration.[13]

In a study headed by P. S. Bernstein, researchers obtained 200 human eyes within 24 hours after being donated to an eye bank. The eyes were dissected to determine the levels of carotenoids in eye tissues. The researchers found that nearly all tissues in the eye had measurable levels of lutein, zeaxanthin, and their by-products. Also present were small amounts of beta-carotene, alpha-carotene, lycopene, and other carotenoids.

Carotenoids in eye tissues are likely to have various functions. As an example, lutein and zeaxanthin in the iris may filter out destructive wavelengths of blue light, and they may function as antioxidants and phototoxic filters in the macula. Also, the presence of high levels of carotenoids in the ciliary (lens) of the eye, a tissue not exposed to intense light, suggests that they may be involved in antioxidant protection of this tissue.

In studying more than 110,000 men and women, researchers at Harvard University in Cambridge found that those who consumed the most foods rich in lutein and zeaxanthin were less likely to develop age-related cataracts than those who ate the least. Foods rich in these carotenoids include dark green leafy vegetables (spinach, broccoli, kale, collard greens, mustard greens), winter squash, corn, and peppers. Consuming at least three weekly servings of these vegetables seems to offer protection.[14]

Researchers have found that lutein supplements can increase the density of the macular pigment, which is one sign of healthy eyes. In a study published in the *Journal of the Science of Food and Agriculture*, a research team asked 5 patients with cataracts and 5 patients with age-related macular degeneration to take lutein ester capsules (from natural compounds found in vegetables and fruit) 3 times a week for an average duration of 26 and 13 months, respectively. Each capsule contained 15 mg of lutein esters and 3.3 mg of vitamin E.[15]

The research team reported that visual acuity in the cataract patients improved by an average of 40 to 50%, which approached normal. Tolerance of glare also improved. Four patients with macular degeneration, who remained in the study, reported stabilized or improved vision. No side effects were recorded.

Volunteers with the highest intakes of folic acid (a B vitamin) and vitamin C were less likely to develop cataracts, according to researchers at Tufts University in Boston. In the study, 78 volunteers who had a cataract in at least one lens had their diets analyzed for concentrations of vitamin A, total carotene, vitamin B_1, vitamin B_2, vitamin B_{12}, vitamin B_6, vitamin B_3, folic acid, vitamin D, vitamin C, and vitamin E.[16]

Cortical cataracts may be partially reversed with vitamin E supplements, according to a study of 25 patients with nuclear cataracts (located near the center of the lens) and 25 patients with cortical cataracts (found toward the outside of the lens). All were scheduled to have the cataracts surgically removed. Before surgery, 12 volunteers in each group were given 100 mg/day of vitamin E or a placebo for 1 month. The researchers said that the vitamin E levels increased and free-radical damage decreased in the lenses of those getting the vitamin.[17]

Also, cortical lens opacity decreased by almost 40% among those getting the vitamin, suggesting a reversal of their condition. For those getting vitamin E, nuclear lens opacity (due to sunlight exposure) decreased by 14%. The study found that cortical cataracts or cloudiness of the lens of the eye, which can result in blindness, may be partially reversed with vitamin E, and that it is thought that more vitamin E was able to reach the cortical lens than the nuclear lens.

During the day, the lens of the eye is exposed to ultraviolet radiation from sunlight, and this generates cell-damaging free radicals. One of the side effects of this exposure is cataract, an opacity in the lens of the eye that interferes with vision and is often associated with diabetes.[18]

In a study published in *Ophthalmology*, a research team evaluated the dietary habits, vitamin supplement usage, and blood levels of vitamin E in 764 volunteers in what was called the Lens Opacities Case-Control Study. Eye lenses of the participants were photographed at the beginning of the study, and follow-up eye exams were scheduled.

It was found that those who took vitamin E supplements had a 57% lower risk of developing cataract, especially after 5 years of supplementation, when compared to volunteers who did not take the vitamin. Also, those with high blood levels of vitamin E had a 42% lower risk of developing cataract. Those who took multivitamin supplements, which contained vitamin E, had a 31% lower risk of developing the disease.

The authors of the article pointed out that cataract is an age-related problem, and that surgery to replace the lens of the eyes is the most frequently performed surgical procedure in the United States. Further, vitamin E and other antioxidants could reduce the number of these operations and reduce eye-related health care costs, they added.

The results of this study, when placed in the context of other studies, says Joel A. Simon, M.D., of the San Francisco V.A. Medical Center in California, is that it is biologically plausible that oxidative damage (damage by oxygen) may lead to cataract formation and that the antioxidants could potentially diminish the risk. However, rather than measure blood levels of vitamin C, it might be more prudent to underscore the public health importance of fresh fruit and vegetable consumption, he said. A vitamin C supplement (250 to 500 mg/day) may also be reasonable for the potential prevention of cataract, cardiovascular, and other diseases, he added.[19]

The prevalence of cataract increases from about 5% at age 65 to about 50% in those older than 75, according to Allen Taylor, M.D., of Tufts University in Boston. The disability and cost for age-related cataract in the United States is between $5 and $6 billion a year. Delaying cataract formation by about 10 years would reduce the incidence of visual disability from cataract by about 45%.[20]

Allen added that risk factors for cataract include light exposure, high energy radiation, exposure to high levels of oxygen, smoking, and reduced levels of antioxidants. For example, optimum levels of vitamin C appear to be 250 mg/day. This would bring close-to-saturating levels of vitamin C in the blood and provide protection against cataract. Poor education and lower socioeconomic status also increase the risk of cataract, he added.

In studying 2,900 people, ranging in age from 49 to 97, higher intakes of protein, vitamin A, vitamin B_3, vitamin B_1, and vitamin B_2 were associated with a reduced risk of nuclear cataract, reported Robert G. Cumming, M.D. Polyunsaturated fatty acid intake was associated with a reduced risk of cortical cataract, he said.[21]

Researchers evaluated 3,089 people between the ages of 43 and 86 for cataract incidence during a 5-year study. Compared with those who did not take multivitamins or supplements of vitamins C and E, the 5-year risk for any cataract was 60% lower among those who, during follow-up, reported the use of supplements containing vitamins C and E for more than 10 years.[22]

Taking multivitamins during that period reduced the risk for nuclear and cortical cataracts, but not for posterior subcapsular cataracts, which involve the cortex at the posterior pole of the lens. Lifestyle and dietary changes did not alter the outcome of the study.

A research team at the University of Stockholm in Sweden studied a 35-year-old male who had posterior subcapsular cataract, severe atopic eczema, asthma, and an inflamed cornea. He was treated with 600 mcg/day of selenium, 1,200 mg/day of vitamin E, 80 mg/day of vitamin B_6, 15 mg/day of vitamin B_2, and 2,000 mg/day of vitamin C. When the treatment began, vision in the right eye was 2/10, and 3/10 in the left eye. Three months later, vision in the right eye was 4/10, and 7/10 in the left eye. Five months later, the vision in the right eye remained at 4/10, but had increased to 8/10 in the left eye.[23]

The researchers said that in less than two months of treatment, all signs of severe atopic dermatitis had vanished and there were no signs of asthma. They believe that it is prudent to try selenium and vitamin E in other kinds of cataracts, such as senile and diabetic cataract. The authors also feel that the use of selenium as sodium selenite or selenomethionine can be safely used without adverse side effects, assuming the patient has normal kidney function.

It has been shown that cataract lenses from smokers contain more cadmium than those from nonsmokers, according to researchers at the University of Oxford in England. Smokers with or without cataract have higher cadmium levels in their blood, and smokers have lower levels of vitamin C, vitamin E, and beta-carotene. Lower blood levels of these vitamins might explain the increased risk for developing cataracts, they added. Tobacco leaves contain significant amounts of cadmium, a toxic metal.[24]

Researchers in Milan, Italy, studied 207 patients with cataracts and 706 without the disease, and found a protective effect from some vegetables, fruit, folic acid, and vitamin E. An increased risk of cataract was found with elevated levels of salt and fat intake in the diet.[25]

How to Deal with Diabetic Retinopathy

Patients with diabetes, hardening of the arteries, and high blood pressure are at risk of developing a form of retinopathy, a disease that affects blood vessels in the eye's retina. In both diabetic retinopathy and hypertensive retinopathy, the blood vessels may leak blood into the retina. In atherosclerotic retinopathy, the blood vessels are apt to thicken.[26]

In a study involving Pycnogenol, a brand of French maritime pine bark extract, researchers gave 20 men and women with retinopathy 50 mg, three times daily, of the extract or a placebo for 2 months. In a separate phase of the study, 20 patients were given the same dosage of Pycnogenol. Eye exams were given before and after supplementation.

Following the study, researchers found that patients given the supplement showed improvements in visual acuity and no decrease in retinal function. All of the patients reported some degree of improvement, while the retinopathies in those given placebos progressively worsened during the study. The supplement—available over the counter—is thought to be effective by quenching free radicals and by strengthening blood vessel walls.

Another prospective study demonstrated that blood levels of magnesium are inversely related to the occurrence or progression of retinopathy. Physicians are reminded that magnesium intake may be of significant benefit in patients with impaired glucose tolerance or who have beginning states of Type 2 diabetes. People at risk for magnesium deficiency also include those on drugs such as thiazide and loop diuretics, or those with inadequate nutrition or alcohol intake, according to the Dutch researchers.[27]

Increased magnesium excretion in the urine of diabetics may be due to poor glycemic control (glycosuria), hyperinsulinism (high insulin levels in the blood), a possible kidney defect, or inadequate nutrition. However, magnesium supplements can improve insulin sensitivity. For example, when 500 mg/day of magnesium were given to patients over a 21-week period, this reduced insulin requirements without changing glycemic control. It has been found that patients with severe diabetic retinopathy have lower blood levels of magnesium, compared with patients without the eye problem.

A study at the Chiba University School of Medicine in Japan evaluated 104 Type 2 diabetics for lipoprotein-A and hemoglobin A1C. The researchers also studied other indicators related to retinopathy. It was reported that lipoprotein-A is thought to be more damaging than low-density lipoprotein cholesterol (LDL, the bad kind). It has been reported that raised blood levels of lipoprotein-A are also an independent risk factor for coronary heart disease, and pose a ten times greater risk for heart disease than raised levels of LDL.[28]

There is a relationship between diabetic retinopathy and plasma homocysteine levels, according to an article in *Diabetes Care*. Homocysteine is a generally benign amino acid, a natural product of the synthesis

In a study involving Pycnogenol, a brand of French maritime pine bark extract, researchers gave 20 men and women with retinopathy 50 mg, three times daily, of the extract or a placebo for 2 months. Researchers found that patients given the supplement showed improvements in visual acuity and no decrease in retinal function. All of the patients reported some degree of improvement, while the retinopathies in those given placebos progressively worsened during the study.

and breakdown of proteins. However, when homocysteine builds up in the bloodstream, it can increase the risk of various disorders, especially heart attack, stroke, and blood clots.[29]

In the study, 69 patients with Type 1 diabetes, with blood pressure readings of 140/90, were free of cardiovascular disease, and 34 did not have retinopathy. It was found that 20 had non-proliferative diabetic retinopathy and 10 had proliferative diabetic retinopathy. Proliferative retinopathy is a disorder of the small blood vessels of the retina of the eye.

A number of studies have reported that homocysteine levels can often be lowered with 5 g/day of folic acid; 100 mg/day of vitamin B_6; 1,000 mcg/day of vitamin B_{12}; 500 mg/day of betaine hydrochloride, a supplemental form of hydrochloric acid; and 1,000 mg/day of phosphatidyl-choline (another name for lecithin).[30]

How to Deal with Macular Degeneration

Antioxidants help to protect the human macula from destruction by oxygen free radicals, which are generated through normal oxygen metabolism. The free radicals can be increased by environmental stressors such as certain wavelengths of light and chemicals, according to David A. Newsome, M.D., of the Retinal Institute of Louisiana at New Orleans. Oral ingestion of antioxidants can increase blood levels of these nutrients, and there is increasing evidence that antioxidants can slow vision loss in macular degeneration.[31]

Newsome says that macular degeneration is one of the "wear and tear" diseases due to oxygen stress. The macula is an oxygen-rich environment in which the metabolic rate is high; this generates a significant amount of free radicals, which can damage tissue by their continuous search for missing electrons. (Free radicals are oxygen molecules with an unpaired electron. This imbalance makes them highly reactive, and they are constantly striving to connect with other molecules. In so doing, they will attack any part of the body, thus contributing to heart disease, cataracts, aging, etc.)

The eye, especially the macula, contains various key naturally occurring antioxidants such as vitamin C, vitamin E, beta-carotene, zinc, selenium, and copper, and antioxidant systems such as catalase, superoxide dismutase, glutathione peroxidase (which involves selenium, zinc, and copper), glutathione reductase (which includes vitamin B_2), metallothionein (which includes zinc), and retinal dehydrogenase (which also includes zinc).

Older people are more susceptible to macular degeneration and tend to eat a diet that is not rich in antioxidants, Newsome said. For example, there are few dietary sources for antioxidants such as zinc, though rich sources include meat, which many older people may not like or be able to afford. Also, older people have reduced intestinal absorption of nutrients, which begins with a lowered output of stomach acid, and this reduces the bioavailability of many of these nutrients.

In a study from the National Cataract Study Group, it was found that there was an approximate 35% reduction in cataract formation in those with higher levels of antioxidants. Newsome and his colleagues have reported a reduction in vision loss among those with macular degeneration who ingested zinc.

Using data from the third National Health and Nutrition Examination Survey (NHANES III), a research team reported in the *American Journal of Epidemiology* the relationship between lutein and zeaxanthin levels and age-related macular degeneration (AMD) among 8,222 men and women. The researchers used photographs of the volunteers' eyes, as well as dietary and blood levels of the two carotenoids.[32]

It was reported that overall results found no relation of dietary or blood lutein or zeaxanthin levels in the early or late stages of age-related macular degeneration. But, among those between the ages of 40 and 79 and with the highest dietary levels of the two nutrients, they had a 90% lower risk of pigment abnormalities in the retina, which is an early indicator of the disease. Those between the ages of 60 and 79, who consumed the highest amounts of lutein and zeaxanthin, had a similar 90% lower risk for late stage age-related maculopathy or AMD.

Outside of supplements, plant pigments are the only source of these nutrients. The researchers added that a growing body of evidence suggests that the two carotenoids help to maintain the health of the retina and vision.

Since carotenoids help to protect plants from dangerous free radicals, which are generated by exposure to oxygen and light, researchers theorized that these antioxidants can also protect human beings when they consume carotenoids found in fruits and vegetables. Researchers have determined that lutein and zeaxanthin form the yellow macular pigment found at the center of the retina. This pigment filters out deleterious blue wavelengths of light and may reduce the amount of free radicals. It has been known for some time that age-related macular degeneration, the leading cause of blindness in the elderly, is related to lower amounts of macular pigment.

Additional research shows that increased dietary intake of lutein-containing foods or lutein supplements increases blood levels of the carotenoid, thereby increasing macular pigment density. However, the normal diet may not contain sufficient amounts of lutein, and lutein ester supplements (a common form of lutein) can be used to optimize levels of the nutrient in the eye.[33]

Another study is consistent with existing research which shows that high levels of lutein and zeaxanthin in the retina greatly reduce the risk of age-related macular degeneration (AMD), and that low levels are not a consequence of the disease. Generally, levels of the two carotenoids were lower in all three concentric sections of the retinas from those who had AMD.

In analyzing the retina, the researchers found that eyes containing the largest amount of the two nutrients were 82% less likely to have AMD. This came after the research team analyzed lutein and zeaxanthin levels in the retinas from 56 eye donors with AMD, and 56 eye donors without the disease. Each eye was segregated into three concentric sections centered around the fovea, the central part of the eye where the largest deposits of the two carotenoids are found.[34]

To ascertain whether or not lutein supplements can increase the macular pigment density, researchers asked 8 men, ranging in age from 18 to 50, to take 10 mg of lutein from marigold flowers for 12 weeks. The supplemental lutein increased lutein levels in both blood and eyes, and during the 12-week study, lutein levels went up five times in the blood and the macular pigment density increased by 19 to 22%. As we know, lutein and zeaxanthin seem to filter out harmful blue wavelengths and protect against free-radical damage, which could lead to macular degeneration.[35]

Researchers have determined that lutein and zeaxanthin protect eye cells from damaging free radicals; however, this protection was most noticeable when the carotenoids were combined with vitamin C and E and other antioxidants. The antioxidants protected the carotenoids from being damaged by free radicals.[36]

In a study involving 16 volunteers, ranging in age from 27 to 54, it was found that high consumption of lutein from vegetables such as spinach and kale may reduce the risk of macular degeneration. The study group had been diagnosed with retinitis pigmentosa or other forms of retinal degeneration, which can contribute to blindness. The 16 volunteers were given 40 mg/day of lutein for 9 weeks, followed by a maintenance dose of 20 mg/day for 17 weeks. Ten other volunteers received 500 mg/day of docosahexaenoic acid (DHA), B vitamins, and digestive enzymes.[37]

The research team reported that, based on vision tests and comments by the volunteers, visual acuity or sharpness of vision and field of vision improved significantly among those taking lutein. The improvements were recorded after 2 to 4 weeks of supplementation and then leveled off at 6 and 14 weeks. Interestingly, improvement in visual acuity was some four times greater among those with blue eyes and dark eyes. Some of the volunteers also said that they could adapt better to light and darkness, had improved color perception, and experienced reduced glare from light.

Tobacco smoke contains large numbers of free radicals, which increase the risk of eye disorders, heart disease, and other problems, according to a recent study. Nonsmokers are also at risk, since second-hand smoke lowers blood levels of total carotenoids, beta-carotene, alpha-carotene, and cryptoxanthin, but not other carotenoids, vitamin A, or vitamin E. Smokers had lower levels of all of these nutrients.[38]

In a study of 3,600 patients, ranging in age from 55 to 80, from 11 medical centers, volunteers were given one of the following supplements or a placebo for an average of 6 years: 1) a multivitamin formula containing 500 mg of vitamin C, 400 IU of vitamin E, and 15 mg of beta-carotene daily; 2) 80 mg/day of zinc and 2 mg/day of copper; or 3) a combination of the just-mentioned vitamins, plus zinc and copper.[39]

Those with the highest risk of advanced age-related macular degeneration experienced the greatest benefit, with the combination of vitamins and zinc reducing the rate of visual acuity loss by 27%. In effect, the antioxidant/zinc combo reduced the overall risk of AMD by 28%. While the vitamins and zinc reduced the risk of this potentially dangerous eye disorder, the effect was most pronounced when the vitamins and mineral were given together. The copper did not seem to affect the outcome.

In two studies involving 21,157 male physicians[40] and 31,843 registered female nurses,[41] it was found that cigarette smoking is an independent risk factor for age-related macular degeneration. Smoking reduces plasma concentrations of several micronutrients that act as antioxidants and may provide protection against macular degeneration.

Vitamin E, as an antioxidant, is instrumental in increasing resistance to age-related macular degeneration. The progressive development of AMD is thought to be influenced by oxidative stress, that is, free-radical damage, according to an article in *Mechanisms of Ageing and Development.*[42]

In the study, a research team evaluated blood levels of nutrients in 25 men and women with AMD, and compared them to a control group of 15 volunteers without the disease. The participants were 60 years of age. It was found that the patients with AMD had significantly lower blood levels of vitamin E and zinc. It was also found that those with AMD had greater exposure to sunlight, which increases free-radical damage to the eyes.

Many studies support the use of vitamin E in preventing macular degeneration. One of these studies involved tabulating diets, blood levels of nutrients and visual health of more than 2,500 people. After analyzing the ratio of vitamin E to blood fats, such as cholesterol, it was reported that those with the greatest concentrations of vitamin E were 82% less likely to develop macular degeneration. People with higher levels of blood fats may be able to protect themselves by increasing their vitamin E intake.[43]

A low-fat diet (less than 25% of the calories as fat) can help to improve the vascular system and may lessen the contributions of vascular disease to the neovascular or wet form of acute macular degeneration, according to G. E. Bunce, M.D., in the *Journal of Nutritional Biochemistry*. In addition, keeping diabetes under control or reducing glucose intolerance can inhibit lens glycosylation. Excess sugar in the diet can promote osmotic swelling and increase oxidant stress, he said. In fact, diabetes can increase cataract prevalence three- to fourfold in those 65 years of age and younger. Smoking and exposure to high-energy radiation can also harm the eyes, he added.[44]

To protect the eyes, Bunce suggests taking antioxidant defenses such as copper, iron, manganese, zinc, selenium, and vitamin B_2; consuming free-radical scavengers such as vitamins E and C and beta-carotene; consuming antioxidants that help to absorb UV light, including beta-carotene, lutein, and zeaxanthin; reducing fat intake to less than 25%; and reducing the risk of Type 2 diabetes by being less than 20% overweight, exercising and reducing calories.

Benefits can be achieved with 200 to 400 IU/day of vitamin E; 100 to 250 mg/day of vitamin C; and 25 mg/day of beta-carotene. Dark green vegetables such as spinach, peppers, and broccoli, are especially helpful, Bunce said.

References

1. "Eye Care and Retinopathy," American Diabetes Association, 1660 Duke St., Alexandria, Va. 22314, 1997.

2. Tapley, Donald F., M.D., et al. *The Columbia University College of Physicians and Surgeons Complete Home Medical Guide*. New York: Crown, 1985, p. 669.

3. Cellini, M., et al. "The Use of Polyunsaturated Fatty Acids in Ocular Hypertension. A Study with Blue-on-Yellow Perimetry," *Acta Ophthalmology Scandinavia*, 1999, pp. 54–55.

4. Virno, M., et al. "Oral Treatment of Glaucoma with Vitamin C," *The Eye, Ear, Nose and Throat Monthly* 46: 1502–1508, Dec. 1967.

5. Filina, A. A., and N. A. Sporova. "Effect of Lipoic Acid on Tyrosine Metabolism in Patients with Open-Angle Glaucoma," *Vestn. Oftalmol.* 107(3): 19–21, May-June 1991.

6. Samples, J. R., et al. "Effects of Melatonin on Intraocular Pressure," *Current Eye Research* 7(7): 649–653, 1988.

7. Linner, E. "The Pressure Lowering Effect of Ascorbic Acid in Ocular Hypertension," *Acta Ophthalmology* 47 (III): 685–689, 1969.

8. Taylor, Allen, M.D., and Thomas Nowell. "Oxidative Stress and Antioxidant Function in Relation to Risk for Cataract," *Advances in Pharmacology* 38: 515–536, 1997.

9. Hankinson, S., et al. "Nutrient Intake and Cataract Extraction in Women: A Prospective Study," *British Medical Journal* 305: 335–339, 1992.

10. Obrosova, I., et al. "Diabetes-Induced Changes in Lens Antioxidant Status, Glucose Utilization and Energy Metabolism: Effect of DL-alpha-Lipoic Acid," *Diabetiologia* 41: 1442–1450, 1998.

11. Brown, L., et al. "A Prospective Study of Carotenoid Intake and Risk of Cataract Extraction in U.S. Men," *American Journal of Clinical Nutrition* 70: 517–524, 1999.

12. Hammond, B. R., Jr., et al. "Carotenoids in the Retina and Lens: Possible Acute and Chronic Effects on Human Visual Performance," *Archives of Biochemistry and Biophysics* 385: 41–46, 2001.

13. Bernstein, P. S., et al. "Identification and Quantification of Carotenoids and Their Metabolites in the Tissues of the Human Eye," *Experimental Eye Research* 72: 215–223, 2001.

14. "Cataracts, Lutein and Zeaxanthin," *Tufts University Health and Nutrition Letter* 17(10): 1, Dec. 1999.

15. Olmedilla, B., et al. "Lutein in Patients with Cataracts and Age-Related Macular Degeneration: A Long-Term Supplementation Study," *Journal of the Science of Food and Agriculture* 81: 904–909, 2001.

16. Jacques, P., et al. "Vitamin Intake and Senile Cataract," *Journal of the American College of Nutrition* 6: 435, 1987.

17. Seth, R. K., et al. "Protective Function of Alpha-Tocopherol Against the Process of Cataractogenesis in Humans," *Annals of Nutrition and Metabolism* 43: 268–289, 1999.

18. Leske, M. C., et al. "Antioxidant Vitamins and Nuclear Opacities," *Ophthalmology* 105: 831–836, 1998.

19. Hamilton, Kirk. "Cataract and Vitamin C." *Clinical Pearls*. Sacramento, Calif.: I.T. Services, 2000, pp. 90–91. Also, Simon, Joel A., M.D. "Serum Ascorbic Acid and Other Correlates of Self-Reported Cataract Among Older Americans," *Journal of Clinical Epidemiology* 52(12): 1207–1211, 1999.

20. Taylor, Allen, M.D. "Nutritional and Environmental Influences on Risk for Cataract," *Nutritional and Environmental Influences on the Eye* 4: 53–93, 1999.

21. Cumming, R. G., et al. "Diet and Cataract: The Blue Mountain Eye Study," *Ophthalmology* 107(3): 450–456, March 2000.

22. Mares-Perlman, J. A., et al. "Vitamin Supplement Use and Incident Cataracts in Population-Based Study," *Archives of Ophthalmology* 118: 1556–1563, Nov. 2000.

23. Ahlrot-Westerlund, Britt, M.D., and Ake Norrby. "Cataracts, Vitamin E and Selenomethionine," *ACTA Ophthalmology,* April 1988, pp. 237–238.

24. Harding, John J. "Cigarettes and Cataract: Cadmium Or a Lack of Vitamin C," *British Journal of Ophthalmology* 79: 199–201, 1995.

25. Tavani, Alessandra, Sc.D., et al. "Food and Nutrient Intake and Risk of Cataract," *Annals of Epidemiology* 6: 41–46, 1996.

26. Spadea, L., and E. Balestrazzi. "Treatment of Vascular Retinopathies with Pycnogenol," *Phytotherapy Research* 15: 219–223, 2001.

27. de Valk, H. W. "Magnesium in Diabetes Mellitus," *Netherlands Journal of Medicine* 54: 139–146, 1999.

28. Morisaki, Nobuhiro, et al. "Lipoprotein(a) Is a Risk Factor for Diabetic Retinopathy in the Elderly," *Journal of the American Geriatric Society* 42: 965–976, 1994.

29. Vaccaro, O., et al. "Plasma Homocysteine and Its Determinants in Diabetic Retinopathy," *Diabetes Care* 23(7): 1026–1027, July 2000.

30. Hoffman, Ronald L., M.D. *Intelligent Medicine.* New York: Simon & Schuster, 1997, p. 282.

31. Newsome, David A., M.D. "Role of Antioxidants in Macular Degeneration: An Update," *Ophthalmic Practice* 12(4): 169–171, 1994.

32. Mares-Perlman, J. A., et al. "Lutein and Zeaxanthin in the Diet and Serum and Their Relation to Age-Related Maculopathy in the Third National Health and Nutrition Examination Survey," *American Journal of Epidemiology* 153: 424–432, 2001.

33. Landrum, J. T., and R. A. Bone. "Lutein, Zeaxanthin and the Macular Pigment," *Archives of Biochemistry and Biophysics* 385: 28–40, 2001.

34. Bone, R. A., et al. "Macular Pigment in Donor Eyes With and Without AMD: A Case-Control Study," *Investigative Ophthalmology and Visual Science* 42: 235–240, 2001.

35. Berendschot, T. T., et al. "Influence of Lutein Supplementation on Macular Pigment, Assessed with Two Objective Techniques," *Investigative Ophthalmology and Visual Science* 41: 3322–3326, 2000.

36. Rozankowska, M. B., et al. "Interaction of Carotenoids with Other Antioxidants in Protection of the Retina Against Oxidative Damage," *Investigative Ophthalmology and Visual Science* 41(Suppl.): S601, 2000.

37. Dagnelie, G., et al. "Lutein Improves Visual Function in Some Patients with Retinal Degeneration: A Pilot Study Via the Internet," *Optometry* 71: 147–164, 2000.

38. Alberg, A. J., et al. "Household Exposure to Passive Cigarette Smoking and Serum Micronutrient Concentrations," *American Journal of Clinical Nutrition* 72: 1576–1582, 2000.

39. The Age-Related Eye Disease Study Research Group. "A Randomized, Placebo-Controlled, Clinical Trial of High-Dose Supplementation with Vitamins C and E, Beta-Carotene and Zinc for Age-Related Macular Degeneration and Vision Loss," *Archives of Ophthalmology* 119: 1417–1436, 2001.

40. Christen, William G., Sc.D., et al. "A Prospective Study of Cigarette Smoking and Risk of Age-Related Macular Degeneration in Men," *Journal of the American Medical Association* 276(14): 1147–1151, Oct. 9, 1996.

41. Seddon, Johanna M., M.D. "A Prospective Study of Cigarette Smoking and Age-Related Macular Degeneration in Women," *Journal of the American Medical Association* 276(14): 1141-1146.

42. Belda, J. I., et al. "Serum Vitamin E Levels Negatively Correlate with Severity of

Age-Related Macular Degeneration," *Mechanisms of Ageing and Development* 107: 159–164, 1999.

43. Delcourt, C., et al. "Age-Related Macular Degeneration and Antioxidant Status in the POLA Study," *Archives of Ophthalmology* 117: 1384–1390, 1999.

44. Bunce, G. E. "Nutrition and Eye Disease of the Elderly," *Journal of Nutritional Biochemistry* 5: 66–77, 1994.

12 Take Care of Your Feet

Foot problems usually happen when there is nerve damage in the feet or when circulation to feet and legs is poor. The feet of diabetics should be checked daily and any serious problems should be referred to a health care provider. The suggestions given here are to ensure that feet are properly cared for in the hope of preventing amputation. Large doses of vitamin E can often prevent amputation. Magnesium, capsaicin, and Pycnogenol are other natural supplements that provide protection to diabetics. Acupuncture may be another option.

Foot problems usually happen when there is nerve damage in the feet and when blood flow is poor, according to the American Diabetes Association of Alexandria, Virginia. About one in five diabetics who enter the hospital have foot problems. It is important that diabetics inspect their feet daily, and ask for professional help if they get a foot injury. A health care provider should check the feet of diabetics at least once yearly.[1] Here are the typical problems to look for:

Skin Changes: Diabetes can cause feet to become very dry, and the skin may peel or crack. That is because the nerves that control sweating in the feet are no longer working. After bathing, dry the feet and seal in the moisture that remains with a thin coat of a lubricant, such as petroleum jelly, unscented hand cream, or other emollient. Do not put oil or cream between the toes, since moisture can cause an infection. Do not soak feet.

Calluses: Calluses build up faster on the feet of diabetics. Using a pumice stone daily will keep calluses under control. It is best to use a pumice stone on wet skin, and apply lotion after using the pumice stone. If calluses are not trimmed, they get very thick, break down, and result in foot ulcers (see below). Diabetics should not cut calluses or corns themselves, since this can lead to open sores and infection. This is best done by a professional. Do not remove calluses or corns with chemical agents, since they can burn the skin.

Foot Ulcers: These ulcers generally occur over the ball of the foot or at the bottom of the big toe. Ulcers can form on the sides of the foot, often caused by poorly fitting shoes. Even if ulcers do not hurt, they should be examined by a health care provider, since neglected foot ulcers can result in infections and a possible loss of a limb.

A health care provider should x-ray the feet of a diabetic to ensure that the bones are not affected. They can also cut out any dead and infected tissue. Diabetics should keep off of their feet, since walking on an ulcer will make it larger and force an infection deeper in the foot. High blood sugar levels make it difficult to fight an infection. If the ulcer is not healing and circulation is poor, the doctor may suggest a vascular surgeon. After the foot ulcer heals, it is still necessary to treat the foot carefully, since scar tissue under the healed wound will break down easily.

Diabetics should wear special shoes after the ulcer has healed to protect the area and prevent the ulcer from returning. Diabetics are more prone to get foot ulcers if they are over 40 years old, have had a foot ulcer before, have had diabetes-related changes in their eyes, or have kidney disease, nerve damage, or poor blood circulation to the feet.

Neuropathy: While it can hurt, diabetic nerve damage (neuropathy) can lessen the ability to feel pain, heat, and cold. Loss of feeling often means that the diabetic may not feel a foot injury. For example, they might have a tack or stone in their shoe and walk all day without feeling it. Therefore, they may not notice a foot injury until the skin breaks down and becomes infected. Nerve damage can also lead to deformities of the feet and toes, causing the toes to curl up. Those with deformed feet should not force them into regular shoes, but ask their health care provider about special therapeutic shoes.

Poor Circulation: Poor circulation (blood flow) can make the feet less able to fight infection and to heal. That's because diabetes causes blood vessels of the foot and leg to narrow and harden. It is possible to control some of the things that cause poor blood flow, such as to stop smoking,

How to Care for Your Feet

1. Keep blood sugar under control.
2. Wash feet daily. Dry them carefully, especially between toes.
3. Check feet daily for sores, calluses, red spots, cuts, swelling, and blisters. To see the bottom of feet, use a mirror or ask someone for help.
4. Do not put feet in hot water. First test to see how hot it is.
5. If feet are cold, wear socks.
6. Do not cut off blood flow to the feet by wearing garters or other such garments.
7. Do not use over-the-counter chemicals on corns, calluses, or warts, since they are usually too strong for diabetics, and they can burn the feet.
8. Cut toenails straight across and file the edges. Do not rip off hangnails.
9. Wear flat shoes that fit the feet.
10. If there is no sensation in the feet, ask the health care provider for advice on proper shoes.
11. Consider wearing comfortable walking shoes daily.
12. Check inside shoes before putting them on, to see that they do not contain pebbles, nails, or other sharp objects. Also check to see that the lining is not torn or rough.
13. Socks should not have seams or other bumpy areas. Do not wear mended socks. Put socks on gently to prevent ripping a toenail. Select padded athletic socks to protect the feet.
14. Do not walk barefoot. It is possible to burn or cut a foot and not notice it. Keep slippers bedside to use when getting up during the night.
15. Do not smoke.
16. See a health care provider at the first sign of infection or inflammation.

since smoking makes arteries harden faster. Also, it is important to keep blood pressure and cholesterol under control.

If feet are cold, there is a tendency to warm them. However, if the feet cannot feel heat, they can be burned with hot water, hot water bottles, or heating pads. To keep feet warm, wear warm socks. Exercise is also good for poor circulation, since it stimulates blood flow to the legs and feet. Walk in sturdy, comfortable shoes, but do not walk with open sores on the feet.

Some people feel pain in their calves when walking fast, up a hill, or on a hard surface. This is called intermittent claudication. Stopping to rest every so often should end the pain. Those who have this problem should stop smoking.

Amputation: Diabetics are more likely to have a foot or leg amputated than others. That's because diabetics often have artery disease, which reduces blood flow to the feet. Diabetics are also prone to nerve damage, which reduces sensation. These problems make it easy to get ulcers and infections that may lead to amputation. The biggest threat to a diabetic's feet is smoking, since this affects the small blood vessels. This causes decreased blood flow to the feet and makes wounds heal more slowly. Amputation is often prevented by improving blood flow to feet and legs.

There are two systems in the feet that seem to go wrong with diabetics, according to Neil M. Scheffler, D.P.M. One is the circulatory system and the other is the nervous system. Problems range from relatively minor ones, such as discomfort, to major ones, including the need for amputation of the leg.[2]

There are three types of diabetic neuropathy, or a disorder of the nerves, Scheffler said. Motor neuropathy affects the muscles, which change the function and shape of the foot. Autonomic neuropathy often inhibits the ability of the foot to sweat, so that feet can become very dry and the skin may crack. Sensory neuropathy prevents the foot from feeling sensations, and this is the form that causes the most trouble, Scheffler added.

Doctors who see patients with diabetic neuropathy have various options, Scheffler said. Doctors can prescribe various drugs, or they may opt for topical creams such as those containing capsaicin, which is derived from hot peppers. Acupuncture is often recommended.

Writing in *The Summary*, a periodic newsletter published by Evan V. Shute, M.D., and his colleagues at the Shute Clinic in London, Ontario, Canada, John K. MacKenzie, M.D., a Canadian physician, told the story of a 70-year-old Halifax fisherman who had been severely diabetic for many years and was taking large doses of insulin daily. When MacKenzie saw the man, he was suffering from extensive ulceration of the left foot with gangrenous changes including the toes. The man was urged to check into a hospital where his blood sugar could be monitored and his leg possibly amputated if it could not be saved.[3]

The man refused to go to the hospital, but at MacKenzie's suggestion, he agreed to take large oral doses of vitamin E. The man, whose daily habit was to sit in the kitchen with his left leg supported on a kitchen chair, became fully ambulatory and the ulcerative area completely healed, MacKenzie reported. The areas of blackish discoloration disappeared and his grossly swollen foot soon became a match for the other foot.

Shute tells the story of a steelworker who had dropped hot slag on his foot 11 months before. He had a dermatitis condition that would not heal. The patient was given 400 IU/day of vitamin E, and a vitamin E ointment was topically applied. The foot and the dermatitis healed in 13 days.[4]

Also in *The Summary*, Shute tells the story of a 59-year-old woman with ulceration on the right foot. A diabetic, she was taking no medication when she came to the hospital in a small town in Pennsylvania. The doctors immediately gave her insulin and 800 IU/day of vitamin E. Then they packed the ulcerated area with cotton saturated with vitamin E. Two months later, all wounds were healed.[5]

Shute relates another success story with vitamin E. Buerger's disease is a chronic disease of the arteries and veins. Eventually, a gradual thrombosis or narrowing of the blood vessels interferes with the blood supply to the affected area, and gangrene results.[6] Shute recounts the story of F. Gerloczy, a Hungarian doctor, who discusses the effects of vitamin E on various circulatory disorders. He gave the vitamin in enormous doses—up to 24,000 IU daily—and had spectacular results in 10 cases of thrombosis of the arteries, 16 cases of thrombophlebitis, and 12 out of 15 cases of Buerger's disease.

Shute said that Buerger's disease is the sinister and usually hopeless condition in which circulation in legs becomes so bad that recovery is impossible and amputation is necessary. However, he said, vitamin E saves many such legs. At the time of his newsletter (1972), there were only 13 papers in the medical literature attesting to that fact.

Poor Circulation: Writing in *Phytomedicine*, a research team reported that while their study did not focus on diabetes, they said that poor blood supply in the veins is a condition which increases blood pressure in the veins and sluggish blood flow in the legs. Common signs of chronic venous insufficiency are varicose veins, a heavy feeling in the legs, and swelling.[7]

In the first phase of their trial, the researchers gave 20 volunteers either a placebo or 100 mg of Pycnogenol three times daily for 2 months. In the second phase, another 20 volunteers received the same amount of Pycnogenol, which is a French maritime pine bark extract that has been shown to reduce platelet aggregation (the stickiness of platelets).

In the first phase of the study, a sense of heaviness in the legs was reduced by 60% in those given the extract, and leg swelling went down 74%. In the second phase, heaviness and swelling went down by 44% and 53%, respectively. The researchers attributed the improvement to the supplement's antioxidant or blood-vessel strengthening effect, or both.

Writing in the *Journal of Nutritional Medicine*, S. E. Browne wrote that intravenous magnesium sulfate has been used in cardiovascular disease for the past 60 years. He initially used magnesium sulfate intramuscularly and then intravenously in his practice in 1958 for patients with gangrene, leg ulcers, Raynaud's disease, chilblains, and intermittent claudication.[8]

For acute myocardial infarction (heart attack), Browne gives 5,000 units of IV Heparin along with 8 mmol (millimole, or one-thousandth of a gram-molecule) of magnesium. In a soft water area (where magnesium is in short supply), 6 of 7 patients with claudication (pain in their legs) were markedly improved by intravenous or intramuscular magnesium sulfate. In a hard water area (rich in magnesium), 14 of 25 patients with claudication showed marked improvement after intravenous magnesium and of 8 patients with leg ulcers, 5 healed quickly after failing to respond to other measures.

Further, 17 patients with minor inflammation in a vein were free of pain, tenderness, and inflammation, with only residual hardness observed after 2 weeks of treatment, and an additional 7 were fully recovered after 3 or 4 weeks of treatment; 1 patient did not improve. Four patients with deep vein thrombosis (blood clots) showed rapid improvement on intravenous magnesium given in addition to anticoagulant therapy. (Since Browne's article is lengthy, anyone interested in this approach should read the entire article.)

Gangrene: Gangrene, which is a dangerous complication of diabetes, is the result of the death of tissue, usually because of a loss of blood supply. This can affect a small area of the skin, a finger, or a large portion of a limb such as a leg. Pain can be felt in the dying tissue, but once the tissues are dead, they become numb and can turn black. A bacterial infection can develop, which causes gangrene to spread and give off an unpleasant odor. Often there is redness, swelling, and oozing pus around the affected area.[9]

There are two types of gangrene. With dry gangrene there is usually no bacterial infection. The deprived area simply dies because its blood supply is blocked. This type, which does not spread to other tissues, can be caused by diabetes, hardening of the arteries, thrombosis, an embolism, or frostbite. An embolism is the obstruction of a blood vessel, especially an artery, by a blood clot, air bubble, cancer cells, fat, bits of bacteria, a foreign body, or other cause, which is carried by the bloodstream until it lodges in and obstructs a blood vessel.

Wet gangrene forms when dry gangrene or a wound becomes affected by bacteria. A virulent form of the disease—gas gangrene—is caused by a dangerous strain of bacteria that destroys muscles and produces a foul-smelling gas. This type of gangrene has caused millions of deaths during war.

To treat dry gangrene, circulation must be improved to the affected area before it is too late. Medications can be prescribed to prevent wet gangrene from developing. If wet gangrene develops, amputation of the affected area is usually unavoidable. Some of the adjacent living tissue may also have to be removed.

References

1. "Foot Care," American Diabetes Association, Alexandria, Va. Undated.

2. Scheffler, Neil M., D.P.M. "Diabetic Neuropathy," *Diabetes Wellness Letter* 6(10): 4, 8, 2000.

3. Adams, Ruth, and Frank Murray. *Improving Your Health with Vitamin E.* New York: Larchmont Books, 978, pp. 43–44.

4. Ibid., pp. 120ff.

5. Ibid., p. 122.

6. Ibid., pp. 135–136.

7. Petrassi, C., et al. "Pycnogenol in Chromic Venous Insufficiency," *Phytomedicine* 7: 383–388, 2000.

8. Browne, S. E. "The Case for Intravenous Magnesium Treatment of Arterial Disease in General Practice: Review of 34 Years of Experience," *Journal of Nutritional Medicine* 4: 169–177, 1994.

9. Clayman, Charles B., M.D., medical editor. *The American Medical Association Home Medical Encyclopedia.* New York: Random House, 1989, pp. 474–475.

13 Take Care of Your Kidneys

Kidney failure is a serious complication of diabetes, which often requires dialysis or a kidney transplant. Kidney disease may be slowed by reducing high blood pressure, lowering cholesterol levels, and reducing the amount of protein in the diet, among other things. Since restricting protein in the diet can lead to malnutrition, the diet of diabetics should be monitored by a physician or dietician. Patients undergoing dialysis may also have nutritional deficiencies, some of which are outlined in this chapter.

Kidney failure is a serious potential complication for long-standing diabetes, according to *The Columbia University College of Physicians and Surgeons Complete Home Medical Guide.* The kidneys are complex, highly efficient organs for filtering waste materials from the blood for disposal from the body. As an example, each of the two kidneys contains more than 1 million nephrons, which are minute filtering systems. Damage to the small blood vessels in the nephrons can lead to progressive kidney failure, which is characterized by the excretion of protein and other nutrients in the urine.[1]

As diabetes also enhances the kidney's vulnerability to infections, diabetics should be aware of any symptoms of kidney or urinary tract infections (flank pain, difficult or burning urination, urgent need to urinate, blood in the urine) and should consult their doctor at once.

The *Guide* added that improved treatments of kidney failure, notably melodialysis using an artificial kidney and replacement of diseased kidneys with transplants, have enhanced the outlook for patients with advanced diabetic kidney disease (diabetic nephropathy). However, these measures do not cure the disease, and studies have reported that kidneys transplanted in patients with poorly controlled diabetes will develop diabetic nephropathy in a few years. Bringing elevated blood glucose into the normal range can reduce kidney damage.

At Washington University School of Medicine at St. Louis, Missouri, Saulo Klahr, M.D., said that the progression of kidney disease may be slowed by reducing high blood pressure, lowering cholesterol levels, reducing the amount of protein in the diet or reducing protein in the urine, and reducing the amount of immune cells in the kidney. Reducing animal protein levels decreases blood pressure and plasma flow within the glomerulus (a small grouping of capillaries in the kidney). Protein restriction is also thought to affect immune function, he said.[2]

Since dietary protein intake can increase blood flow to the kidneys, decreasing the amount of protein in the diet can reduce the blood flow to the kidney, according to Ping H. Wang, M.D., of the University of California at Irvine. This seems to provide a protective effect on a variety of kidney diseases. While previous studies have not consistently shown the efficacy of dietary protein restriction in reducing the risk of kidney disease progression, his study clearly shows that by lowering the amount of protein intake, the risk of end-stage kidney disease (the need for dialysis) can be reduced by 30% in most diabetic and nondiabetic patients, he said.[3]

Since the significant side effect of restricting protein is malnutrition, the patient should be closely followed by a physician and dietician. A low-protein diet for people with kidney disease should consist of 0.6 g per kilogram of body weight. This is safe for a majority of patients, he added.

"I would routinely recommend people with impaired kidney function to start a low-protein diet," Wang said. "However, because the risk of malnutrition may be increased in those who had a significant amount of protein excretion in their urine (more than 10 g/day), this patient group would not be good candidates for dietary protein restriction therapy."

Researchers, using a diabetic rat model, have found that there is an increased level of thiobarbituric acid reactive substances (TBARS) and activity of the enzyme superoxide dismutase and CM5-Px in the kidney during the progression of diabetes. The susceptibility of the kidney to oxidative stress, found early in diabetes, may be an important factor in the development of diabetic nephropathy.[4] TBARS are toxic molecules that can damage the kidneys.

A study by A. Hanck, M.D., in Basel, Switzerland, evaluated the vitamin status of 6 patients, ranging in age from 45 to 66, and 4 other volunteers, 28 to 40 years of age, who, due to nephropathy caused by analgesics or diabetes, underwent Continuous Ambulatory Peritoneal Dialysis (CAPD). Compared to healthy controls, vitamins B_1, B_6, C, and folic acid in the blood were in the lower range of normal, while vitamin A and B_{12} amounts in the blood were elevated. After supplementing with 8 mg of B_1, 8 mg of B_2, 10 mg of B_6, 50 mg of nicotinamide (B_3), 10.9 mg of calcium pantothenate (pantothenic acid), 30 mcg of biotin, 2 mg of folic acid, and 100 mg of vitamin C, given twice daily over 7 weeks, the levels of B_6 and C were normalized and the levels of folic acid greatly increased. However, levels of B_1 and B_2 remained unchanged. Pantothenic acid, biotin, and folic acid are B vitamins.[5]

During the 13-week study, levels of vitamins A and B_{12}, which were not supplemented, tended to normalize. The results of the trial show that increasingly efficient methods of dialysis lead to a growing loss of nutrients, whereby even substances regarded as insoluble in water are eliminated. This can lead to depleted body stores and malfunction, especially during long-term dialysis patients. Hanck recommends 30 mg of B_1, 10 to 50 mg of B_6, 0.5 to 1 mg of folic acid, and 100 to 200 mg of vitamin C twice daily.

Diabetics with kidney failure must endure dialysis, with a machine that filters their blood, or have a kidney transplant if a donated kidney can be found. Without dialysis, harmful levels of toxins can build up in their bodies.

Kidney dialysis patients are subject to painful muscular contractions in their legs. These cramps disrupt sleep, among other things. However, as reported in *Nephrology, Dialysis Transplantation*, researchers advised 60 dialysis patients to follow one of four daily supplement regimens for 8 weeks: 1) 400 mg of vitamin E, 2) 250 mg of vitamin C, 3) a combination of both vitamins, or 4) a placebo or look-alike pill.[6]

The patients taking a combination of vitamin E and vitamin C reaped the greatest benefits: a 97% reduction in leg cramps. When taken alone,

Since dietary protein intake can increase blood flow to the kidneys, decreasing the amount of protein in the diet can reduce the blood flow to the kidney, according to Ping H. Wang, M.D., of the University of California at Irvine. His study clearly shows that by lowering the amount of protein intake, the risk of end-stage kidney disease (the need for dialysis) can be reduced by 30% in most diabetic and nondiabetic patients, he said.

vitamin E and vitamin C resulted in 54% and 61% reductions in leg cramps, respectively, while the placebo brought only a 7% reduction in symptoms.

Malnutrition, mentioned above, is one of the main factors in the death and disability of dialysis patients, according to Richard Schmicker, M.D., in Berlin, Germany. Food restriction, adequate protein and energy intake, electrolyte (mineral) balance, and vitamin intake are important when beginning dialysis, he said.[7]

Because of deficiencies, he suggested that dialysis patients may need to take supplements of vitamin C (100 mg/day), vitamins B_1 and B_2 (between 1.5 and 1.6 mg/day), and vitamin B_6 (10 to 20 mg/day). Folic acid may need to be supplemented at 1 mg/day. Vitamin A may not be needed, since it is often higher in dialysis patients, he said.

In a study in Rome, Italy, it was reported that of the 48 chronic hemodialysis patients, coenzyme Q10 levels were abnormally low in 62% of the cases. Reduced levels of coenzyme Q10 may increase the risk of oxidative damage in patients with chronic uremic poisoning who are undergoing hemodialysis.[8]

Michael T. Pedrini, M.D., and colleagues at the University of California at Irvine also agree that restricting dietary protein effectively slows the progression of both diabetic and nondiabetic kidney diseases. They evaluated the effects of a low-protein diet on chronic kidney disease in 1,413 volunteers from five studies of nondiabetic renal (kidney) disease and 108 patients in five studies with Type 1 diabetics. In five studies involving Type 1 diabetes, a low-protein diet significantly slowed the increase in urinary albumin levels or the decline in other parameters. Albumin is one of a number of water-soluble proteins that are found in blood plasma.[9]

At Schneider Children's Hospital in New Hyde Park, New York, researchers pointed out that the kidney plays a significant role in maintaining taurine balance, an amino acid that acts as an antioxidant in the body. It can prevent the oxidizing of fats in capillaries and tissues in the kidney that are exposed to high glucose and other conditions. In experimental tests, dietary taurine ameliorates kidney disease, including refractory nephrotic syndrome (which does not respond to traditional treatment) and diabetic nephropathy.[10]

References

1. Tapley, Donald F., M.D., et al. "Diabetes and Other Endocrine Disorders," *The Columbia University College of Physicians and Surgeons Complete Home Medical Guide.* New York: Crown, 1985, pp. 474ff.

2. Klahr, Saulo, M.D. "Progression of Kidney Disease May Be Preventable," *Kidney 90/Medical News Report* 7(4): 6–7, July/August 1990.

3. Hamilton, Kirk. "Renal Disease, Diabetes and Protein Restriction," *The Experts Speak.* Sacramento, Calif.: I.T. Services, 1997, p. 115. Also, Wang, Ping H., M.D. "The Effect of Dietary Protein Restriction on the Progression of Diabetic and Nondiabetic Renal Disease: A Meta-Analysis," *Annals of Internal Medicine* 124(7): 627–632, April 1, 1996.

4. Kakkar, Rakesh, et al. "Antioxidant Defense System in Diabetic Kidney," *Life Sciences* 60(9): 667–679, 1997.

5. Hanck, A., M.D. "Vitamin Intake Under CAPD," *Niren-Und Hochdruckkrankheiten* 21 (Suppl. 1): S64–S69, May 1992.

6. Khajehdeni, P., et al. "A Randomized, Double-Blind, Placebo-Controlled Trial of Supplementary Vitamins E, C and Their Combination for Treatment of Hemodialysis Cramps," *Nephrology, Dialysis Transplantation* 16: 1448–1451, 2001.

7. Schmicker, Richard. "Nutritional Treatment of Hemodialysis and Peritoneal Dialysis Patients," *Artificial Organs* 19(8): 837–841, 1995.

8. Triolo, Luigi, M.D., et al. "Serum Coenzyme Q10 and Uremic Patients and Chronic Hemodialysis," *Nephron* 66: 153–156, 1994.

9. Pedrini, Michael T., M.D., et al. "The Effect of Dietary Protein Restriction on the Progression of Diabetic and Nondiabetic Renal Diseases: A Meta-Analysis," *Annals of Internal Medicine* 124(7): 627–632, April 1, 1996.

10. Trachtman, H., and J. A. Sturman. "Taurine: A Therapeutic Agent in Experimental Kidney Disease," *Amino Acids* 11: 1–13, 1996.

14 Take Care of Your Thyroid Gland

The thyroid gland, located in front of the neck, releases two powerful hormones, T3 and T4, which increase the uptake of oxygen, the rate at which fats and carbohydrates are metabolized for energy, and the basal metabolic rate, which is a measure of the energy expended during respiration, circulation, and other processes. Some people are diagnosed with hypothyroidism, which means insufficient production of thyroid hormone. Others suffer from hyperthyroidism, which is an overproduction of the hormone.

Many diabetics have hypothyroidism, which leads to weakness, itching, constipation, muscular pains, elevated blood fats, poor wound healing, hardening of the arteries and gangrene, among other things. Thyroid therapy corrects the problem with hypothyroidism and protects diabetics from hardening of the arteries and other complications. In addition, proper amounts of thyroid hormone are necessary for the body to maintain proper levels of blood sugar, especially for Type 2 diabetics.

An organ of the endocrine system, the thyroid gland is located in the neck, just below the voice box. It consists of two lobes, one on each side of the windpipe and joined by a narrow portion of tissue called isthmus.

Thyroid tissue is made up of two types of secretory cells—follicular cells and parafollicular cells (C cells). Follicular cells are made up of hollow, spherical follicles, which secrete the iodine-containing hormones thyroxine (T4) and triiodothyronine (T3). Inside the follicles is a semifluid, colloid substance that is essential for the production of T4 and T3.[1]

Parafollicular cells are found singly or in groups in the spaces between the follicles. These cells secrete the hormone calcitonin. Between the follicles are a number of blood capillaries, which are small lymphatic vessels, and connective tissue.

T4 and T3 hormones play a significant role in controlling body metabolism. For example, calcitonin acts with parathyroid hormone (produced by the parathyroid gland) to regulate calcium balance in the body. By regulating metabolism, the two hormones release energy from nutrients or use energy to create other substances, such as proteins. In children, the two hormones are essential for normal physical growth and mental development. The secretion of T4 and T3 is controlled by a hormonal feedback system that involves the pituitary gland and hypothalamus in the brain.

"Insufficient thyroid hormone production is known as hypothyroidism," states the *American Medical Association Home Medical Encyclopedia.* "Symptoms include tiredness, dry skin, hair loss, weight gain, constipation and sensitivity to cold. Overproduction of thyroid hormones—hyperthyroidism—causes fatigue, anxiety, palpitations, sweating, weight loss, diarrhea and intolerance to heat."

It was the late Broda O. Barnes, M.D., in his landmark book, *Hypothyroidism: The Unsuspected Illness,* who highlighted the many health problems due to low thyroid function. Concerning diabetes, he called it an "iceberg" disease, in that it involves more than sugar in the blood; that is, sugar in the blood is only the tip of the iceberg. Today, diabetics are not so much troubled by metabolic crises, but may suffer from the complications of diabetes—from blindness, kidney and nervous disease, skin infections, and above all, degenerative changes in the heart and blood vessels.

Diabetics have twice the rate of coronary heart disease as nondiabetics, and at the famed Joslin Clinic in Boston, Massachusetts, 46.5% of diabetic deaths have been due to atherosclerotic heart disease. Further, as many as 77% of diabetic deaths are due to blood vessel disease of one type or another, he said.[2]

"The complications of diabetes are much like the manifestations of hypothyroidism," Barnes continued. "Many diabetics do, in fact, have low thyroid function. I am not the first to observe that the complications of diabetes, particularly the atherosclerotic complications (hardening of the arteries), are not due to the disturbance in carbohydrate metabolism but to something else. And that something else could well be hypothyroidism. I believe that thyroid therapy for people with low thyroid function who have not yet developed diabetes may do much to prevent appearance of the disease."

Barnes discussed a paper by C. D. Eaton, M.D., a Detroit physician, in a report in *The Journal of the Michigan Medical Society* in 1954. After dealing with hundreds of diabetics, Eaton said that the symptoms of hypothyroidism and diabetes are quite similar, except for the disturbance in carbohydrate metabolism that occurs in diabetes. The patients with both complications suffered from one or many of such symptoms as weakness, itching, constipation, somnolence, muscular pains, elevated blood fat levels, susceptibility to infections, poor healing of wounds, premature hardening of the arteries, and gangrene.

While controlling the sugar level in diabetic patients, Eaton found that the other symptoms persisted. And when he determined the incidence of hypothyroidism in diabetic patients with the basal metabolic rate, he found that even though that test is not very sensitive and may miss many cases of low thyroid function, it established that hypothyroidism was more frequent in diabetics than in nondiabetics.

When Eaton began giving thyroid therapy in small doses to his hypothyroid diabetic patients, he found that the thyroid had no direct influence on diabetes. But when sugar metabolism was controlled by insulin or diet or other measures, it *remained controlled* when thyroid doses were added.

Eaton also noted that there were fewer problems with blood clots in the arteries, which he interpreted as being due to improved circulation and less pooling and stagnation of blood. In addition, as a result of increased circulation in the extremities, there was less gangrene, even in those with hardening of the arteries.

"All of the diabetic patients I have personally treated to date have run subnormal basal temperatures and have had symptoms of hypothyroidism, and with thyroid therapy they have had not only relief of the hypothyroidism symptoms but have shown no detectable progression in atherosclerosis," Barnes added.

The size of a proper starting dose of thyroid therapy will vary with the age and size of the patient, Barnes said. A child under 3 years of age will usually not need more than one-quarter grain daily. By age 6, one-half grain may be used in the beginning; a teenager or adult may be safely started on one grain daily; for overweight people, two grains may be used, but larger doses are not needed initially. The starting dose should be used for about two months, and perhaps increased after that. Those who have

Basal Body Temperature Test to Check Your Thyroid Status

1. Before going to sleep, shake down a thermometer to below 95° F and place it near your bed.

2. Upon waking, place the thermometer in your armpit for 10 minutes. Do not move about, but rest with your eyes closed.

3. After 10 minutes, record the temperature and date.

4. Record the temperature on successive mornings at the same time. Menstruating women should perform the test on the second, third, and fourth days of menstruation.

The correct basal body temperature should be between 97.6 and 98.2° F. It will register below the normal reading of 98.6, since you are taking your temperature under the arm rather than orally or anally. Show the readings to your physician to determine if you have hypothyroidism.

Source: Julian Whitaker, M.D. *Dr. Whitaker's Guide to Natural Healing.* Rocklin, Calif.: Prima Publishing, 1995, pp. 282–283.

had a heart attack should not begin therapy for at least two months after the incident, then the starting dose should not be more than one-half grain a day. The basal temperature (see chart) can serve as an excellent guide not only to the need for thyroid therapy, but also to determine the proper thyroid dosage, Barnes said.

Proper levels of thyroid hormone are necessary for the body to maintain proper levels of blood sugar, explain Ronald Klatz, D.O., and Robert Goldman, M.D. Therefore, hypothyroidism may be implicated in diabetes, especially Type 2 diabetes, which is a condition in which the body has difficulty in regulating blood sugar levels.

Basically, the thyroid allows us to convert glucose into energy, but in cases of hypothyroidism, glucose cannot be utilized, resulting in glucose waste and hypoglycemia. Hypoglycemia causes the excretion of adrenaline, which causes toxicity of the circulatory system. These circulatory problems are common in diabetics, but they can be reduced or avoided with thyroid supplements. The authors added that thyroid supplements have also been shown to reverse other symptoms of diabetes, and in some cases, have reversed Type 2 diabetes.[3]

The medical treatment for hypothyroidism involves taking desiccated thyroid or synthetic thyroid hormone, according to Michael Murray, N.D., and Joseph Pizzorno, N.D. While synthetic hormones are popular, physicians, especially naturopathic physicians, usually prefer desiccated natural thyroid, complete with all the thyroid hormones, not just thyroxine. The thyroid extracts sold in health food stores are required to be free of thyroxine in order to prevent such serious problems as heart disturbances, insomnia, and anxiety. The health food store products may provide support for those with mild hypothyroidism, the authors said.[4]

"It is important to nutritionally support the thyroid gland by avoiding goitrogens and insuring adequate intake of key nutrients required in the manufacture of thyroid hormone. For this reason, most health food store thyroid products also contain supportive nutrients such as iodine, zinc and tyrosine," the authors added.

Goitrogenic agents, which produce goiter, include: 1) members of the cabbage family—cabbage, turnip, rutabaga, kale (cooking usually inactivates the goitrogenic agent); 2) milk from cows that have eaten plants containing goitrogens; 3) raw soybeans; 4) thiocyanate containing drugs for high blood pressure; 5) arsenic; and others.

Thyroid hormone or extract is the sixth most commonly prescribed drug in the United States, according to *Family Practice News*. Unfortunately, some elderly patients were placed on thyroid in excessively high amounts years ago in the absence of primary thyroid gland failure. A low thyroid stimulating hormone may be indicative of inappropriate thyroid suppression therapy or atrial fibrillation, the publication added.[5]

Researchers in Brazil evaluated 12 hyperthyroid patients and 7 hypothyroid patients to determine their zinc levels. They found that hyperthyroid patients showed a marked zinc loss, with maintenance of serum zinc due to probable tissue depletion of the mineral and lower zinc incorporation into their tissues after being given a zinc supplement. The findings were probably due to the catabolic state of hypothyroidism. Catabolism is the breaking down of complex chemical compounds into simpler ones, such as glycogen into carbon dioxide and water. For the hypothyroid volunteers, there was a definite zinc deficiency with lower intestinal absorption of the mineral.[6]

Subclinical hypothyroidism (too low to be diagnosed by conventional tests) is found in more than 10% of women over 60, thus increasing serum lipids and lowering the threshold for developing major depressive disorders, according to Kenneth A. Weeber, M.D., of the San Francisco-Mount Zion Medical Center in California. Subclinical thyrotoxicosis (excessive amounts of thyroid hormone) is a state in which there is normal serum T4 but with a level of thyroid-stimulating hormone (TSH) that is undetectable in an individual who is not ill. Subclinical thyrotoxicosis is sometimes associated with reduced bone mineral density in postmenopausal women and a threefold relative risk for the development of atrial fibrillation (irregular heart beat).[7]

Inadvertent excess hormone in the treatment of hypothyroidism can result in subclinical hypothyroidism, according to *Family Practice News*. It has been estimated that, even in thyroid disease clinics, excessive doses may occur in about 20% of the patients. The cardiovascular system does not tolerate subclinical hyperthyroidism, and there is evidence for increased heart rate and contractility associated with subclinical hyperthyroidism. The publication added that atrial fibrillation is a symptom of subclinical hyperthyroidism, along with arrhythmias and premature atrial beats. Contractility refers to the ability of a muscle to shorten or become reduced in size or developing increased tension.[8] Subclinical hyperthyroidism is when a patient does not have a full-blown case of hyperthyroidism, or overactive thyroid gland.

Smoking appears to have a goitrogenic (or goiter-producing) effect, apparently from the action of thiocyanate and other compounds found in cigarette smoke, according to researchers in Pisa, Italy. This is especially important for people who live in iodine-deficient areas. Smokers have a high prevalence of Graves' disease (an autoimmune disease of the thyroid gland), as well as Graves' ophthalmology (increased water in the eye as a result of hyperthyroidism).[9]

References

1. Clayman, Charles B., M.D. *The American Medical Association Home Medical Encyclopedia.* New York: Random House, 1989, pp. 985ff.

2. Barnes, Broda O., M.D., and Lawrence Galton. *Hypothyroidism: The Unsuspected Illness.* New York: Thomas V. Crowell Co., 1976, pp. 214ff.

3. Klatz, Ronald, D.O., and Robert Goldman, M.D. *Stopping the Clock.* New Canaan, Conn.: Keats Publishing, 1996, p. 175.

4. Murray, Michael, N.D., and Joseph Pizzorno, N.D. *Encyclopedia of Natural Medicine.* Rocklin, Calif.: Prima Publishing, 1998, p. 562.

5. Bates, Betsy. "Improper Thyroid Hormone Therapy Often Missed," *Family Practice News,* Jan. 15, 1996, p. 22.

6. Pimenta, W. P., et al. "The Assessment of Zinc Status by the Zinc Tolerance Test and Thyroid Disease," *Trace Elements in Medicine* 9(1): 34–37, 1992.

7. Weeber, Kenneth A., M.D. "Subclinical Thyroid Dysfunction," *Archives of Internal Medicine* 157: 1065–1068, May 26, 1997.

8. Cooper, Catherine. "Overtreating Hypothyroidism Is An Easy, Insidious Mistake," *Family Practice News,* June 1, 1993, p. 5.

9. Bartalena, Luigi, et al. "Cigarette Smoking and the Thyroid," *European Journal of Endocrinology* 133: 507–512, 1995.

15 Cholesterol: Friend or Foe?

Although cholesterol is essential for human health, a small number of people have inherited a condition in which they do not metabolize the fat-like substance and must take steps to lower it. This is especially timely for diabetics in order to avoid a heart attack or stroke.

HDL-cholesterol is the beneficial kind that offers protection against coronary artery disease. LDL-cholesterol is the harmful kind and must be kept in check.

It is also important to control triglycerides, another fat, which are discussed in another chapter. However, since triglycerides are often studied with cholesterol, many useful substances for lowering triglyceride levels are dealt with here.

Before embarking on a drug-laden regimen for lowering cholesterol in the blood, ask your physician about the numerous natural approaches, with few if any side effects, such as: vitamin B_3, lecithin, oat bran, garlic, Lactobacillus acidophilus, rhubarb stalk fiber, walnuts, almonds, pistachios, barley bran, chromium, omega-3 fatty acids, red yeast rice, psyllium, and numerous others.

Cholesterol is an important constituent of body cells, and it is involved in the formation of hormones and bile salts, as well as in the transport of fats in the bloodstream to tissues throughout the body, according to the *American Medical Association Home Medical Encyclopedia*. Most of the cholesterol in the blood is made by the liver from foods, especially saturated fats. However, some cholesterol is absorbed directly into the bloodstream from cholesterol-rich foods, such as eggs and dairy products.[1]

Cholesterol and triglycerides (the most abundant fats in the body) are transported through the body in the form of lipoproteins. These particles are made up of cholesterol and lipoproteins, and an outer wrapping of phospholipids and apoproteins (carrier proteins). The most abundant cholesterol in the blood is high-density lipoproteins (HDL-cholesterol), which seems to protect against arterial disease. It is referred to as "good" cholesterol. If most cholesterol in the blood is low-density lipoprotein cholesterol (LDL, the "bad" cholesterol) or very low-density lipoprotein cholesterol, the risk of developing disease is increased.

"The level of cholesterol in the blood is influenced by diet, heredity and metabolic diseases such as diabetes mellitus," the publication stated. "There is overwhelming evidence that a high blood cholesterol level increases the risk of developing atherosclerosis (accumulation of fatty tissue on the inner lining of arteries) and with it the risk of coronary heart disease and stroke."

While we are constantly bombarded in the media with details of how cholesterol is killing us, the eminent heart surgeon Michael E. DeBakey, M.D., states that only about 30% of his heart patients have any form of abnormality in their cholesterol. He added that the majority of heart patients have perfectly normal cholesterol levels and have been eating most anything they want without dietary restrictions.

While DeBakey has not ruled out the importance of diet, he has said that it is not the specific cause of heart disease. "We don't know the cause and we need to take a much saner attitude towards diet in relation to the disease, since it is obvious that diet, as far as 65 to 70% of the patients are concerned, has not been related or associated with the disease in our experience."[2]

Joseph L. Goldstein, M.D., and Michael S. Brown, M.D., of the University of Texas Southwestern Medical School at Dallas, state the cause of high cholesterol levels is abnormal cholesterol *synthesis,* that is, how it is made. The key seems to be the enzyme that controls the rate of cholesterol synthesis. The genetic defect underlying inherited high cholesterol is in the gene that makes fat-proteins that usually exert feedback control over the enzyme, they added.

Cholesterol is, after all, needed by the body. Mark D. Altschule, M.D., points out that cholesterol is the material from which cortisone and other adrenal gland hormones are derived. During exercise, cholesterol can serve as a source of energy. The fatty substance is oxidized to carbon dioxide and water like any other source of energy (sugar, fat, etc.), and it is

How to Measure Cholesterol

Cholesterol in the blood is measured as milligrams per deciliter, with a deciliter equivalent to 100 ml or 3.3 oz. of blood.

200 mg/dl or below	Desirable
200 to 239 mg/dl	Borderline high
240 mg/dl or above	High; ask physician for recommendations

Low-Density Lipoprotein Cholesterol (LDL)

100 mg/dl or less	No treatment needed
100 mg/dl to 130 mg/dl	Diet, exercise, lifestyle changes
130 mg/dl and over	Diet, exercise, lifestyle changes, medication

High-Density Lipoprotein Cholesterol (HDL)

40 mg/dl or more	No treatment needed
60 mg/dl	Ideal for protecting against heart disease

Triglycerides

150 mg/dl	No treatment needed
400 mg/dl and over	High, ask physician for recommendations

changed by the body into bile constituents (yes, gallstones are almost pure cholesterol). Digestion would be difficult without bile salts to emulsify fats in the digestive tract so they can be absorbed into the body. Cholesterol is present in every body cell, and it may help to regulate the transport of nutrients and waste products in and out of the body.

Ordinary diets are likely to supply 600 to 900 milligrams of cholesterol daily, according to the U.S. Department of Agriculture. A "low cholesterol" diet usually provides about 300 milligrams of cholesterol each day. The USDA added that studies have not shown convincingly that the reduction of dietary cholesterol in the general population reduces the frequency of hardening of the arteries; however, people with atherosclerosis usually have higher blood cholesterol levels than those without the disease.

Blood levels of cholesterol are elevated in diabetes, during periods of weight gain or low thyroid activity, and with other conditions of depressed metabolism. Cholesterol is elevated by several dietary factors, including calories in excess of energy needs, high intakes of fat, especially certain saturated fatty acids and dietary cholesterol; by high protein intakes, such as animal proteins and those high in the sulfur-containing amino acids (methionine and cystine); and by choline and rapidly absorbed sugars.[3]

High cholesterol levels in the blood can be lowered by relatively high intakes of linoleic acid and perhaps by other polyunsaturated fatty acids, by high intakes of nicotinic acid (vitamin B_3), by dietary starches in place of sugars, and by strict vegetarian-type diets, as well as by stepped-up energy metabolism, such as regular exercise, thyroid hormone, and other agents that speed up metabolism.[4]

Surprisingly, meat is not necessarily high in cholesterol, according to William C. Sherman, Ph.D. A standard serving (100 g or 3-1/2 oz.) of beef, pork, or lamb has only about 70 mg of cholesterol. Veal is a little higher at about 90 mg/serving. Liver is relatively high in cholesterol, around 300 mg/serving, and kidney has 345 mg in an average serving.

To lower cholesterol levels, Roger Williams, Ph.D., of the University of Texas at Austin, suggested consuming more lecithin. Lecithin has soap-like characteristics and is a powerful emulsifying agent; its presence in the blood tends to dissolve cholesterol deposits. When there is substantially more lecithin in the blood than cholesterol—a ratio of 1:2 to 1 is said to be favorable—the actual amount of cholesterol can be high without the blood plasma getting milky or showing a tendency to produce fatty deposits, he said. Lecithin reduces cholesterol absorption by 36.7% at a dose of 700 mg, and by 34.4% at a dose of 300 mg.[5]

According to Teh C. Huang, D.V.M., the body favors saturated fats over unsaturated fats in the normal, healthy condition. In fact, body tissues utilize more saturated fats than polyunsaturated fats of about 3:1. There are often recommendations for a 1:1 ratio, but it is unnatural to change our bodies' composition, he added.

John Yudkin, M.D., a British nutritionist, said that the flap over cholesterol and its relation to heart disease began in 1913 when a Russian scientist named Anitschkow fed rabbits very large quantities of cholesterol and noticed deposits in the rabbits' arteries and called it arteriosclerosis. "Let me say in parentheses that there is still some argument as to the relevance of this change to arteriosclerosis (hardening of the arteries) in man."

Yudkin cites another paper the Russian published in 1914. "It's not a tirade but a warning on his own experiments to those who have taken his work to imply that all that is important in man in causing arteriosclerosis and heart disease is the amount of cholesterol in the diet and consequently in the blood," Yudkin continued.

Yudkin went on to say that Anitschkow got the effect with his rabbits by feeding them *huge* quantities of cholesterol, while the amount of cholesterol that people ingest is very much less. Nobody could possibly eat the sorts of amounts that he gave his rabbits, Yudkin continued. (Rabbits are vegetarians and would have trouble metabolizing cholesterol-rich diets.) "So Anitschkow was very anxious to prevent people—unsuccessfully as it turns out—from saying that what we must do in order to prevent arteriosclerosis in man is to limit the consumption of cholesterol," Yudkin said. (Yudkin blamed the high rates of heart disease in Western countries on the high white sugar diets.)

Eggs are certainly maligned by the health establishment, yet, if they only had vitamin C, they would be the perfect food. They do not contain vitamin C because the hen manufactures what she needs. Meanwhile, a large egg contains between 250 and 275 mg of cholesterol.

"The egg is truly Nature's masterpiece," according to the U.S. Department of Agriculture. "It is a prepackaged container of many important nutrients needed by every member of the family. Eggs are especially valued for the amount and high quality of the protein they contain. In fact, egg protein is so near perfect that scientists often use it as a standard to measure the protein in other foods."

Eggs also provide significant amounts of vitamin A, iron, and riboflavin (vitamin B_2), and they are one of the few foods that contain natural vitamin D. Eggs contribute smaller amounts of many other nutrients, such as calcium, phosphorus, and thiamine (vitamin B_1).

"The nutrients are unevenly distributed within the egg," the USDA said. "Egg yolk, little more than one-third of the edible part, contains the fat, vitamin A, thiamine and nearly all of the calcium, phosphorus and iron in the egg and considerable protein and riboflavin. Egg white is much higher than egg yolk in water content. The white contains protein and riboflavin—not so much as an equal weight of egg yolk, but, because there is nearly twice as much white as yolk, more than half the total protein and riboflavin in an egg are in the white."

If you were to avoid all the cholesterol you could in your diet, your body would still manufacture cholesterol at a fairly steady rate and in a relatively profuse amount. It has been shown repeatedly that the less cholesterol a person eats, the more his body produces. It has also been shown that the normal person's body will rid itself of just about the same amount of cholesterol as that eaten, according to the National Commission on Egg Nutrition in Illinois.

For those who don't metabolize the cholesterol in eggs properly, this could cause hardening of the arteries and lead to heart attack and stroke, major health problems for diabetics.

It has been estimated that between 5 and 13% of the population has inherited a condition in which they do not metabolize cholesterol properly and must take measures to lower it in the blood. But as we will see, there are numerous ways of lowering cholesterol naturally without resorting to drugs. There are hundreds of articles in medical journals that show how this can be done; here are just a few of them.

Niacin, B₃: At Bowman Gray School of Medicine in Winston-Salem, North Carolina, 28 men with normal cholesterol levels, but with low plasma concentrations of HDL-cholesterol, were randomly selected to receive increasing doses of niacin (vitamin B_3) up to 3,000 mg/day or no vitamin for 12 weeks; then the men took the opposite treatment, and of the group, 15 completed the study.[6]

The vitamin treatment brought a 14% decrease in total cholesterol; a 40% decrease in triglycerides; and an 18% decrease in LDL-cholesterol and a 30% increase in HDL-cholesterol, which we know is the "good" cholesterol. Since the large dose of niacin can cause flushing, physicians should supervise the dosages.

The crystalline niacin was given in incremental doses starting at 125 mg/t.i.d. (three times a day). The dose was doubled after that first week to 250 mg/t.i.d., and then doubled after the second week to 500 mg/t.i.d. Following the third week, the dose went to 1 g/b.i.d. (twice a day), and after the fourth week to 1 g/t.i.d., if tolerated. If the patient could not tolerate the higher doses, the amounts were reduced.

In a double-blind trial at Duke University Medical Center at Durham, North Carolina, researchers studied 399 male and female volunteers, ranging in age from 21 to 75. During the test, 173 were randomly selected to receive Niaspan, a time-release niacin (B_3), at doses increasing from 1,000 to 2,000 mg at bedtime, or gemfibrozil (a lipid-lowering drug) at 600 mg twice daily.

During the study, 82% of the 88 volunteers given the niacin and 80% of the 85 given gemfibrozil completed the study. The research team reported that Niaspan at 1,500 and 2,000 mg versus the drug raised HDL-cholesterol levels 21 and 26%, respectively. The 2,000 mg dose was given once daily and was well tolerated.[7]

A study at Brookhaven Memorial Hospital Medical Center, Patchogue, New York, studied 22 men and 1 woman, between the ages of 41 and 80, who had hardening of the arteries. They were given either 600 mg of gemfibrozil orally, twice daily, or time-release nicotinic acid (a form of vitamin B_3), starting at 100 to 250 mg three times daily. This amount was eventually increased to 1,500 to 3,000 mg/day for 3 months. For those who tolerated the therapy, HDL-cholesterol increased by 15% while taking the drug, by 35% while taking vitamin B_3, and by 45% while taking a combination of the two substances.[8]

In a study involving 4 men and 6 women with moderately high cholesterol levels, they substituted 20% of their daily caloric intake with pistachio nuts for 3 weeks. It was found that there was a reduction in total cholesterol, an increase in HDL-cholesterol, a decrease in total cholesterol/HDL ratio and a decrease in LDL/HDL ratio.

Pistachios: In a study involving 4 men and 6 women with moderately high cholesterol levels, they substituted 20% of their daily caloric intake with pistachio nuts for 3 weeks. It was found that there was a reduction in total cholesterol, an increase in HDL-cholesterol, a decrease in total cholesterol/HDL ratio, and a decrease in LDL/HDL ratio. There was a slight reduction in triglycerides and LDL-cholesterol. Blood pressure and weight were unchanged.[9]

Omega-3 Oils: At the Hospital of Valdinievole in Pescia, Italy, 16 patients with high blood levels of fats were given 1 gram of omega-3 fatty acids daily for 90 days. This brought a decrease in blood triglyceride and cholesterol levels, and an increase in HDL-cholesterol. There were minimal side effects.[10]

Psyllium Fiber: In a study involving 197 volunteers, James W. Anderson, M.D., and colleagues gave them 5.1 g of psyllium (a high-fiber plant substance), compared with 51 people who took a cellulose placebo twice daily for 26 weeks. The participants had high blood levels of cholesterol and followed the American Heart Association Step 1 diet for 8 weeks. The researchers found that serum total and LDL-cholesterol were 4.7 and 6.7% lower in the psyllium group than in the placebo group after 24 to 26 weeks. The use of 5.1 g of psyllium twice daily brought net reductions in serum total and LDL-cholesterol (the "bad" kind) in both men and women.[11]

Bran: At Texas A&M University at College Station, researchers evaluated 79 men and women whose mean age was 48.2 years; all had high cholesterol levels. They were given 20 g of cellulose, 3 g of barley oil extract, or 30 g of barley bran flour daily. Barley bran flour significantly lowered total serum cholesterol, as did the barley oil following 30 days of treatment. LDL-cholesterol went down 6.5% with the addition of barley bran flour, and 9.2% with the barley oil. LDL-cholesterol did not go down significantly in the cellulose group. HDL-cholesterol dropped appreciably in the cellulose and barley bran flour group, but not with the barley oil.[12]

A research team at the University of California, Davis Medical Center and Sutter Heart Institute in Sacramento, California, gave participants 84 g/day of rice bran, oat bran, or rice starch placebo to their usual low-fat diet. Serum cholesterol went down significantly in the rice bran and oat bran groups by 8.3 and 13%, respectively. There was no change in the placebo group. The researchers attributed the change to a lowering of LDL-cholesterol by 13.7% in the rice bran group and 17.1% in the oat bran group. There was no significant change in triglycerides, HDL-cholesterol, or apoprotein-A readings.[13]

Nuts: Australian researchers evaluated 16 men, average age of 41, who consumed a diet containing 36% of calories from fat for 9 weeks. In the first 3 weeks, the diet was supplemented with raw peanuts at 50 g/day, coconut cubes at 40 g/day, and a coconut confectionery bar at 50 g/day. During the following 3 weeks, the diet was supplemented with monounsaturated fatty acid-rich raw almonds at 84 g/day, equivalent to 46 g fat, and in the following 3 weeks, the diet was supplemented with polyunsaturated fatty acid-rich walnuts at 68 g/day, equal to 46 g of fat. There was a 7 and 10% reduction in total and LDL-cholesterol after supplementation with almonds, and a 5 and 9% reduction after eating walnuts.[14]

Plant Fiber: At the University of Alberta, Edmonton, Canada, a research team studied 10 men with high cholesterol levels who consumed 27 g of ground rhubarb stalk fiber daily for 4 weeks. This brought an 8% lowering of total serum cholesterol and a 9% lowering of LDL-cholesterol. HDL-cholesterol remained unchanged. One month after the fiber was stopped, total and LDL-cholesterol returned to the same levels as at the beginning of the study.[15]

In two controlled studies, involving some 250 volunteers, Cholestin, which is derived from red yeast rice, lowered blood levels of LDL-cholesterol by 20 to 30%. The recommended dose at 2.4 g/day contains 4.6 mg of lovastatin, a constituent in the rice.[16]

Garlic: A Medline search from 1966 to 1991, which reviewed twenty-eight studies on the use of garlic and blood cholesterol levels, found that patients treated with garlic consistently showed a greater reduction in total cholesterol compared to those given a placebo. A meta-analysis of the trials (a compilation of the data) estimated that cholesterol levels dropped 23 mg/dl. The average drop in total cholesterol in the blood was about 9%.[17]

Chromium: Researchers at Oklahoma State University at Stillwater studied 42 elderly volunteers, 60 years of age or older, who were given 150 mcg/day of chromium or a placebo. This brought a reduction in LDL-cholesterol. HDL-cholesterol, triglycerides, and glucose were unchanged.[18]

Acidophilus: At the V.A. Medical Center in Lexington, Kentucky, James W. Anderson, M.D., and colleagues gave 29 volunteers 200 ml/day of *Lactobacillus acidophilus* for 3 weeks. In a second, double-blind study, patients consumed fermented milk (yogurt) containing *L. acidophilus* or a placebo fermented milk for 4 weeks.[19]

The fermented milk brought a 2.4% reduction in serum cholesterol levels, while the *L. acidophilus* reduced serum cholesterol by 3.2%. Combined analysis of both trials showed a 2.9% reduction in serum cholesterol concentrations. Anderson pointed out that a 1% drop in blood cholesterol levels is associated with a 2 to 3% reduction in risk of coronary artery disease, and that regular consumption of yogurt containing an appropriate strain of *L. acidophilus* may reduce coronary heart disease by 6 to 10%.

Grains and Pulses: A study involving 30 Type 2 diabetics used a cereal-pulse mix, given for 1 to 2 months, which was beneficial in controlling hyperglycemia and hyperlipidemia. The pulse mix, per 100 g, contained 52 g wheat grits, 20 g soybean, 6.5 g red gram dhal, 6.5 g lentil, 3.25 g black gram dhal, 3.25 g guar seed, 1.6 g fenugreek, 0.3 g turmeric, 0.15 g asafetida (a gum resin of various Oriental plants related to the carrot family), and 0.15 g toasted cumin seeds. The mix, per 100 g, contained 287 calories, 45.6 g carbohydrate, 16.87 g protein, 4.13 g fat, and 1.68 g fiber. The mix lowered total cholesterol, LDL-cholesterol, triglycerides and HDL-cholesterol.[20]

A 98-day study at Illinois State University at Normal, evaluated 29 sedentary men with high cholesterol levels, who ranged in age from 38 to 70. Following a 2-week adjustment period on a low-fat, controlled diet, the volunteers were given either a low-fat controlled diet plus 20 g of corn bran supplement, or a low-fat controlled diet with 20 g of wheat bran supplement.

The low-fat diet significantly lowered all the lipid parameters except for HDL-cholesterol. The corn fiber supplement brought an additional lowering of serum cholesterol, triglyceride, and VLDL-cholesterol concentrations. The corn and wheat fiber did not significantly alter LDL-cholesterol and HDL-cholesterol concentrations; however, the researchers agreed that supplementing a low-fat diet with corn bran is an effective way of reducing serum lipid concentrations in men with elevated cholesterol readings.[21]

Dietary Recommendations: On May 15, 2001, the National Cholesterol Education Program, which is coordinated by the National

Heart, Lung and Blood Institute in Washington, D.C., published guidelines which suggested that the number of Americans who should be using diet to lower their cholesterol levels should be increased from 52 to 65 million, and the number of people who should be prescribed cholesterol-lowering drugs should go up from 13 to about 36 million. It was recommended that diabetics monitor their cholesterol levels in order to avoid a heart attack.[22] An abbreviated version of the 200-page report appeared in the May 16 issue of the *Journal of the American Medical Association*.[23,24]

The recommendations were hardly new, since we have known for some time that we should keep total cholesterol at 200 mg/dl or below, eat a diet low in saturated fats and cholesterol, increase physical activity, and lose weight if overweight.

What was new was that many of the members of the panel that issued the guidelines have close ties with the drug companies that produce the leading cholesterol-lowering drugs. With these conflicts of interest, one wonders how these panel members and their colleagues can keep a straight face while urging Americans to take more cholesterol-lowering drugs, which often have debilitating side effects, rather than the numerous natural solutions, some of which are detailed here.

References

1. Clayman, Charles B., M.D., medical editor. *The American Medical Association Home Medical Encyclopedia.* New York: Random House, 1989, p. 275.

2. Murray, Frank. *Program Your Heart for Health.* New York: Larchmont Books, 1977, pp. 210ff, 262ff.

3. Coons, Callie Mae. *Food, Yearbook of Agriculture,* 1959.

4. Ibid.

5. Ostlund, R. E., et al. "Sitostanol Administered in Lecithin Micelles Potently Reduces Cholesterol Absorption in Humans," *American Journal of Clinical Nutrition* 70: 826–831, 1999.

6. King, James M., M.D., et al. "Evaluation of Effects of Unmodified Niacin on Fasting and Postprandial Plasma Lipids and Normolipidemic Men with Hypoalpha Alipoproteinemia," *American Journal of Medicine* 97: 323–331, Oct. 1994.

7. Guyton, J. R., et al. "Extended-Release Niacin vs. Gemfibrozil for the Treatment of Low Levels of High-Density Lipoprotein Cholesterol," *Archives of Internal Medicine* 160: 1177–1184, April 24, 2000.

8. Zema, M. J. "Gemfibrozil, Nicotinic Acid and Combination Therapy in Patients with Isolated Hypoalphalipoproteinemia: A Randomized, Open-Label, Crossover Study," *Journal of the American College of Cardiology* 35(3): 640–646, March 1, 2000.

9. Edwards, K., et al. "Effect of Pistachio Nuts on Serum Lipid Levels in Patients with Moderate Hypercholesterolemia," *Journal of the American College of Nutrition* 18(3): 229–232, 1999.

10. Saba, Paolo, et al. "A Pilot Study of the Effects of Omega-3 Polyunsaturated Fatty Acids on Blood Lipids in Hyperlipidemic Patients," *Current Therapeutic Research* 55(4): 408–415, April 1994.

11. Anderson, J. W., et al. "Long-Term Cholesterol-Lowering Effects of Psyllium As An Adjunct to Diet Therapy in the Treatment of Hypercholesterolemia," *American Journal of Clinical Nutrition* 71: 1433–1438, 2000.

12. Lupton, Joanne, R., Ph.D. "Cholesterol-Lowering Effect of Barley Bran Flour and Oil," *Journal of the American Dietetic Association* 95: 65–70, 1994.

13. Gerhardt, Ann L., and Noreen B. Gallo. "Full-Fat Rice Bran and Oat Bran Similarly Reduce Hypercholesterolemia in Humans," *Journal of Nutrition* 128: 865–869, 1998.

14. Abbey, Mavis, et al. "Partial Replacement of Saturated Fatty Acids with Almonds or Walnuts Lowers Total Plasma Cholesterol and Low-Density Lipoprotein Cholesterol," *American Journal of Clinical Nutrition* 59: 995–999, 1994.

15. Goel, Vinti, Ph.D., et al. "Cholesterol Lowering Effects of Rhubarb Stalk Fiber in Hypercholesterolemic Men," *Journal of the American College of Nutrition* 16(6): 600–604, 1997.

16. Zoler, M. L. "Cholestin Cuts Serum Cholesterol by 20%-30%," *Family Practice News,* May 15, 1999, pp. 30–31.

17. Warshafsky, S., et al. "Effect of Garlic on Total Serum Cholesterol: A Meta-Analysis," *Annals of Internal Medicine* 119(7/Part I): 599–605, Oct. 1, 1993.

18. Hermann, J., et al. "Effects of Chromium Supplementation on Plasma Lipids, Apolipoproteins and Glucose in Elderly Subjects," *Nutrition Research* 14(5): 671–674, May 1994.

19. Anderson, J. W., and S. E. Gilliland. "Effect of Fermented Milk (Yogurt) Containing Lactobacillus Acidophilus L1 on Serum Cholesterol in Hypercholesterol Humans," *Journal of the American College of Nutrition* 18(1): 43–50, 1999.

20. Mani, U. V., et al. "Long-Term Effect of Cereal-Pulse Mix (Diabetic Mix) Supplementation on Serum Lipid Profile in Non-Insulin Dependent Diabetes Mellitus Patients," *Journal of Nutritional and Environmental Medicine* 7: 163–168, 1997.

21. Shane, Jan M., et al. "Corn Bran Supplementation of a Low-Fat Controlled Diet Lowers Serum Lipids in Men with Hypercholesterolemia," *Journal of the American Dietetic Association* 95(1): 40–45, Jan. 1995.

22. "NCEP Issues Major New Cholesterol Guidelines," NIH News Release, May 15, 2001.

23. Cleeman, James I., M.D., et al. "Executive Summary of the Third Report of the National Cholesterol Education Program (NCEP) Expert Panel on Detection, Evaluation and Treatment of High Blood Cholesterol in Adults (Adult Treatment Panel III)," *Journal of the American Medical Association* 285(19): 2486ff, May 16, 2001.

24. Pace, Brian, M.A., et al. "Cholesterol and Atherosclerosis," *Journal of the American Medical Association* 285(19): 2536, May 16, 2001.

16 Homocysteine: More Dangerous than Cholesterol?

Homocysteine, an amino acid that is related to two others–methionine and cysteine–may be more dangerous than cholesterol in contributing to cardiovascular disease and stroke. Normally benign, homocysteine can build up in the arteries, thereby decreasing the flow of blood and causing serious complications, such as blood clots. Diabetics are especially at risk for having abnormal levels of homocysteine in the blood.

Since a buildup of homocysteine may be related to a deficiency in three B vitamins (folic acid, B_6, and B_{12}), smoking, alcohol, and coffee consumption, the vitamins are being used by numerous researchers to lower homocysteine levels. Betaine and N-acetylcysteine can also lower these levels. A diet containing folic acid–rich fruits and vegetables also provides protection against this potentially serious amino acid, as can a vegan diet with supportive exercise and stress management.

Homocysteine, an amino acid that is involved in the breakdown of proteins, is normally benign and processed by the body, but a rare genetic disorder prevents the processing of the substance, according to Ronald L. Hoffman, M.D. When homocysteine accumulates in the bloodstream, it can increase the risk of heart attack, diabetes, stroke, and blood clots in the lungs or legs. It can also damage the cells lining the arteries. This buildup is independent of cholesterol in the blood, in that a patient can have low levels of cholesterol and still be at high risk for heart disease or stroke, he said.[1]

In his practice in New York City, Hoffman tests for homocysteine in the blood and urine of patients, and reports that high levels can be reduced with folic acid, a B vitamin, at 5 mg/day; vitamin B_6, 100 mg/day; vitamin B_{12}, 1,000 mcg/day; betaine, 500 mg/day; and phosphatidyl-choline, 1,000 mg/day.

Raised blood levels of homocysteine need to be checked because elevated cholesterol may not be an accurate indicator of risk for disease. Homocysteine can damage blood vessel walls and is related to endothelial dysfunction, a constriction of blood vessels that can reduce the flow of blood, according to the *American Journal of Cardiology*.[2]

While excess homocysteine results from low levels of three B vitamins (folic acid, B_6, and B_{12}), various antioxidants may be deterrents. In one instance, a research team elevated homocysteine levels in 10 healthy men and women by giving them supplemental doses of methionine, a dietary amino acid. Homocysteine is derived from methionine when it is broken down from cysteine, another sulfur-containing amino acid. The volunteers also received a placebo, and during the study, they were given 1,200 IU/day of vitamin E, a powerful antioxidant.

The research team found that vitamin E supplements prevented endothelial dysfunction, thereby maintaining normal blood flow. However, it did not alter homocysteine levels. It is apparent that vitamin E can reverse some—but not all—of the consequences of homocysteine, but it definitely plays a role in reducing the risk of coronary heart disease, a major problem for diabetics, they said.

Homocystinuria, in which homocysteine is excreted in the urine, was discovered over 40 years ago when high levels of homocysteine, the oxidized form of the amino acid methionine, was found in the urine of some children with mental retardation, reported David E. L. Wilcken, M.D., of the Prince Henry Hospital in Little Bay, Australia. Three years after this study, the association with severe vascular disease and homocysteine was found to be the usual cause of premature death.[3]

The researchers found that homocysteine is derived from methionine in three steps. In one step, methylcobalamin, folic acid, and betaine are involved. (The authors detail the complicated scientific progression in this reference.)

Writing in the *American Journal of Clinical Nutrition*, Benedicte Chirstensen, et al., said the previous studies have shown that consuming very high doses of unfiltered coffee increases homocysteine and total cholesterol.[4] The research team, from Ulleval University Hospital in Oslo,

Norway, stated that a recent intervention study showed that very high intakes of unfiltered coffee increased plasma homocysteine levels by 10%.

"The effect of coffee on homocysteine could be mediated directly or indirectly by the metabolism of folic acid, vitamin B_6 (pyridoxine) and vitamin B_{12}," the Norwegians said. "Of these, the concentration of serum folate (folic acid) is known to be the strongest determinant of the concentration of plasma homocysteine, whereas the effects of vitamin B_6 and B_{12} are considered to be less important. Indeed, the concentration of vitamin B_{12} was not influenced by coffee consumption in our study."

From their study, the researchers said that abstaining from even commonly consumed amounts of filtered coffee may lower the concentrations of both homocysteine and total cholesterol. However, it is not obvious that the effect on homocysteine is related to alterations in folic acid status.

"If there is interference with folate," they continued, "it may theoretically happen by three different mechanisms: 1) coffee drinkers could have lower intakes of folate-consuming foods; 2) the intake of coffee could interfere with the absorption of folate from the diet: 3) there might be substances in coffee that interfere with folate-homocysteine metabolism."

At the Radcliffe Infirmary, Oxford, England, Robert Clarke, M.D., and associates, studied 1,114 people for 12 weeks concerning the effect of folic acid supplements on homocysteine levels in the blood. Vitamin B_6 and vitamin B_{12} were also added to the mix. It was suggested that daily consumption of 0.5 to 5 mg/day of folic acid in Western populations, along with 0.5 mg/day of vitamin B_{12}, would be expected to reduce homocysteine levels by about one-quarter or one-third.[5]

Clarke found that folic acid–rich foods could lower homocysteine levels by 25%. However, similar effects were seen with 0.5 to 5 mg/day of folic acid supplements. It was also found that vitamin B_{12} at 0.5 mg/day brought an additional 7% reduction in homocysteine in the blood, but 16.5 mg/day of vitamin B_6 had no effect.

At Haukeland University Hospital in Bergen, Norway, a research team evaluated 9,165 people between the ages of 40 and 42. Of these, 2,351 volunteers between the ages of 65 and 67 were considered healthy, and 425 people of varying ages had a lifestyle profile characterized by low folic acid intakes, smoking, and coffee consumption that was associated with a high median total homocysteine concentration.

Those with high folic acid intakes, who were nonsmokers, and had low coffee intake of less than one cup per day, had almost normal homocysteine levels. Coffee consumption revealed an especially strong relationship to homocysteine levels. Smoking also increased levels, the researchers reported.[6]

Elevated homocysteine levels are an increased risk factor for cardiovascular disease, according to a research team in Utrecht, the Netherlands. The study involved 7,983 people, including 104 with a myocardial infarction (heart attack) and 120 with a stroke. The increased risk of stroke or heart attack increased directly with the amount of homocysteine in the blood.[7]

Dutch researchers, in studying 2,435 men and women, between the ages of 20 and 65, for 3 years, found that changing dietary habits can significantly change plasma homocysteine concentrations in the general population. However, in studying all of the B vitamins, this study found that only folic acid had a significant lowering effect on the amino acid.[8]

In a study of 885 men and women, between the ages of 67 and 95, who were part of the Framingham Heart Study, it was found that those who ate the least amount of fruits and vegetables (about 2 servings daily) had higher homocysteine levels in their blood, compared to those who ate the most fruits and vegetables (9 servings per day). The more foods that contained folic acid, the lower the homocysteine levels.[9]

It was reported that women had higher levels of folate than men, generally because women used more vitamin supplements in addition to the folic acid–rich foods. Men got their folic acid from beer, bread, and eggs. (In 1947, scientists in the Framingham Heart Study began collecting health information on more than 5,000 citizens in Framingham, Massachusetts, to understand the risk factors for cardiovascular disease. The study ended in 1971, mainly due to economic reasons.)

Researchers at the University of Bonn in Germany studied 106 volunteers, about 25 years of age, who were divided into three groups. It was found that healthy, young females with normal homocysteine levels who were supplemented for 4 weeks with either 400 mcg/day of folic acid, 2 mg/day of vitamin B_6, or a combination of the two, had reduced plasma homocysteine levels by 17% with the combination therapy. Supplementation with folic acid alone reduced homocysteine levels by 11.5%. However, vitamin B_6 in this study had no effect on plasma homocysteine concentrations.[10]

When researchers evaluated 100 consecutive patients for cardiovascular disease, they found that homocysteine levels in 40 patients with atrial fibrillation (irregular heartbeat) were similar to 60 cardiovascular patients who did not have the irregularity. The patients with atrial fibrillation who had had a stroke, but had recovered, had higher homocysteine levels than those with the heart problem who had never had a stroke. It was also found that, in those who had a stroke with atrial fibrillation, there was a marked increase in homocysteine levels at the end of the seventh decade.[11]

Elevated homocysteine levels seem to be a greater risk factor for mortality in Type 2 diabetics than in nondiabetics, according to Ellen K. Hoogeveen, M.D., Ph.D. Her study involved 2,484 men and women who were between the ages of 50 and 75. She found that the odds ratio for 5-year mortality for high homocysteine levels was 1.34 in nondiabetics and 2.51 in diabetics.[12]

In another study, involving 631 people between the ages of 50 and 75, Hoogeveen reported that a high serum total homocysteine level is a stronger (1.6-fold) risk factor for cardiovascular disease in those with Type 2 diabetes than in those without the disease.[13]

In a trial involving 625 people, between the ages of 50 and 75, Hoogeveen reported that the prevalence of retinopathy (an eye disorder) was 9.8% in those with normal glucose tolerance, 11.8% in those with impaired glucose tolerance, 9.4% in those with newly diagnosed Type 2 diabetes, and 32.3% for those with known Type 2 diabetes. She also found that the prevalence of retinopathy was 10.3% in those without high blood pressure, compared to 16.3% with hypertension. After adjusting for variables, the odds ratio for the relationship between retinopathy (damage to small blood vessels in the eye) and high homocysteine levels was 0.97 in those without diabetes and 3.44 in patients with the disease.[14]

In studying 452 Type 2 diabetics, men and women between the ages of 40 and 74, it was found that total homocysteine levels were higher in men than in women, which correlated with the duration of high blood pressure and systolic blood pressure. Of those with neuropathy (nerve damage) and macroalbuminuria (protein in the urine), 2.2% met the criteria for vitamin B_{12} deficiency and 1% met the criteria for folic acid deficiency. Elevated levels of homocysteine in the diabetics seemed to be due to a combination of vitamin deficiency and reduced kidney function, but were not a predictor of cardiovascular disease. Albuminuria is sometimes a symptom of kidney disease.[15]

Increasing consumption of citrus fruits and vegetables, which are rich sources of folic acid, will improve folate levels in the blood and reduce total homocysteine levels, which may help to prevent cardiovascular disease and neural tube defects in infants, according to researchers at Wageningen Agricultural University in the Netherlands. Their study involved 66 people between the ages of 18 and 45.[16]

Betaine, which is derived from choline, a vitamin B-like substance, is necessary for the recycling of homocysteine back into methionine. As we know, homocysteine is involved in the conversion of methionine into cysteine. When patients with abnormal levels of homocysteine are unresponsive to vitamin B_6, doctors often substitute betaine. Dosages range from 3 g twice daily to 20 g/day. For patients less than 3 years of age, the recommended dose is 100 mg/kg, which can be increased in 100 mg/kg increments. Long-term studies have reported that betaine often prevents serious blood clots.[17]

Researchers in Italy studied 10 healthy volunteers, with a mean age of 73, who had urinary homocysteine levels evaluated after 50 mg/kg of body weight of N-acetylcysteine was given intravenously. It was reported that total plasma homocysteine and cysteine levels fell progressively by 69 and 40%, respectively. The researchers said that intravenous N-acetylcysteine brought an efficient and rapid reduction in homocysteine. They added that this therapy may be an alternative approach in the treatment of those with high homocysteine levels.[18] N-acetylcysteine is a supplement that increases blood levels of glutathione, which can reduce the formation of harmful free radicals.

Elevated homocysteine levels can be lowered to normal levels in almost all cases with simple, safe, and inexpensive treatments with vitamin B_6, folic acid, and betaine, according to M. van den Berg, M.D., and associates at the Free University Hospital in Amsterdam, The Netherlands. The authors recommend a methionine-loading test for screening for high levels of homocysteine in those with an individual risk for hardening of the arteries or blood clots.[19] If methionine, the amino acid, is not converted into cysteine, high levels of homocysteine will result.

When the researchers screened 730 vascular patients, they found that 25 to 33% had peripheral arterial disease, 20 to 28% had cerebrovascular disease, and 15% had coronary artery disease. Factors that may increase homocysteine levels include: 1) deficiencies in vitamin B_6, folic acid, and vitamin B_{12}; 2) kidney failure; 3) excess protein intake; 4) use of a drug such as nitric oxide, methotrexate (a drug used to treat cancer, psoriasis, and rheumatoid arthritis), or anti-epileptic drugs.

The research team added that, with elevated fasting homocysteine levels, folic acid at 0.65 mg/day brought a 40% reduction; 2.5 mg/day, a 37% reduction; 5 mg/day, a 50% reduction; and 10 mg/day, also a 50% reduction. Vitamin B_6 had no effect on homocysteine levels, and vitamin B_{12} had only a modest effect.

The researchers contended that 0.4 mg/day of vitamin B_{12} would be suitable. However, in patients with elevated post methionine challenge hyperhomocysteinemia, vitamin B_6 at 100 mg/day and folic acid at 5 mg/day results in a 50% reduction; vitamin B_6 at 100 to 250 mg/day brought a 40% reduction; and folic acid in 6 patients brought only a 45% reduction in this complication.

In a trial at the Lifestyle Center of America in Sulphur, Oklahoma, 40 people were placed on a strict vegan diet for 1 week. This means no meat, eggs, or dairy products. The study included moderate exercise and stress management, and the volunteers avoided tobacco, alcohol, and caffeinated beverages. Blood levels of homocysteine dropped 13%, with the greatest reduction of more than 20% in those with heart disease. In this study, 63% had diabetes; 60% had high blood pressure; and 43% had high cholesterol levels.[20]

References

1. Hoffman, Ronald L., M.D. *Intelligent Medicine.* New York: Simon & Schuster, 1997, pp. 281–282.

2. Raghuveer, G., et al. "Effect of Vitamin E on Resistance Vessel Endothelial Dysfunction Induced by Methionine," *American Journal of Cardiology* 88: 285–290, 2001.

3. Wilcken, David E. L., and Nicholas Dudman, P.B. "Homocysteinuria and Atherosclerosis," *Molecular Genetics of Coronary Artery Disease, Candidate Genes and Processes in Atherosclerosis* 14: 311–324, 1992; Karger, Basel, Switzerland.

4. Christensen, Benedicte, et al. "Abstention from Filtered Coffee Reduces the Concentrations of Plasma Homocysteine and Serum Cholesterol—A Randomized Controlled Trial," *American Journal of Clinical Nutrition* 74: 302–307, 2001.

5. Clarke, Robert, et al. "Lowering Blood Homocysteine with Folic Acid Based Supplements: Meta-Analysis of Randomised Trials," *British Medical Journal* 316: 894–898, March 21, 1998.

6. Nygard, Ottar, et al. "Major Lifestyle Determinants of Plasma Total Homocysteine Distribution: The Hordaland Homocysteine Study," *American Journal of Clinical Nutrition* 67: 263–270, 1998.

7. Bots, M. L., et al. "Homocysteine and Short-Term Risk of Myocardial Infarction and Stroke in the Elderly: The Rotterdam Study," *Archives of Internal Medicine* 159: 38–44, Jan. 11, 1999.

8. de Bree, A., et al. "Association Between B Vitamin Intake and Plasma Homocysteine Concentrations in the General Dutch Population Aged 20-65," *American Journal of Clinical Nutrition* 73: 1027–1033, 2001.

9. Tucker, Katherine L., Ph.D. "Diet Is Critical in Keeping Homocysteine Levels Low, and Thus Preventing Disease," *Modern Medicine* 65: 11, Feb. 1997.

10. Dierkes, Jutta, et al. "Folic Acid and Vitamin B6 Supplementation and Plasma Homocysteine Concentrations in Healthy Young Women," *International Journal of Vitamin and Nutrition Research* 68: 98–103, 1998.

11. Friedman, H. S. "Serum Homocysteine and Stroke in Atrial Fibrillation," *Annals of Internal Medicine* 13(3): 253–254, Feb. 6, 2001.

12. Hoogeveen, Ellen K., M.D., Ph.D., et al. "Hyperhomocysteinemia Increases Risk of Death, Especially in Type 2 Diabetics: 5-Year Follow-Up of the Hoorn Study," *Circulation* 101: 1506–1511, April 4, 2000.

13. Hoogeveen, Ellen K., M.D., Ph.D., et al. "Hyperhomocysteinemia Is Associated with an Increased Risk of Cardiovascular Disease, Especially in Non-Insulin Dependent Diabetes Mellitus: A Population-Based Study," *Arteriosclerosis, Thrombosis and Vascular Biology* 18: 133–138, 1998.

14. Hoogeveen, Ellen K., M.D., Ph.D., et al. "Hyperhomocysteinemia Is Associated with the Presence of Retinopathy in Type 2 Diabetes Mellitus," *Archives of Internal Medicine* 160: 2984–2990, 2000.

15. Stahler, S. P., et al. "Total Homocysteine Is Associated with Nephropathy in Non-Insulin-Dependent Diabetes Mellitus," *Metabolism* 48(9): 1096–1101, Sept. 1999.

16. Brouwer, I. A., et al. "Dietary Folate from Vegetables and Citrus Fruit Decreases Plasma Homocysteine Concentrations in Humans in a Dietary Controlled Trial," *Journal of Nutrition* 129: 1135–1139, 1999.

17. "Betaine for Homocystinuria," *Medical Letter* 39 (Issue 993): 12, Jan. 31, 1997.

18. Ventura, P., et al. "N-Acetyl-Cysteine Reduces Homocysteine Plasma Levels After Single Intravenous Administration by Increasing Thiols Urinary Excretion," *Pharmacology Research* 40(4): 345–350, 1999.

19. van den Berg, M., and G. H. J. Boers. "Homocystinuria: What About Mild Hyperhomocysteinemia?" *Postgraduate Medicine Journal* 72: 513–518, 1996.

20. "Homocysteine Lowered by Vegan Diet," *Preventive Medicine* 30: 225–233, April 2000.

17 What Are Triglycerides?

High levels of triglycerides, the most abundant fat in the body, and low levels of HDL-cholesterol, the beneficial kind, are closely associated with insulin resistance, which is linked to high blood pressure and elevated fats in the blood. With insulin resistance, diabetics may produce enough insulin, but their bodies do not properly assimilate it. The body needs insulin to remove triglycerides from the blood, and when diabetes is under control, the amount of the fat in the blood is usually kept at the desired level. Raised levels of triglycerides are associated with coronary artery disease and stroke.

Various researchers have equated the high-sugar diet in Western countries with elevated triglyceride levels. However, researchers around the world have found that vitamin B_3, omega-3 fatty acids, magnesium, fenugreek seed powder, and other natural supplements can lower triglyceride levels, as well as the various types of cholesterol.

About three-fourths of the deaths among diabetics are caused by cardiovascular complications, according to the *Columbia University College of Physicians and Surgeons Complete Home Medical Guide.* Those with diabetes have a much higher rate of heart disease and circulatory disorders than the general population. These problems range from an increased risk of heart attacks, strokes, and high blood pressure to impaired circulation involving large and small blood vessels. In addition, arteriosclerosis (hardening of the arteries) and a buildup of fatty deposits (atherosclerosis) appear at an earlier age and advance more rapidly in those with diabetes. High blood levels of cholesterol and triglycerides are found in both male and female diabetics. Women, who often have lower blood fat levels and a lower incidence of heart disease than men, often have very high levels of blood fats when they are diabetic. High blood pressure, which increases the risk of strokes and heart attacks, is also common among diabetics.[1]

How diabetes promotes cardiovascular and circulatory problems is unclear, however, many researchers think the answer lies in the abnormally high blood glucose, the publication said. High blood glucose affects various blood components, especially red blood cells and platelets, and these abnormalities may have a role in the development of hardening of the arteries. Insulin is thought to increase the production of fats in the artery walls, which promotes the buildup of fatty deposits. Since Type 2 diabetics have high levels of insulin—although they do not effectively utilize it—it is thought that this may be a factor in the high degree of fatty deposits in these patients. In Type 1 diabetes, insulin therapy seems to inhibit the atherosclerotic process by normalizing blood sugar, the publication continued.

So what are triglycerides? A pure fat is composed of molecules of glycerol (a trihydroxy alcohol, the same as glycerin), to each of which 1, 2, or 3 fatty acids are linked to form monoglycerides, diglycerides, or triglycerides, respectively, reported *Food: The Yearbook of Agriculture*. Natural fats, as in meats, grains, and nuts, are made up mostly of triglycerides with only trace amounts of the mono- and di- forms and some free fatty acids. Processed fats, such as hydrogenated commercially hardened shortenings, may contain up to 20% monoglycerides and diglycerides.[2]

Type 2 diabetics have usually been hypoglycemic and have been producing large quantities of insulin to deal with their blood sugar for many years before diabetes is diagnosed, according to Robert C. Atkins, M.D. Insulin—which also contributes to obesity (excess glucose—sugar—is converted into triglyceride fat)—is responsible for much damage to the body. Indeed, he said, there is now evidence implicating it as a major cause of hardening of the arteries. That, in fact, is where the linkage between blood sugar disorders and cardiovascular illnesses is found, he added.[3]

In evaluating 740 coronary patients at the University of Maryland School of Medicine at Baltimore between 1977 and 1978, 350 with coronary artery disease were recontacted beginning in 1988. It was found that HDL-cholesterol (the good kind) was significantly lower and the triglycerides were higher in patients than in controls. Independent predictors of cardiovascular disease included diabetes, HDL-cholesterol less than 35 mg/dl, and triglycerides greater than 100 mg/dl. It was found that reduced survival rates from coronary artery disease were reported in those with triglyceride levels less than 100 mg/dl, compared with triglycerides over 100 mg/dl. Therefore, the cutoff points established in the National Cholesterol Education Program for elevated triglycerides (over 200 mg/dl) may need to be refined, stated Michael Miller, M.D., and colleagues.[4]

Since cholesterol and triglyceride levels are often measured at the same time, there are a number of natural ways to lower triglyceride levels. Here is a review of some of them. Ways to lower cholesterol levels are dealt with elsewhere in this book.

At the Medical Hospital and Research Center in Moradabad, India, researchers studied 400 patients between the ages of 25 and 63, most of whom were men. In the controlled study, 206 volunteers were given a magnesium-rich diet, while 194 others received their usual diet for 6 weeks. After 6 weeks, there was a significant drop in total serum cholesterol, LDL-cholesterol, and triglycerides in those getting the magnesium-rich diet, HDL-cholesterol went down slightly in the control group, but increased 2.5 mg/dl in the magnesium diet group.[5]

Elevated blood levels of triglycerides are associated with other cardiovascular risk factors, especially reduced levels of HDL-cholesterol, the beneficial kind. However, omega-3 fatty acids from fish oil can effectively reduce blood levels of triglycerides at low doses of l g/day.

Elevated blood levels of triglycerides are associated with other cardiovascular risk factors, especially reduced levels of HDL-cholesterol, the beneficial kind. However, omega-3 fatty acids from fish oil can effectively reduce blood levels of triglycerides at low doses of l g/day.[6]

At the National Institute of Nutrition in Hyderabad, India, defatted fenugreek seed powder (100 mg divided into two equal doses) was given in the diet to 10 Type 1 diabetics, ranging in age from 12 to 37. The therapy was given for two 10-day periods (5 patients each) to see what effect there would be on blood glucose and serum lipid profiles.[7]

The researchers reported that the fenugreek diet significantly reduced fasting blood sugar and improved glucose tolerance, and there was a 54% reduction in daily urinary glucose excretion. Total cholesterol, LDL-cholesterol, VLDL-cholesterol, and triglycerides were significantly reduced, while HDL-cholesterol remained unchanged.

Researchers studied 234 men, between the ages of 36 and 56, who were randomly selected to supplement with 3.8 g/day of EPA (eicosapentaenoic acid), 3.6 g/day of DHA (docosahexaenoic acid), or 4 g/day of corn oil for 7 weeks. It was found that triglycerides decreased 26% in the DHA group and 21% in the EPA group compared with the corn oil group. Both DHA and EPA reduced serum triglycerides, but had different effects on lipoprotein and fatty acid metabolism. The data suggest that omega-3 fatty acids should be taken into consideration when evaluating triglyceride levels.[8]

Thirty-six postmenopausal women, 43 to 60 years of age, were given 8 capsules daily of either placebo oil or omega-3 fatty acids, which contained 2.4 g/day of EPA and 1.6 g/day of DHA for 28 days. This brought a 26% lower serum triglyceride level, a 28% lower overall ratio of serum triglyceride to HDL-cholesterol. The researchers suggested that this therapy could reduce the risk of coronary heart disease in postmenopausal women by 27%.[9]

Norwegian researchers gave 64 healthy male volunteers, ages 35 to 45, either 14 g/day of fish oil concentrate (55% omega-3 fatty acids) or 14 g/day of olive oil for 6 weeks. Plasma fibrinogen was reduced 13%, and blood levels of triglycerides went down 22% with the fish oil supplement. Three weeks after the supplementation ended, both variables were back to where they had been at the beginning of the trial. Plasma fibrinogen is thought to be a more significant and independent cardiovascular risk than total serum cholesterol.[10]

Swedish researchers treated 8 patients with primary high triglyceride levels with 4 g/day of niacin (vitamin B$_3$) for 6 weeks. This reduced apolipoprotein-b by about one-third and triglyceride levels by almost one-half. The vitamin, in the form of nicotinic acid, either reduces VLDL-cholesterol synthesis in the liver, or increases the clearance of large and small VLDLs. HDL-cholesterol also increased.

Patients with high cholesterol levels have elevated amounts of cholesterol, LDL-cholesterol, and apolipoprotein-b.[11] Other researchers have reported that, in studying 1,045 patients who had recently had a heart attack, those who had high levels of apolipoprotein-b were 8 times more likely to have a second heart attack than those with low levels of the protein. Those with elevated levels of apolipoprotein-b had low amounts of apolipoprotein-a, which pushes cholesterol to the liver.[12] Apolipoproteins are ingredients in blood lipoproteins that transport fat and cholesterol through the lymphatic system and bloodstream. There are nine different apolipoproteins (a, b, etc.). Apolipoprotein-a is associated with HDL-cholesterol, the beneficial kind, while apo-b is associated with LDL-cholesterol, the harmful kind.

At University Hospital, Leiden, the Netherlands, researchers gave 9 volunteers with raised triglycerides 1 g/day of fish oil containing 55.7% omega-3 fatty acids and 1 unit of vitamin E oil for 6 weeks, followed by 5 g/day of fish oil for an additional 6 weeks. The 5 g/day of fish oil brought a significant increase in omega-3 fatty acid content in VLDL-cholesterol, LDL-cholesterol and decreases in serum triglycerides, VLDL-triglycerides and VLDL-cholesterol concentrations of 54, 56 and 40%, respectively. As is often the case with fish oil therapy, the LDL-cholesterol (the harmful kind) went up by 23%.[13]

As reported in *Atherosclerosis*, 16 Type 2 diabetics with raised triglyceride levels, between the ages of 40 and 75, took 3 capsules daily of fish oil (containing 2.5 g/day of omega-3 fatty acids) or a placebo (containing 3 g/day of olive oil) for 2 months, and then for the last 4 months they took a dose of 1.7 g/day of omega-3 fatty acids or 2 g/day of olive oil. There was no improvement in LDL-cholesterol, but there was a positive effect in lowering triglycerides.[14]

References

1. Tarpley, Donald F., M.D., et al. *The Columbia University College of Physicians and Surgeons Complete Home Medical Guide.* New York: Crown, 1985, p. 481.

2. Leverton, Ruth M. "Amino Acids," *Food: The Yearbook of Agriculture.* Washington, DC: U. S. Department of Agriculture, 1959, p. 76.

3. Atkins, Robert C., M.D. *Dr. Atkins' Health Revolution.* Boston: Houghton Mifflin Co., 1988, pp. 83–89.

4.. Miller, Michael, M.D., et al. "Normal Triglyceride Levels and Coronary Artery Disease Events: The Baltimore Coronary Observational Long-Term Study," *Journal of the American College of Cardiology* 31(6):1252–1257, May 1988.

5. Singh, R. B., et al. "Can Dietary Magnesium Modulate Blood Lipids?" *Journal of the American College of Nutrition* 9(5):527/Abstract 23, 1990.

6. Roche, H. M., and M. J. Gibney. "Effect of Long-Chain-3 Polyunsaturated Fatty Acids on Fasting and Postprandial Triglyceride Metabolism," *American Journal of Clinical Nutrition* 71(Suppl.):232S–237S, 2000.

7. Sharma, R. D., et al. "Effect of Fenugreek Seed on Blood Glucose and Serum Lipids in Type 1 Diabetes," *European Journal of Clinical Nutrition* 44:301–306, 1990.

8. Grimsgaard, Sameline, et al. "Highly Purified Eicosapentaenoic Acid and Docosahexaenoic Acid in Humans Have Similar Triglyceride Lowering Effects But Divergent Effects on Serum Fatty Acids," *American Journal of Clinical Nutrition* 66:6149–659, 1997.

9. Stark, K. D., et al, "Effect of a Fish-Oil Concentrate on Serum Lipids in Postmenopausal Women Receiving and Not Receiving Hormone Replacement Therapy in a Placebo-Controlled, Double-Blind Trial," *American Journal of Clinical Nutrition* 72:389–394, 2000.

10. Flaten, Hugo, et al. "Fish Oil Concentrate: Effects on Variables Related to Cardiovascular Disease," *American Journal of Clinical Nutrition* 52:300–306, 1990.

11. Tornvall, Per, et al. "Normalization of Composition of Very Low Density Lipo-proteins in Hypertriglyceridemia by Nicotinic Acid," *Atherosclerosis* 84:219–227, 1990.

12. "Heart Attack," *New Scientist* 162(2187):25, May 22, 1999.

13. Hau, Man-Fai, et al. "Effects of Fish Oil on Oxidation on Resistance of VLDL in Hypertriglyceridemic Patients," *Arteriosclerosis, Thrombosis and Vascular Biology* 16:1197–1202, 1996.

14. Patti, L., et al. "Long-Term Effects of Fish Oil on Lipoprotein Subfractions and Low Density Lipoprotein Size in Non-Insulin Dependent Diabetic Patients with Hypertrigly-ceridemia," *Atherosclerosis* 1h6:361–367, 1999.

18 Hyperglycemia—Too Much Blood Sugar

If your blood sugar level is above 250 mg/dl or is at or above 180 mg/dl at the same time of day for three consecutive days, you are said to have hyperglycemia, or high blood sugar. High blood sugar levels over time can lead to diabetic complications that can damage blood vessels and nerves. Elevated blood sugar levels can also lead to diabetic ketoacidosis. When the body does not have enough insulin and is starved for glucose, it burns stored fat to fuel cells. This causes a buildup of ketones, which are by-products of fat metabolism. High amounts of ketones can poison the blood and bring on coma. Too much glucose in their blood can leave a person weak and groggy, and can even impair driving. A variety of popular drugs, such as beta-blockers, corticosteroids, nasal decongestants, oral contraceptives, thiazide diuretics, and others can cause hyperglycemia.

If your blood glucose level is above 250 mg/dl or is at or above 180 mg/dl at the same time of day for three days in a row, you are considered to have hyperglycemia (high blood sugar), according to Robert H. Phillips, Ph.D. Elevated blood sugar levels may lead to diabetic ketoacidosis, which is generally associated with Type 1 diabetes, or hyperglycemic hyperosmolar syndrome (elevated blood sugar), which is related to Type 2 diabetes.[1] If high blood sugar levels last for several years, this can lead to diabetic complications such as damage to blood vessels and nerves. When the body, without enough insulin, is starved of glucose, it begins to burn stored fat to fuel cells. This leads to a buildup of ketones, which are by-products of fat metabolism. High amounts of ketones are toxic, causing the blood to become highly acidic. This results in diabetic ketoacidosis (DKA).

There are a number of causes of hyperglycemia, according to Phillips. These include eating the wrong foods, eating too much of the right foods, lack of exercise, psychological and emotional stress, illness or injury, and taking too much or too little medication. Warning signs of hyperglycemia include frequent urination, excessive thirst, frequent or excessive hunger, blurred vision, fatigue, and confused thinking.

Although Type 2 diabetes is often described as a disease of insulin resistance, it is hyperglycemia rather than hyperinsulinemia (high insulin levels) that appears to be the primary defect, reported Matthew C. Riddle, M.D., of Oregon Health Sciences University at Portland. When hyperglycemia is uncontrolled, it plays a significant role in driving disease progression.[2]

Riddle added that when glucose is reduced, beta-cell responses to glucose and other stimuli become almost normal. Beta cells in the pancreas produce insulin. At the same time, reductions in excess glucose in muscle and adipose tissues may improve insulin sensitivity, that is, bring it near a more normal state. Vigorous early treatment with insulin may allow enough recovery of insulin secretion and action to allow dietary or oral therapy to maintain control, at least for a time.

The progression of Type 2 diabetes is driven by declining beta-cell functions and increasing insulin resistance, Riddle added. The cause of the decline in beta-cell function is unknown, but it seems to be related to accumulation of amyloid material (a waxy translucent substance) in the beta-cell mass as well as a reduction in that mass.

Declining rates of beta-cell function appear to be a function of age, Riddle said. While the decline in rates of insulin secretion during the initial stages of diabetes may be due to some defect in the ability of beta cells to sense hyperglycemia, the progressive failure of beta cells is characteristic of the disease process. Although Type 2 diabetes is often characterized as a disease of insulin resistance, some experts, such as Derek LeRoith, Ph.D., of the National Institutes of Health, Bethesda, Maryland, consider the defect in insulin secretion to be at least as important.

Blood sugar levels generally rise within 30 to 60 minutes after eating starchy foods, according to Robert A. Ronzio, Ph.D. The levels then return to a baseline within 3 to 5 hours as starch is digested to glucose and absorbed. If the blood sugar level remains high, a prediabetic or a diabetic condition may result. This is because the pancreas may not synthesize enough insulin or the cellular mechanisms responding to insulin may be defective.[3]

Sustained high blood sugar levels promote the bonding of glucose to proteins, including hemoglobin, Ronzio said. Thus, the resulting proteins do not function normally, and their gradual accumulation may contribute to the organ deterioration associated with uncontrolled diabetes.

Fifteen male patients from a hospital in Mexico City, who had suffered a heart attack 6 to 24 months before and had significant coronary artery blockage, were compared to 15 age-matched controls, reported *Archives of Medical Research*. The researchers found that the insulin sensitivity index was significantly lower in the patients with coronary heart disease than in the healthy controls.[4] Insulin sensitivity is the preferred state, in which cells remain receptive to the action of insulin.

It was also found that patients with coronary heart disease had high insulin levels. It is suggested that abnormal levels of insulin in the blood may play a role in hardening of the arteries through altered fat metabolism, impaired clotting of blood, high blood pressure, and damage to blood cells.

Italian researchers evaluated 60 diabetics with liver damage, ranging in age from 45 to 70, who were receiving insulin and had been diagnosed with high levels of insulin in their blood. For their liver problem, the patients received either 600 mg/day of silymarin (from milk thistle) or no herb for 6 months. Following 6 months of therapy, the silymarin-treated patients had the mean levels of fasting glucose (glucose in the blood following no food for 8 hours or more), daily blood glucose, daily glycosuria (urinary excretion of carbohydrates), glycosylated hemoglobin (glucose in red blood cells), daily insulin needs, fasting insulinemia (amount of insulin circulating in the blood), blood malondialdehyde (a marker for fatty acid oxidation), and basal and glucagon-stimulated C-peptide counted. These readings were significantly lower than in the untreated patients and lower than when the study began.[5]

The researchers said that the results suggested that silymarin can reduce the oxidation of fats in liver cells of diabetic patients with liver disease and that it can decrease the production of insulin and thus the need for insulin shots. Silymarin is apparently effective by restoring the blood membranes of liver cells and increasing the sensitivity of insulin cells. The researchers added that the silymarin therapy should continue for longer than 6 months in order to identify the point at which the biochemical benefits cease to exist.

At the 61st Scientific Sessions of the American Diabetes Association in Philadelphia in 2001, Daniel J. Cox, Ph.D., of the

University of Virginia Health Systems at Charlottesville, and colleagues, presented data which showed that hyperglycemia can slow mental capacity. Too much glucose in the blood can leave a person weak and groggy and even impair driving.[6]

In the study, the research team recruited 105 Type 1 diabetics and monitored their blood sugar levels and studied their mental clarity. For one month, the volunteers recorded their physical condition on a hand-held computer and documented such high blood sugar symptoms as headache, dry mouth, and need to urinate. The researchers found that when concentrations of blood sugar were low, test scores were predictably worse than normal. But high levels seemed to impair mental capacity also.

Blood sugar levels are considered normal at 80 to 240 mg/dl of glucose of blood. During the study, a reading of 270 mg/dl or slightly higher corresponded with a 10% decline on the mental tests. That reading dropped 25% when the reading was 300 mg/dl. It was also reported that high blood sugar amounts caused patients to take longer in performing their self-tests when glucose was normal.

In a separate study, Cox and his associates reported that hypoglycemia (low blood sugar) hampers driving ability. In comparing driving records of 1,000 diabetics, the researchers said that Type 2 diabetics were no more likely to get into accidents, but Type 1 diabetics were involved in about twice as many collisions. Cox added that diabetics should spread their insulin intake over the day to avoid sudden dips in blood sugar.

In studying 2,808 men and 3,560 women, between the ages of 45 and 74, vitamin C blood levels were significantly higher in those with hemoglobin A1C levels less than 7%, compared with diabetics or those who had undiagnosed high blood glucose levels with hemoglobin A1C more than 7%. Hemoglobin A1C is formed when glucose is attached to hemoglobin molecules. Increasing blood levels of vitamin C through dietary means may be a significant way for the public to reduce the prevalence of diabetes, the researchers said.[7]

A number of popular drugs can elevate glucose levels (hyperglycemia) and thereby lead to diabetes, according to Beatriz Luna, Pharm.D., of Campbell University School of Pharmacy at Bules Creek, North Carolina, and colleagues at other North Carolina facilities. These drugs include beta-blockers, thiazide diuretics, corticosteroids, niacin, Pentamidine, and others.[8] "Of recent interest are the increasing numbers of reported cases of new-onset diabetes mellitus in patients receiving treatment with protease inhibitors or atypical antipsychotic agents," Luna said.

Elevated blood glucose concentrations can have significant consequences, especially in high-risk populations, Luna continued. In the setting of hyperglycemia, granulocyte (white blood cell) activity can be impaired, which compromises the normal immunological response and the host's capacity to resist infection. In addition, hyperglycemia inhibits the development of granulation tissue, thus impairing the wound healing process. A recent meta-analysis (composite of several studies) reported that cardiovascular readings increased continuously with glucose levels higher than 75 mg/dl in nondiabetic patients.

Luna said that 82 patients treated with clozapine, a neuroleptic drug used to treat schizophrenia, were studied to determine the incidence of treatment-related impaired glucose tolerance and diabetes in patients without a prior diagnoses of diabetes. At the end of the 5-year study, about 30% of the patients were diagnosed with Type 2 diabetes.

"Recent findings continue to support the theory that patients receiving beta-blocker treatment (for high blood pressure) may be at increased risk for developing hyperglycemia and subsequent diabetes mellitus, although some data suggest that the newer beta-blocking agent caredilol does not pose the same risk and may improve insulin sensitivity," Luna added.

While drug interactions may vary from person to person, there are a number of these medications that cause hyperglycemia, according to Seymour L. Alterman, M.D., and Donald A. Kullman, M.D. These include calcium channel blockers, corticosteroids, isoniazid, nasal decongestants (epinephrine-like drugs), oral contraceptives, dilantin, rifampin, thiazide diuretics, and nicotinic acid.[9]

References

1. Phillips, Robert H., Ph.D. *Coping with Diabetes.* New York: Avery/Penguin-Putnam, 2000, pp. 110–111.

2. Riddle, Matthew C., M.D. "Impaired Insulin Secretion and Risk of Progressive Hyperglycemia." Paper read at American Diabetes Association 60th Annual Scientific Session, June 9–13, 2000, San Antonio, Texas.

3. Ronzio, Robert A., Ph.D. *The Encyclopedia of Nutrition and Good Health.* New York: Facts on File, Inc., 1997, p. 235.

4. Ariza, C., et al. "Hyperinsulinemia in Patients with Coronary Heart Disease in Absence of Overt Risk Factors," *Archives of Medical Research* 28(1); 115–119, 1997.

5. Velussi, M., et al. "Silymarin Reduces Hyperinsulinemia, Malondialdehyde Levels and Daily Insulin Need in Cirrhotic Diabetic Patients," *Current Therapeutic Research* 53(5): 533–545, 1993.

6. Seppa, Nathan. "Thinking Blurs When Blood Sugar Strays," *Science News* 160(3): 47, July 21, 2001.

7. Sargeant, L. A., et al. "Vitamin C and Hyperglycemia in the European Prospective Investigation into Cancer-Norfolk (EPIC-Norfolk) Study: A Population-Based Study," *Diabetes Care* 23(6): 726–732, June 2000.

8. Luna, Beatriz, Pharm.D., and Mark N. Feinglos, M.D. "Drug-Induced Hyperglycemia," *Journal of the American Medical Association* 286(16): 1945–1948, Oct. 24/31, 2001.

9. Alterman, Seymour L., M.D., and Donald A. Kullman, M.D. *How to Prevent, Control and Cure Diabetes.* Hollywood, Fla.: Frederick Fell Publishers, 2000, p. 96.

19 Hypoglycemia—Too Little Blood Sugar

Hypoglycemia (low blood sugar) is roughly the opposite of diabetes. In diabetes, the body does not produce enough insulin, which helps the body to use sugar and other carbohydrates, so the levels of sugar become so high that sugar overflows the urine. For low blood sugar, the body glands manufacture too much insulin, so that blood sugar levels are too low most of the time.

Hypoglycemia can be caused by taking too much diabetes medicine or other drugs; eating too little, not eating at all, or eating too many refined carbohydrates; exercising too strenuously; and drinking alcohol without eating. Symptoms include being tired, shaky, hungry, nervous, confused, et cetera.

Hypoglycemia can be controlled by following the diet and nutrition suggestions in this chapter. The hypoglycemic should eat often, providing meals and snacks are high-protein and low-carbohydrate. Beware of the foods on the no-no list, such as potatoes, pasta, rice, macaroni, noodles, sugar-containing foods, coffee, grapes, raisins, plums, figs, dates, and others.

When Ruth Adams and I were researching a book, *Is Low Blood Sugar Making You a Nutritional Cripple?*, I asked the Food and Drug Administration in Washington, D.C., for the names of several doctors who specialized in hypoglycemia or low blood sugar. They referred me to a prominent researcher in Pittsburgh, Pennsylvania, who proceeded to tell me that there was no such thing as low blood sugar. At the time, Ruth and

Is Your Blood Sugar Low? Some Symptoms of Hypoglycemia

If you answer "yes" to five or more of these questions, perhaps you should ask your doctor for a Glucose Tolerance Test.

1. Does your mind go blank at times?

2. Are you forgetful?

3. Do you occasionally have difficulty concentrating?

4. Do you lose your temper easily?

5. Do you have difficulty in controlling your emotions?

6. Are you very impatient?

7. Do certain things irritate you?

8. Are you depressed or "blue?"

9. Are you nervous?

10. Are you very tense?

Source: Patrick Quillin, Ph.D., R.D. *Healing Nutrients.* New York: Vintage Books/Random House, 1987, p. 215.

I were just beginning to know respected holistic doctors who used diet and megavitamin therapy to treat disease, and we just assumed that the Pittsburgh doctor had his head buried deeply in the sand.

Writing in the Introduction of the book, Robert C. Atkins, M.D., said, "The commonest condition I am called upon to treat in my private practice of internal medicine is low blood sugar. I know this to be true because I perform Glucose Tolerance Tests on every new patient and the results of this testing actually do show that the majority of my patients do not have normal curves, but, instead, have findings consistent with the diagnosis of low blood sugar. More to the point, I know this because I place these patients on my own version of an anti-hypoglycemia diet with megavitamin therapy, and the majority of them improve dramatically in regard to the various presenting complaints for which they sought help."[1]

Atkins said that, at a Las Vegas medical convention, the prevalence of low blood sugar was under discussion, and every physician who reported doing glucose tolerance testing routinely also commented on the extreme frequency with which he found hypoglycemia. There were, of course, dissenters, he added, but in every case they were doctors who did not routinely perform the test.

Hypoglycemia is roughly the opposite of diabetes. In Type 1 diabetes, the body does not produce enough insulin (which helps the body to use sugar and other carbohydrates) so that levels of sugar become so high that sugar may overflow into the urine. Low blood sugar is exactly the opposite. The body glands manufacture too much insulin, so that blood sugar levels are entirely too low most of the time. Since many important functions of the body (chiefly those involving the nerves and the brain) depend on sugar in the blood, they may actually become sugar-starved in such a condition.

Obviously, such a state may have serious consequences. A typical hypoglycemic victim is an emotional "yo-yo," strung out on a chemical reaction he cannot control, with reactions so severe they frequently resemble insanity.

The diabetic may be given a manufactured insulin to make up for the secretion he cannot produce. If he gives himself too large a dose, he may suffer from insulin shock, perspiration, nervousness and anxiety, trembling, fatigue, and in the worst case scenario, possibly death. If the low blood sugar patient goes too long on an inadequate diet or too long without eating, he may induce much the same kind of condition in himself. Or the symptoms may take on a number of violent and bizarre forms. In any case, diabetes and hypoglycemia may be the aftermath of several years of low blood sugar levels.

"If these disasters are caused by too little sugar in the blood, the best diet to overcome them would seem to be a diet rich in sugar," we reported. "In the early days of experimentation, doctors used to give their patients sugar when they found that hypoglycemia was present. They gave them candy or glucose tablets to eat whenever they felt the symptoms of low blood sugar returning. For a time this seemed to work, until, gradually, the patients found that they needed the sugar supplements almost all the time. If they did not have the supplements handy, the unpleasant and dangerous symptoms returned shortly after meals."

It was then determined that perhaps the same diet prescribed for diabetics would work for hypoglycemics. Sure enough, a diet high in protein, with sugars and starches omitted or cut to a minimum, and with a moderate amount of fat, steadied the wild swings in blood sugar readings so that the badly affected patient could eventually go from breakfast to lunch without any symptoms, and from lunch to dinner without any complications.

The spacing of meals is important to a hypoglycemic, as it is to the diabetic. He must eat frequently. In the diet prescribed by Seale Harris, M.D., and made famous in the book, *Body, Mind and Sugar,* the low blood sugar patient must take 4 ounces of fruit juice or an orange or grapefruit immediately upon arising, eat a high-protein breakfast, take 4 ounces of juice 2 hours after breakfast, have a high-protein lunch, then drink 8 ounces of milk 3 hours after lunch, and 4 ounces of juice an hour before dinner. Following a high-protein dinner, he must take 8 ounces of milk within 2 to 3 hours, then 4 ounces of milk or a small handful of nuts every 2 hours until bedtime.

A high-protein meal can consist of meat, eggs, fish, milk, cheese and other high-protein foods in normal quantities, plus all vegetables except potatoes and some fruits. The vegetable foods can be cooked or raw. Only

Typical Symptoms of Hypoglycemia

In the early stages of the disease, the patient may experience recurring feelings of light-headedness, usually at mid-morning and late afternoon.

Later the symptoms may be many, but some of the most common complaints are fatigue or exhaustion, headaches, heart palpitations, muscular aching or twitching, prickling or tingling of the skin, excessive sweating, gasping for breath, trembling, dizziness, weak spells, fainting, double or blurred vision, cold hands and feet, craving for sugar, hunger, chronic indigestion, and nausea.

Psychological symptoms are confusion, absent-mindedness, indecisiveness, loss of memory and/or concentration, irritability, moodiness, restlessness, insomnia, fears, nightmares, paranoia, anxiety, and depression.

one slice of bread or toast can be eaten at any meal, and spaghetti, rice, macaroni, and noodles are forbidden. Salad greens, mushrooms, and nuts can be eaten as freely as desired.

For beverages, any unsweetened fruit or vegetable juice (except grape or prune juice), weak tea, decaffeinated coffee, coffee substitutes, club soda, and distilled liquors are allowed.

Absolutely forbidden on the diet are candy, cake, pie, pastries, sweet custards, puddings, and ice cream; caffeine (strong tea, coffee, or soft drinks containing caffeine); potatoes, grapes, raisins, plums, figs, dates, bananas, wines, cordials, cocktails and beer, pastas and, of course, sugar. Of course, potatoes, grapes, raisins, plums, bananas, figs, et cetera, are excellent foods; they are just not recommended for anyone with low blood sugar.

It is easy to see that the daily routine followed by millions of people creates nutritional cripples insofar as blood sugar levels are concerned. Those who eat no breakfast, or take only coffee and something sweet—like a doughnut or a Danish—then light up a cigarette, have started a vicious cycle that can endanger their health.

Speaking at a meeting of the International College of Angiology in 1974, Benjamin Sandler, M.D., said that the fundamental cause of anginal syndrome and myocardial infarction (heart attack) is a sharp fall in the blood sugar to hypoglycemic levels in nondiabetics and to similar hypo- glycemia levels in diabetics. In the nondiabetic, these attacks occur when blood sugar levels plunge way down; in the diabetic, they occur when blood sugar levels fall relatively low.

In an earlier book, I detailed the story of Virginia Woolf, the gifted British writer and author of *Mrs. Dalloway* and other novels, who commit- ted suicide in 1941 at the age of 59. In *Beginning Again*, the third volume of her husband's autobiography in which Leonard Woolf shares some details of their life, the information suggests Virginia was suffering from hypoglycemia and serious vitamin and mineral deficiencies. Leonard Woolf said that the mental illness that pursued Virginia through her adult life played a large part in both their lives and was the ultimate cause of her death. They went to many doctors for an answer to her poor health, and she was finally diagnosed with neurasthenia, which is described as an emotional and psychic disorder with fatigability, lack of motivation, feel- ings of inadequacy, and psychosomatic symptoms.

"If Virginia lived a quiet vegetative life, eating well, going to bed early and not tiring herself mentally and physically, she remained perfectly well,"

Leonard said. "But if she tired herself in any way, if she was subjected to any severe physical, mental or emotional strain, symptoms at once appeared which in the ordinary person are negligible and transient, but with her were serious danger signals. The first symptoms were a peculiar headache low down at the back of the head, insomnia, and a tendency for the thoughts to race. If she went to bed and lay doing nothing in a darkened room, drinking large quantities of milk and eating well, the symptoms would slowly disappear and in a week or 10 days she would be well again."

Leonard said Virginia suffered from manic-depressive illness. In the manic stage she was wildly excited: her mind raced and she talked incessantly. At the height of the attack she had delusions and heard voices. In the depressive stage that followed, she was "in the depths of melancholia and despair; she scarcely spoke, refused to eat, refused to believe that she was ill and insisted that her condition was due to her guilt; at the height of this stage she tried to commit suicide . . . in 1941 she drowned herself in the river Ouse."

Leonard Woolf reported that one of the most troublesome symptoms of Virginia's breakdown was her refusal to eat. At almost every meal, someone had to sit beside her for an hour or more, trying to persuade her to eat a few mouthfuls. Left alone, she ate very little, and it was with great difficulty that she could be induced to drink even a glass of milk regularly every day.

Virginia Woolf was born in 1882, and during her lifetime not much was known about vitamins, which were first isolated in 1911 (vitamin B_1). Even less was known about hypoglycemia. At the time, mental illness was considered a form of demon-possession or else a Freudian nightmare brought about by psychotic and guilt-ridden associations with family and friends.

In his book, *Fighting Depression*, Harvey Ross, M.D., a Los Angeles psychiatrist, tells the story of Mitch, an 11-year-old boy with hypoglycemia and schizophrenia, who talked to his deceased grandfather, set fires in his room, attacked his sisters, and sometimes ate 60 candy bars a day, many stolen from neighborhood stores. The level of sugar in his blood decreased when he ate carbohydrates, leaving him with too little sugar to nourish his nervous system. Hypoglycemia patients like Mitch, Ross said, are often overweight and undernourished.[2]

To treat the boy, Ross put Mitch on a high-protein, low-carbohydrate diet with small meals and frequent in-between-meal snacks, rich in protein. After each meal, Mitch took 500 mg of vitamin B_3 (niacin), 500 mg of vitamin C, 100 mg of pyridoxine (vitamin B_6), 100 mg of pantothenic acid (a B vitamin), 200 IU of vitamin E, and a multiple B-complex tablet. While these doses are large for a child, most are water-soluble and pass out of the system in urine and feces during the day.

"Mitch began to respond almost immediately," Ross said. "Within the first week he became calm and was able to concentrate. I increased the niacin dosage to 1,000 mg after each meal. I had purposely started him on a lower dose because niacin can cause flushing of the skin and itching. But the larger doses made him nauseous, which is also a common problem. I see it in about 20% of my patients. I switched him to niacinamide, another form of vitamin B$_3$, and the nausea subsided. After one month, Mitch began to lose weight and his schoolwork improved. I increased his vitamin C intake to 1,000 mg three times daily. He continued to improve, although he still disrupted his class from time to time and argued with his parents. I supplemented his diet with l-glutamine, an amino acid that appears to benefit brain nutrition."

During an interview with his parents conducted over the course of three months, they told Ross that Mitch was doing well. None of his perceptual distortions had recurred. He was still losing weight, and his ability to concentrate continued to improve. Two problems remained. He became weak if he did not eat, a common symptom of hypoglycemia. And he continued to wet the bed, a persistent problem his parents had failed to mention initially.

"Mitch and his vitamins are going to be together for a long time," Ross continued. "If his symptoms do not reappear, he will continue his present treatment for several years. Then I will reduce the doses slowly to see if he can function normally with less vitamins. Although Mitch's case is not a classic case of depression, it serves to illustrate the problems that low blood sugar can cause," Ross added.

In a study reported in the *Journal of Internal Medicine*, two groups of Type 2 diabetics (14 and 10 in each group) and 12 Type 1 diabetics were evaluated in a 4-week trial. The first group consumed wholemeal bread with butter and meat, while the second group was given uncooked corn starch. The researchers found that the uncooked corn starch, eaten at bedtime, was similar to nighttime glucose intake following insulin replacement, with a peak in blood glucose after four hours. Therefore, uncooked corn starch at bedtime may be a reasonable way to prevent a glycemic decline during the night following insulin intake.[3]

Hypoglycemia can be divided into three general causes, according to Martin L. Budd, N.D., DO. They are: 1) high sugar diet leading to hyperinsulinism (high levels of insulin); 2) hypoadrenalism-stress (sluggish adrenal glands); and 3) alimentary or surgical-gastric surgery leading to rapid stomach emptying or "dumping syndrome." Reactive hypoglycemia almost always is accompanied by a personality disorder, he said. Many patients with symptoms of anxiety, irritability, depression, fatigue, sugar-craving, and premenstrual syndrome (PMS) have shown improvement or complete remission with nutritional treatment, he added.[4]

Oral medications for Type 2 diabetics that stimulate the pancreas to produce insulin—the sulfonylureas and repaglinide—need to be used exactly as prescribed to prevent hypoglycemia, according to Porter Shimer. This condition occurs when glucose levels drop too low—below 70 mg/dl—which produce symptoms that can include dizziness, nervousness, sleepiness, or suddenly feeling hungry. In fact, hypoglycemia can develop when too much medication has been taken for the amount of glucose present in the blood.[5]

A research team at the Royal Bournemouth Hospital in Dorset, England, reported that those who ingest moderate amounts of caffeine may develop hypoglycemic symptoms if plasma glucose levels fall into the low normal range. This might occur after eating a large amount of carbohydrates. In the study, the initial caffeine load was about 400 mg of caffeine.[6]

Researchers at the Second Affiliated Hospital, Hunan Medical University in China, studied 38 diabetics, ranging in age from 20 to 70; of these, 33 were Type 2 diabetics and 5 were Type 1. Each was given 0.1 g/day of the mineral lithium. The researchers found that the mineral appeared to have a hypoglycemic effect in addition to oral hypoglycemic agents and insulin.

Blood glucose levels went down significantly in the patients with mild symptoms treated only with lithium, although fasting blood glucose did not change significantly. The hypoglycemic effect of lithium may result from the metabolism of glucose, such as promoting the absorption of glucose and glycogenesis (the formation and storage of glycogen).[7]

In his book, *Dr. Whitaker's Guide to Natural Healing*, Julian Whitaker, M.D., reported that chromium is known for its role in the glucose tolerance factor. The mineral works closely with insulin in facilitating the uptake of glucose into the cells. Without chromium, he said, insulin's action is blocked and glucose levels are elevated. Therefore, chromium is a critical nutrient in diabetes as well as hypoglycemia. In one study, 8 female patients with hypoglycemia were given 200 mcg/day of chromium for 3 months and had a reduction of their symptoms of hypoglycemia. In addition, glucose tolerance test results were improved and the number of insulin receptors on red blood cells were increased.[8]

"Although there is no Recommended Daily Allowance for chromium, it appears that we need at least 200 micrograms each day in our diet," Whitaker says. "Chromium levels can be depleted by refined sugars, white flour products and lack of exercise. I believe the individual with hypothyroid should supplement the diet with 200 to 400 micrograms of chromium each day. Chromium polynicotinate, chromium picolinate and chromium-enriched yeast are the best forms."

Julian Whitaker, M.D., reported that chromium is known for its role in the glucose tolerance factor. The mineral works closely with insulin in facilitating the uptake of glucose into the cells. Without chromium, he said, insulin's action is blocked and glucose levels are elevated. Therefore, chromium is a critical nutrient in diabetes as well as hypoglycemia.

A study in the *International Journal of Sports Medicine* showed that eating carbohydrates prior to exercise after a morning fast and also ingesting carbohydrates after 4 hours of food deprivation can cause hypoglycemia in exercisers. It is recommended that carbohydrates should be taken 15 to 60 minutes before exercise, and the amount should be at least 70 grams.[9]

In the study, 19 cyclists ingested 50 g of glucose dissolved in water around noon, after having a normal breakfast, followed by 30 minutes of rest and then 40 minutes of cycling at 60% of a predetermined maximal power output. Pre-exercise carbohydrate ingestion after a 4-hour fast can induce hypoglycemia, the researchers said.

Angina pectoris (heart attack) may be induced by spontaneous hypoglycemia and by hypoglycemia induced by increased insulin administration, reported the *American Heart Journal.*[10]

Hypoglycemia may be related to aggressive behavior. Perhaps the most aggressive and hostile people in the world are the Qolla, who live around Lake Titicaca between Peru and Bolivia, reported Carl C. Pfeiffer, Ph.D., M.D. The incidence of fights, theft, rape, and murder among them is staggering. On a visit to the region, Ralph Bolton, a California ethnographer, found that 55% of the men in a sample tested suffered from mild to severe hypoglycemia, and this was probably the cause of the Qolla's hyperaggression.[11]

Perhaps hypoglycemia is at the root of much of the anti-social and aggressive personal behavior in the United States, Pfeiffer said. No one can say for certain, but hypoglycemia and schizophrenia have been found to occur in juvenile delinquents and in convicted offenders.

"Hypoglycemia is one of the most important causes of exhaustion, chronic nervous fatigue, depression and irritability, and it prevents many from achieving happy, productive lives," Pfeiffer added. "It affects different people in varied ways and no two cases are exactly alike. None of the symptoms are specific to hypoglycemia, and their wide variety and common nature complicate diagnosis. When no physical or mental malfunction can be found, the patient should be checked for this disorder. Hypoglycemia affects more women than men, and the highest incidence is between the ages of 30 and 40. Hypoglycemia is more likely to be found in the person with a family history of obesity, diabetes, mental illness and alcoholism."

The major cause of hypoglycemia, Pfeiffer said, is thought to be the tremendous amounts of sugar (sucrose) and other refined carbohydrates and stimulants (caffeine, nicotine, etc.) ingested, especially in the United States. The body's biochemical processes cannot handle this tremendously increased load of sugar. It initially seems ironic that excess sugar consumption can cause low blood sugar, but this is precisely what may happen, he said.

Hypoglycemia can be controlled simply by diet and nutrient therapy, Pfeiffer added. The hypoglycemic can lead a normal or near-normal healthy life. A total improvement can be maintained, but the patient is seldom cured. He or she must follow the diet, or gradually the old symptoms will recur. A further worsening of the hypoglycemia or progression toward diabetes may be indicated in the successive glucose tolerance tests, each time the hypoglycemia patient falls by the wayside and then starts again on his low-carbohydrate diet, Pfeiffer said.

Writing in the *South African Medical Journal*, G. Borok reported that excess consumption of refined foods, especially sugar, and not eggs, bacon, or butter leads to ischemic heart disease. Excess consumption of any food leads to hyperglycemia with resultant hyperinsulinemia. Insulin converts glucose to glycogen and glycerols, which lowers blood sugar levels, and adrenaline is released to help maintain blood sugar levels, and a vicious cycle is begun.

What Nutrients Can Alleviate Hypoglycemia?

1. Beta-carotene and vitamin D capsules (500 and 400 IU daily).

2. Vitamin C (500 mg with or after each meal).

3. B Complex (50 mg, three times daily).

4. Fish oil capsules (1,000 mg three times daily).

5. Digestive enzymes, if necessary.

6. GTF chromium or chromium picolinate (200 mcg, three times daily).

7. St. John's wort polyphenol complex (one daily).

8. Soy food shake for breakfast.

Source: Earl Mindell, R.Ph., Ph.D. *Earl Mindell's Vitamin Bible for the Twenty-First Century.* New York: Warner Books, 1999, p. 300.

Borok said that all foods are broken down into simple sugars, but this can be done in a slow, steady rate in their whole forms. Refined sugars and foods (disaccharides) are broken down before absorption to monosaccharides and glucose by the amylase in the saliva. They are easily available for energy storage, but elevated blood sugar levels can lead to hypoglycemia.[12]

In an article in the *Journal of the American Geriatric Society*, M. J. Roberts said that corrective diet therapy has prevented or diminished attacks of spontaneous angina pectoris that are related to hypoglycemia. It is suggested that myocardial glucopenia (hypoglycemia) is the initial event resulting in ischemic heart disease.[13]

References

1. Adams, Ruth, and Frank Murray. *Is Low Blood Sugar Making You a Nutritional Cripple?* New York: Larchmont Books, 1970, pp. 5ff.

2. Ross, Harvey, M.D. *Fighting Depression.* New York: Larchmont Books, 1975, pp. 78ff.

3. Axelsen, M., et al. "Bedtime Uncooked Cornstarch Supplement Prevents Nocturnal Hypoglycemia in Intensively Treated Type 1 Diabetic Subjects," *Journal of Internal Medicine* 245: 229–236, 1999.

4. Budd, Martin L., N.D., DO. "Hypoglycemia and Personality," *Complementary Therapies in Medicine* 2:142–146, 1994.

5. Shimer, Porter. *New Hope for People with Diabetes.* Roseville, Calif.: Prima Publishing/ Random House, 2001, p. 78.

6. Kerr, David, N.D., et al. "Effect of Caffeine on the Recognition and Responses to Hypoglycemia in Humans," *Annals of Internal Medicine* 119: 799–804, 1993.

7. Hu, M., et al. "Assisting Effects of Lithium on Hypoglycemia Treatment in Patients with Diabetes," *Biological Trace Elements Research* 60: 131–137, 1997.

8. Whitaker, Julian, M.D. *Dr. Whitaker's Guide to Natural Healing.* Rocklin, Calif.: Prima Publishing, 1995, p. 281.

9. Knipers, H., et al. "Exercise Ingestion of Carbohydrates and Transient Hypoglycemia During Exercise," *International Journal of Sports Medicine* 20: 227–231, 1999.

10. Harrison, T. R., et al. "Glucose Deficiency as a Factor in the Production of Symptoms Referable to the Cardiovascular System," *American Heart Journal* 26(2): 147–163, 1943.

11. Pfeiffer, Carl C., Ph.D., M.D. *Mental and Elemental Nutrients.* New Canaan, Conn.: Keats Publishing, 1975, pp. 380ff.

12. Borok, G. "Is Butter Bad for You?" *South African Medical Journal* 72: 227, Aug. 1, 1987.

13. Roberts, H. J. "The Role of Diabetogenic Hyperinsulinism in Nocturnal Angina Pectoris, With Special Reference to the Etiology of Ischemic Heart Disease," *Journal of the American Geriatric Society* 15(6): 545–555, 1967.

20 The Glycemic Index—What It Reveals about Blood Sugar

Developed by David Jenkins in 1981, the glycemic index measures the rise in blood sugar after eating a certain food compared to the blood sugar rise caused by glucose. Any carbohydrate will bring a rise in blood sugar. Foods are rated up to 100, and those with the highest ratings (potatoes, white bread, rice, cornflakes, etc.) are not suitable foods for diabetics.

In Type 1 and Type 2 diabetes, low-glycemic-index diets, when compared with high-glycemic-index diets of similar nutrient composition, bring improvements in glucose and lipid metabolism. Evidence suggests that the glycemic index of one's diet may be the most important dietary factor in preventing (or generating) Type 2 diabetes.

The glycemic index is a ratio that measures the rise in blood sugar after eating a certain food compared to the blood sugar rise caused by glucose. Glucose (blood sugar) has been arbitrarily assigned a glycemic index of 100, which is similar to the boiling point of water at 100 degrees Centigrade and its freezing point at zero, reported Eberhard Kronhausen, Ed.D.[1]

Any carbohydrate will cause a rise in blood sugar, and foods with a high glycemic index (meaning they raise it fast) include processed breakfast cereals, breads, root vegetables (yams, sweet potatoes, potatoes, and carrots), and most canned foods. The magnitude of blood glucose

Glycemic Index of Selected Foods

All values are given in comparison to sucrose, with a glycemic index of 100.

Breads		Bran Chex	58	Pineapple	52
French	95	All Bran	42	Orange	43
Wholemeal	72			Apple	36
White	70	**Potatoes**		Peach	28
Barley	65	Various kinds	80–100		
Rye	65			**Rice**	
Sourdough	57	**Dairy Foods**		Low amylose,	
Pumpernickel	41	Ice cream, full fat	61	white or brown	70–90
Heavy mixed grain	30–45	Yogurt, low fat, fruit	33	High amylose,	
		Milk, skim	32	Basmati, etc.	50–60
Breakfast Cereals		Milk, full fat	27		
Cornflakes	84			**Legumes**	
Cheerios	83	**Fruits**		Baked beans, canned	48
Rice Krispies	82	Watermelon	72	Lentils	28
Cream of Wheat	66	Pawpaw	58	Soybeans	18
Muesli	66	Banana	53		

Source: Janette Brand-Miller, Ph.D., and Kaye Foster-Powell, B.Sc. "Diets with Low Glycemic Index: From Theory to Practice," *Nutrition Today* 34(2): 66, March/April 1999. (The Glycemic Index was developed in 1981 by David Jenkins.)

response depends on the type of food and the form in which it is consumed. For example, spaghetti produces a smaller rise in blood glucose than wholemeal or white bread, since the glycemic index for pasta is only 40% of white bread and roughly 60% that of wholemeal bread.

Pureed vegetables and fruits provide a more pronounced glucose response than do whole or cut-up vegetables and fruits. As an example, a whole apple produces less of a blood glucose response and has a lower glycemic index than apple puree. Apples, oranges, and grapefruit, with their fiber, have a lower index than juices made from these fruits. Cooked fruits and vegetables produce higher blood glucose response than do raw apples or carrots.[2]

A study evaluated the role of the glycemic index in diabetes and found that, in eleven medium- to long-term studies, all but one showed positive findings with regard to the relationship between the absorption values reflected in the glycemic index and diabetes, according to researchers at the University of Sydney in Australia. A low-glycemic-index diet reduced glycosylated hemoglobin by 9%, fructosamine by 8%, urinary C-peptides by 20%, and day-long blood glucose by 16%. The fructosamine test measures the glycation of a protein in the blood that has a shorter half-life than hemoglobin. C-peptide levels indicate how much insulin the body is making. On average, cholesterol was reduced 6% and triglycerides by 9%.[3]

The researchers found low-glycemic index diets to be very "user friendly." Of 44 foods evaluated, there was often no difference in glycemic index values between sweetened and non-sweetened foods. For example, the glycemic index of tropical fruits ranged from mango at 51 to watermelon at 72; in breakfast cereals from 43 to 90; in beverages, from orange juice at 53 to an orange soft drink at 68; in dried fruits, from apricots at 30 to sultanas (seedless grapes) at 61. They went on to say that dairy products with added sugar had a higher glycemic index than those without. Fat reduces the glycemic response to foods.

"In subjects with Type 1 and Type 2 diabetes, low-glycemic index diets, in comparison with high-GI diets of similar nutrient composition, lead to improvements in glucose and lipid metabolism," according to Janette Brand-Miller, Ph.D., and Kay Foster-Powell, B.Sc.: "In eight well-designed long-term studies using a cross-over design, the low-GI diet reduced glycosylated proteins by an average of almost 14% over periods ranging from two to 12 weeks."[4] Glycosylation refers to the joining of glucose (sugar) to the hemoglobin protein in red blood cells.

They further said that "recent epidemiologic evidence indicates that the GI of the diet may be the most important dietary factor in preventing Type 2 diabetes. Two large-scale prospective studies . . . showed that diets with a high glycemic load increase the risk of developing Type 2 diabetes after controlling for known risk factors such as age and body mass index."

Foods with a low glycemic index are said to be beneficial in relation to the insulin resistance syndrome, according to Elin M. Ostman and colleagues at Lund University in Sweden. Originally, the index was introduced to classify carbohydrate foods according to their effect on how much glucose was in the blood following a meal. Data now suggest that a diet with a low glycemic index improves blood glucose control, the blood lipid profile, and blood clotting activity, suggesting a therapeutic role in the treatment of disease related to insulin resistance, the researchers said. Epidemiologic studies also suggest that such a diet may reduce the risk of Type 2 diabetes and heart attack.[5]

"Today, there is an international consensus regarding the nutritional relevance of the Glycemic Index concept," the authors continued. "In dietary recommendations from the Food and Agricultural Organization and the World Health Organization, an increased consumption of low-glycemic index foods is strongly advocated. Pasta, legumes and products based on whole cereal grains are examples of commercially available low-glycemic index foods. Unfortunately, most breakfast cereals and conventional bread products belong to the group of foods that elicit high metabolic responses. It is known that the use of whole cereal grains and sourdough fermentation in bread making produces bread products with lower Glycemic Indexes."

In the Swedish study, lactic acid in fermented milk products (such as yogurt) did not lower the glycemic and insulinemic indexes. The latter refers to the amount of insulin circulating in the blood. In spite of low glycemic indexes of 15 to 30, all of the milk products produced high insulinemic indexes of 90 to 98, which were not significantly different from the insulinemic index of the bread that was studied. Also, the addition of yogurt and pickled cucumber to a breakfast with a high-glycemic-index bread significantly lowered after-eating levels of glycemia and insulinemia (abnormal amounts of insulin in the blood) compared with the reference meal. In contrast, the addition of regular milk and fresh cucumber had no favorable effect on the metabolic responses.

In a 6-year study involving more than 65,000 women, it was found that those who consumed diets high in carbohydrates from white bread, potatoes, white rice, and pasta had two-and-one-half times the risk for Type 2 diabetes than participants who ate a diet rich in high-fiber foods such as whole wheat bread and whole grain pasta, according to Walter Willett, Ph.D., of the Harvard School of Public Health in Boston, Massachusetts.[6]

He added that low-fiber carbohydrates, such as pasta, behave like white sugar during digestion, and that fiber helps to reduce the rate of carbohydrate absorption. Enriched white flour is nutritionally stripped of its nutrients. For example, of the 15 key nutrients in white flour—including vitamin E—only 5 equal or surpass levels found in whole wheat flour, he said. Unground whole wheat is even better than ground whole wheat.

Willett said in studying the blood glucose levels in 16 adults with diabetes who had eaten breads made with varying ratios of whole grains and millet flours, the higher proportion of whole grains (unmilled grains), the lower the blood glucose. He added that ground whole wheat has a similar effect on blood sugar levels as white flour, but not as much as unground

kernels. People should eat as many whole grains in a coarse form as possible, and if the first word in the ingredient list is not "whole," other grains
should be selected, he said.

In the study by Jenkins of the glycemic index of 62 commonly eaten
foods and sugars, these were given individually to groups of 5 to 10 healthy
fasting volunteers. Blood glucose levels were monitored over 2 hours. The
largest rises were seen with vegetables, of about 70%; and lower rises were
from breakfast cereals at 65%, cereals and biscuits at 60%, fruit at 50%,
dairy products at 35%, and dried legumes at 31%. There were obviously
great variations within food groups, and there was a significant negative
relationship between fat and protein and after-meal glucose rise, but not
with fiber or sugar content.[7]

It was found that sugars such as glucose, maltose, and sucrose produce large increases in blood sugar levels, whereas fructose (fruit sugar) is
metabolized without insulin and causes minimal increases, even in diabetics. Foods that are high in sticky fiber or foods that are resistant to
forming a jelly-like consistency show slower rates of digestion and absorption. These foods may be called low-glycemic-index foods. In a study of 44
foods containing simple sugars, it was reported that there was no difference in the glycemic index between the sweetened and unsweetened products.

At the University of Toronto in Canada, researchers said that it is generally thought that foods high in viscous fiber or antinutrients result in
slower rates of digestion and absorption, and that these are low-glycemic
index foods. Increased meal frequency reduces after-dinner insulin and
glucose responses in those with Type 2 diabetes and in nondiabetic volunteers, and it lowers serum concentrations of LDL-cholesterol and
apoprotein-B. Increased meal frequency may also slow small intestinal
absorption in diabetes, hyperlipidemia, and obesity, the researchers said.

Eating foods that are low in the glycemic index, along with eating
smaller portions more frequently, can lower the glycemic response, the
researchers said.[8] Lipoprotein-B is a single protein found in LDL-cholesterol,
which allows LDL to attach itself to cells. LDL-cholesterol, the so-called bad
kind, is associated with cardiovascular disease by way of oxidation and free
radical damage. When LDL becomes oxidized, it can clog arteries and lead
to cardiovascular disease.[9]

Potatoes have a high glycemic value, regardless of variety, cooking
methods, and maturity, reported a research team from the University of
Sydney in Australia. New potatoes have a low glycemic index, probably

due to differences in their starch content as compared to mature potatoes. In their study, the glycemic values ranged from 65 for canned new potatoes to 101 for boiled potatoes. The average size of the tuber was found to correlate with the glycemic index, the research team said.[10]

At the King Fahd Central Hospital in Gizan, Saudi Arabia, researchers evaluated the glycemic index for 11 common foods that were consumed by 55 Indian volunteers with Type 2 diabetes. It was found that the glycemic index was low (13 to 26) for Bengal gram, banana, apple, groundnuts, and milk; high (72 to 95) for wheat chapati, millet bread, and potato; rice, sago, and white bread registered intermediate values (55 to 64). Foods with a low glycemic index resulted in a low insulin response.[11]

Researchers at the University of Toronto in Canada studied the effect of extruded rice noodles on digestibility and glycemic response in healthy volunteers and Type 2 diabetics. The extrusion process reduced the starch digestibility by 15%, and thereby the glycemic index in healthy volunteers consuming the foods by 36%. In the diabetics, the reduction of glycemic index was about 24%. The researchers suggested that the low glycemic response to high amylose and rice noodles suggests that these foods may be beneficial to diabetics (and nondiabetics). Amylose is a component of starch characterized by its glucose content.[12]

A study reported in the *New Zealand Journal of Medicine* evaluated the glycemic index of 28 carbohydrate foods in 29 healthy females and 18 males, compared with 3 females with Type 2 diabetes and 9 male diabetics. There were no statistically significant differences between the glycemic index foods tested in both groups. Carbohydrates rich in soluble fiber had the lowest glycemic index, but other factors are involved.

For example, a low glycemic index is registered in foods that are rich in fat as well as carbohydrate, or when fructose contributes significantly to the total carbohydrate content. Thus, fruits high in glucose, such as grapes, have a higher glycemic index than fructose itself.[13] Whole grains have a lower glycemic index than when the cereal is extensively processed and the cellular structure altered. Whole fruits have a lower glycemic index than pureed forms, in spite of a similar content of total sugars.

A group at the University of Baroda in India studied the glycemic index and triglyceride levels in 30 Type 2 diabetics, who were given 50 g portions of four cereal-green leafy vegetable combinations traditionally consumed in India. The foods were rice in the form of flakes and puffs; wheat bhakari (wheat flour kneaded, rolled out, and shallow fried); wheat bhakari stuffed with fenugreek; and spinach leaves.[14]

The puffed rice and wheat bhakari showed a higher glycemic response than when the group was given 50 g of glucose. Rice flakes and wheat bhakari stuffed with green leafy vegetables had a lower glycemic response; puffed rice had a higher glycemic response when compared with rice flakes and rice alone, because puffing involves parching while flaking involves pounding. The parching probably alters structural changes in the rice and may be responsible for the increased glycemic response to puffed rice. Pounding flattens the rice kernels and may be responsible for the lowering of the glycemic response.

Eight healthy volunteers were studied for the glycemic index and insulin response from 12 rice products at the University of Sydney in Australia. The products were brown and white versions of three commercial varieties of rice, a waxy rice, a converted rice, a quick-cooking brown rice, puffed rice cakes, rice pasta, and rice bran. The glycemic indexes of the products ranged from 64 to 93, with glucose as the standard at 100.

The high amylose rice gave a lower glycemic and insulin index than the normal-amylose and waxy-rice varieties. As might be expected, the converted rice and most of the other rice products had high glycemic indexes. Insulin indices correlated positively with the glycemic index. Many rice products should be classified as high glycemic index foods, the authors said. However, the high amylose rice varieties may have a potential value in low glycemic diets.[15]

References

1. Kronhausen, Eberhard, Ed.D., et al. *Formula for Life.* New York: William Morrow and Co., 1989, pp. 306ff.

2. Murray, Michael, N.D., and Joseph Pizzorno, N.D. *Encyclopedia of Natural Medicine.* Rocklin, Calif.: Prima Publishing, 1998, p. 415.

3. Miller, Janette, et al. "Importance of Glycemic Index in Diabetes," *American Journal of Clinical Nutrition* 59 (Suppl.): 747S–752S, 1994.

4. Brand-Miller, Janette, Ph.D., and Kaye Foster-Powell, B.Sc. "Diets With a Low Glycemic Index: From Theory to Practice," *Nutrition Today* 34(2): 64–72, March/April 1999.

5. Ostman, Elin M., et al. "Inconsistency Between Glycemic and Insulinemic Response to Regular and Fermented Milk Products," *American Journal of Clinical Nutrition* 74: 96–100, 2001.

6. Foltz-Gray, Dorothy. "Against the Grain?" *Hippocrates,* Nov. 1997, pp. 54–61.

7. McLaren, D. S. "Not Fade Away—The Glycemic Index," *Nutrition* 16: 151–152, 2000.

8. Jenkins, David J. A., et al. "Low Glycemic Index: Lente Carbohydrates and Physiological Effects of Altered Blood Frequency," *American Journal of Clinical Nutrition* 59(Suppl.): 706S–709S, 1994.

9. Ronzio, Robert A., Ph.D. *The Encyclopedia of Nutrition and Good Health.* New York: Facts on File, Inc., 1997, p. 273.

10. Soh, N. L., and J. C. Brand-Miller. "The Glycemic Index of Potatoes: The Effect of Variety, Cooking Method and Maturity," *European Journal of Clinical Nutrition* 53: 249–254, 1999.

11. Banzal, Sudodh, et al. "Glycemic Index of, and Insulin Response to, Some Food Items Consumed by Indians," *Medical Science Research* 25: 529–531, 1997.

12. Panlasigui, Leonara N., Ph.D., et al. "Extruded Rice Noodles: Starch Digestibility and Glycemic Response of Healthy and Diabetic Subjects with Different Habitual Diets," *Nutrition Research* 12: 1195–1204, 1992.

13. Perry, T., et al. "Glycemic Index of New Zealand Foods," *New Zealand Medical Journal* 113: 140–142, April 28, 2000.

14. Mani, E. V., Ph.D., et al. "Study on the Glycemic Index of Selected Cereals and Cereal-Green Leafy Vegetable Combinations in Non-Insulin-Dependent Diabetes Mellitus Patients," *Journal of Nutritional Medicine* 4: 321–325, 1994.

15. Miller, Janette, et al. "Rice: A High or Low Glycemic Index Food?" *American Journal of Clinical Nutrition* 56: 1034–1036, 1992.

21 Impotence: A Major Problem for Male Diabetics

An estimated 18 million men have erectile dysfunction, or impotence, and it is three times more common in men with diabetes. Impotence is often caused by circulatory problems related to hardening of the arteries. The fatty deposits that often clog arteries of the heart can also build up in the arteries in the penis. Other causes include decreased testosterone levels, prescriptions for high blood pressure, stress, an injury, worry about sexual performance, and other factors.

A number of nutritional approaches are being used to treat impotence. Some of these are zinc, vitamin A, vitamin E, vitamin B_6, ginseng, yohimbine, Ginkgo biloba, golden root, and many others.

Erectile dysfunction—or impotence—is defined as an inability to have and maintain an erection rigid enough for sexual intercourse, reported Marvin E. Levin, M.D., and Michael A. Pfeiffer, M.D., in *The Uncomplicated Guide to Diabetes Complications*. It is estimated that more than 18 million American men are bothered by impotence, and it is three times more common in men with diabetes in any age group.[1]

The Massachusetts Male Aging Study (MMAS) evaluated 1,709 randomly chosen men from the Boston suburbs, and of these, 1,290 (75.5%) completed questionnaires regarding their sexual health. Over half (52%) of the healthy middle-aged men complained of erectile dysfunction. The authors added that the MMAS and other studies show that diabetes in men over 40 years of age is associated with impotence.

Impotence in diabetics may be the result of nerve damage, clogged arteries, decreased testosterone levels, prescriptions for high blood pressure (beta-blockers and diuretics), depression, ulcers, or drugs to prevent vomiting. Also, it is made worse by psychological factors, an injury, blood vessel disease with decreased circulation, and nerve damage. Other factors are stress, fears about aging, and worry about sexual performance.

Although impotence can occur for a number of reasons, in men 40 and older it is often associated with circulatory problems related to hardening of the arteries, according to Kenneth Goldberg, M.D., of the Male Health Center in Dallas, Texas. The same fatty deposits that often clog arteries of the heart can also build up in the tiny arteries in the penis. Therefore, too little blood is available to pump up the spongy cylinders that cause an erection. Also, drugs prescribed to treat high blood pressure and nerve damage caused by diabetes can also cause erectile dysfunction, Goldberg added.[2]

Men with diabetes typically suffer from impotence, first because of poor circulation, and second because of autonomic nerve damage, according to Ronald L. Hoffman, M.D. This complication of diabetes can reduce potency in men as early as in their 30s and 40s.[3]

In the standard workup for lack of erection, a urologist will measure penile blood flow and perhaps perform an angiogram, in which a dye is injected to see how it travels through the bloodstream. Less invasive is the penile Doppler test, in which a ring with a sensor is placed around the penis to test for nocturnal erection. This is a modern form of the old postage stamp test, in which a roll of postage stamps is placed around the flaccid penis at bedtime, and checked the next morning to see if an erection has taken place and the roll of stamps has been separated.

One possible cause of diminished hormones that contributes to impotence is smoking, which leads to large amounts of carbon dioxide in the blood, reducing the hormone levels and contributing to erectile dysfunction, states Robert M. Giller, M.D. Smoking not only affects hormonal levels, but it can clog the penile arteries, causing impotence, even in younger men. One study reported that men as young as 35 suffered from impotence due to smoking; men who smoked a pack of cigarettes a day for 20 years were four times more likely than nonsmokers to become impotent because of clogged arteries, Giller said.[4]

"Some men develop adult-onset diabetes as they age, without knowing it," Giller continued. "If this happens, in addition to impairing the blood flow to the penis, it can wreak havoc with blood sugar levels; this, too, can contribute to impotence."

Another cause of impotence, according to Giller, is illness. For example, men who have had a heart attack worry about sex and its effect on the heart. Actually, regular sexual activity can reduce the risk of another heart attack. Some medications, such as drugs for high blood pressure, can interfere with the autonomic nervous system as well as with the production and action of sex hormones. Blood pressure can often be reduced with natural treatments. Prostate surgery can often impair the ability to achieve erection. Major abdominal surgery can also cause impotence.

Researchers at the University of South Carolina at Columbia studied 3,250 men, ranging in age from 26 to 83, who were without erectile dysfunction at their first office visit. The men were studied for 6 to 48 months, at which time impotence was recorded in 2.2% of them during follow-up. Each mmol/liter of increase in total cholesterol was associated with 1.32 times the risk of erectile dysfunction; every mmol/liter of increase in HDL-cholesterol was associated with 0.38 times the risk.[5] (A millimole [mmol] is one-thousandth of a gram-molecule. A gram-molecule is the amount of an element with a mass in grams equal to its molecular weight. For example, a molecule of water weighs 18.015 g.)

Volunteers with HDL-cholesterol over 1.55 mmol/liter—or 60 mg/dl—had three times the risk of erectile dysfunction. Also, men with total cholesterol over 6.21 mmol/liter—or 240 mg/dl—had 1.83 times the risk as did men with total cholesterol less than 4.65 mmol/liter—or 180 mg/dl. The researchers said that high levels of total cholesterol and low levels of HDL-cholesterol are significant risk factors for developing erectile dysfunction.

A study involving 4,400 Vietnam veterans reported that impotence occurred at a 50% higher rate among current smokers than in nonsmokers or past smokers. The rate of impotence among nonsmokers was 2.2%; 2% for former smokers; and 3.7% for current smokers.[6]

Natural Remedies for Impotence

• Stop smoking.
• If you have high blood pressure or elevated cholesterol, you should try to remedy these problems, as they can affect potency.
• If you suffer from diabetes, hardening of the arteries, or high blood pressure, your impotence could be connected to these problems. Follow appropriate measures to keep them under control.
• Check any medications to see if they affect potency. Ask your doctor to check the *Physicians' Desk Reference* to learn about side effects of your medications.
• If you have had a heart attack or other major illness, discuss with your doctor its effects on your sex life.
• If you have had prostate or abdominal surgery, it's possible you have had nerve or vascular damage that can be reversed. Ask your doctor.
• If you sense that your impotence has a psychological basis (fear of performing), try to get counseling.
• Take 50 mg/day of zinc.
• Take one 40 mg capsule or tablet daily of Ginkgo biloba for up to 6 months. If there are no results, discontinue.
• Take three 5.4 mg tablets daily of yohimbine for about 2 months. If no results, discontinue.

Source: Robert M. Giller, M.D., and Kathy Matthews. *Natural Prescriptions.* New York: Carol Southern Books, 1994.

In a Medline review of 73 articles published between 1966 and 1998, regarding testosterone replacement for erectile dysfunction, the overall response rate was 57%, according to the *Journal of Urology,* which did the review. Men with primary versus secondary testicular failure had a response rate of 64% versus 44%, respectively.[7]

At Massachusetts Medical Society in Boston, researchers reported that millions of men may be suffering from impotence due to the failure to produce nitric oxide. Tests performed on small strips of the corpus cavernosum (erectile tissue in the penis), removed from 21 impotent men at the time of penile prosthesis insertion, showed that the liberation of nitric oxide resulted in rapid and complete relaxation of the tissue.[8]

The nitric oxide was released by adding S-nitroso-N-acetylpenicillamine. The researchers suggested that a possible alternative treatment would be a removable penile patch that delivers an agent which raises nitric oxide levels, according to Jacob Raifer, M.D.

Writing in the *New England Journal of Medicine,* Raifer said that nitric oxide is involved in nerve transmission, leading to smooth muscle relaxation of the corpus cavernosum, which allows for penile erections. Defects in this pathway may lead to some forms of impotence.[9] A colorless, free-radical gas, nitric oxide is involved in the dilation of blood vessels, and is a potent vasodilator. A shortage of the substance may contribute to high blood pressure and the formation of the atherosclerotic plaque.

Men having trouble maintaining an erection might want to try natural remedies before opting for a Viagra prescription, according to Earl Mindell, R.Ph., Ph.D. He recommends 60 mg three times daily of Ginkgo biloba; 2 to 4 capsules daily of a combination of saw palmetto, zinc, and pumpkin seed oil; and 4 to 5 g of arginine, taken 45 minutes before sex. For men over 50, he recommends one tablet, 25 to 50 mg/day of DHEA (dehydroepiandrosterone). DHEA, a steroid hormone, should not be taken by those under 40 unless blood levels of the hormone are low; men over 50 can take 50 mg/day, Mindell said.[10]

Some patients have improved potency and fertility after their zinc and vitamin B_6 deficiencies have been corrected, according to Carl C. Pfeiffer, Ph.D., M.D. Cadmium, a harmful metal, antagonizes zinc and can, in extreme cases, stop the formation of sperm in the testes.[11] Semen contains considerable amounts of zinc and sulfur. Semen is 25% calcium, 14% zinc, 14% magnesium, 0.015% copper, and 3% sulfur. The odor of semen is due to amines such as spermine and spermidine. The vitamin content of semen consists of 13 mg of vitamin C and is 53% inositol, which is related to the B-complex. The main energy source is fructose at 224 mg%.

A study in Hawaii evaluated 25 male volunteers, 40 to 70 years of age, with mild to moderate erectile dysfunction. They were evaluated during a 4-week period when they were given a supplement containing various vitamins, minerals, and herbs. The supplement contained Ginkgo biloba (24% flavone glycosides, 6% terpene lactones), Korean ginseng (30% ginsenosides); American ginseng (5% ginsenosides); and L-arginine (an amino acid); along with vitamins A, C, E, B_1, B_2, B_3, B_6, B_{12}, folic acid, pantothenic acids, and biotin; and the minerals zinc and selenium.[12]

The volunteers were given the supplement twice daily, once in the morning after waking, and once in the evening. Of the 21 men who completed the study, 88.9% improved their ability to maintain an erection during sexual intercourse, and 75% had improved satisfaction with their sex life. There were no side effects reported.

In 1982, a group of physicians at Queens University in Kingston, Ontario, Canada, studied the effect of yohimbine on organic impotence. The study involved 23 patients, ranging in age from 32 to 72, of which almost half were diabetics. The other volunteers had high blood pressure and other circulatory problems and they were taking antihypertensive drugs.[13]

The patients were given 6 mg of yohimbine hydrochloride three times daily for 10 weeks. Since that is virtually the maximum dose, a few of the patients experienced nervousness, unspecified gastric complaints, and mild tremors. They were told to reduce the amount to 2 mg three times daily, and then to increase the amount until they were back to 18 mg/day. All of the volunteers eventually were able to tolerate that amount without further complications. Six of the 23 men were able to experience sustained erections and to resume normal satisfactory sexual relations. Four others reported partial satisfaction. Yohimbine hydrochloride, extracted from the bark of a West African tree, is a stronger version of yohimbe and is FDA approved to treat impotence.

At Valparaiso University in Indiana, researchers recruited 11 men with erectile dysfunction from a urology outpatient clinic at an academic hospital. When yohimbine was given up to 10 mg three times daily, there was no effect in sexually functional men, but mixed effects in the sexual function of men with erectile dysfunction. The herb may have exerted an enhancing effect on sexual desire and improved sexual performance. In this study, and others, the improved erection response was about 20% or higher, reported David L. Rowland, Ph.D.[14]

Foods and Herbs for Erection Problems and Increasing Libido

1. Fava bean (*Vicia faba*): A source of L-dopa, the bean allegedly was used to incite the Roman poet Cicero to passion. An 8- to 16-oz. serving of the beans might be enough to give erection a boost.
2. Ginkgo biloba: In several studies, physicians have obtained good results with 60 to 240 mg/day of a standard ginkgo extract. In one 9-month study, 79% of the men with impotence due to atherosclerotic clogging of the penile arteries reported significant improvement and no side effects.
3. Velvet bean (*Mucuna*, various species): These seeds contain more L-dopa than fava beans and are considered an aphrodisiac.
4. Yohimbe: After taking the herb for 1 month, 14% of the men studied reported restoration of full and sustained erections; 20% reported partial response; there was no improvement in the others.
5. Anise (*Pimpinella anisum*): It has a reputation for increasing male libido.
6. Cardamom (*Elettaria cardamomum*): Arab cultures hold this herb in high esteem for its aphrodisiac qualities. It is often mixed with coffee.
7. Cinnamon (*Cinnamomum*, various species): In a test at the Smell and Taste Research Foundation in Chicago, Illinois, Alan Hirsch, M.D., reported that the smell of cinnamon buns increased blood flow in male medical students.
8. Ginger (*Zingiber officinale*): Saudi researchers suggest that ginger extracts significantly increase sperm motility and quality.
9. Ginseng (*Panax*, various species): Chinese philosophers maintain that ginseng makes an old man young again.
10. Muira puama: One study shows that this little-known herb may be effective in restoring libido and treating erectile dysfunction.
11. Oat (*Avena sativa*): Stallions that are fed wild oats supposedly become friskier and libidinous, which generated the phrase "sowing wild oats."
12. Querbracho (*Aspidosperma quebracho-blanco*): In South America, this herb is considered a male aphrodisiac. It is not recommended for those with high blood pressure.
13. Wolfberry (*Lyciumm chinese*): In one study, men over 59 ate about 50 g of wolfberries a day for 10 days and reported significantly raised testosterone levels.
14. Ashwaganda (*Withania somnifera*): Occasional use, in a tea, is said to increase male libido.
15. Country mallow (*Sida corifolia*): This stimulant herb has a folk reputation as an erection-enhancing aphrodisiac. This herb contains 850 parts per million of ephedrine.
16. Guarana (*Paullinia cupana*): This Brazilian herb contains lots of caffeine and is regarded as an aphrodisiac.
17. Saw palmetto (*Serenoa repens*): This Southeast U.S. herb has been used to treat prostate problems, and was once considered useful for treating impotence and loss of libido.

Source: James A. Duke, Ph.D. *The Green Pharmacy.* Emmaus, Penn.: Rodale Press, 1997.

A study in Brazil evaluated 22 men, with a mean age of 58, who complained of organic erectile dysfunction. The volunteers were treated for 30 days with a placebo and then 30 days with a daily dose of 100 mg of oral yohimbine hydrochloride. Fourteen and 55% of the men reported complete or partial response to the treatment, respectively. Common side effects included anxiety, increase in cardiac frequency, increased urinary output, and headache, but none of the men dropped out of the study. However, the authors said that a single dose would not have any effect on impotence.[15]

Nutrition plays a role in determining sexual impotence, according to Julian Whitaker, M.D. Vegetables, fruits, whole grains, and legumes are key food groups, along with proteins (fish, chicken, turkey, lean cuts of hormone-free meat). Nutrients such as zinc, essential fatty acids, vitamin A, vitamin B_6, and vitamin E are also necessary for healthy sexual function, he said.[16]

Since it is concentrated in semen, frequent ejaculation depletes zinc stores. Zinc is necessary for more enzyme activity than any other mineral. Food sources of zinc include nuts, seeds, legumes, and liver. Other suggestions for preventing impotence, Whitaker said, are:

1. Exercise. The better physical fitness a man can attain, the better his sexuality.

2. Yohimbine. In one study, yohimbine (from the West African tree Pausinystalia johimbe) was successful in 34 to 43% of the cases in increasing blood flow into erectile tissue.

3. Muira Pauma (*Ptychopetalum olacoides*). In one study, men were given 1 to 1.5 g/day of muira extract. Of those with a lack of sexual desire, 3 out of 5 (62%) felt a positive effect within 2 weeks. Of those concerned about erections, 1 in 2 felt the herb was beneficial.

4. Ginkgo biloba. Various studies have shown that this herb is valuable in increasing blood flow and oxygen to many tissues.

Researchers in China, Russia, and the Far East have long used *Rhodiola rosea* (golden root) to ward off fatigue and treat a variety of conditions, such as weak erections. A 3-month clinical trial revealed significant improvement in sexual function and other conditions. In a Russian study, a research team, using experimental animals with diabetes, found that golden root and ginseng increased the blood levels of insulin and decreased the level of glucagon, a hormone that promotes an increase in the sugar content of the blood by accelerating the rate of glycogen breakdown in the liver. Typical dosage of the over-the-counter supplement is one or two capsules, or follow directions on the label.[17]

Since the purpose of this chapter is to discuss possible natural and nutritional approaches to impotence, I won't be dealing with penile implants, injection therapy, hormonal treatments, vacuum devices, topical drugs, bypass surgery, et cetera. These are subjects for the patient to discuss with his urologist.

References

1. Levin, Marvin E., M.D., and Michael A. Pfeiffer, M.D. *The Uncomplicated Guide to Diabetes Complications.* Alexandria, Va.: American Diabetes Association, 1998, pp. 304ff.

2. Feinstein, Alice, editor. *Prevention's Healing with Vitamins.* Emmaus, Penn.: Rodale Press, 1996, p. 334.

3. Hoffman, Ronald L., M.D. *Intelligent Medicine.* New York: Simon & Schuster, 1997, p. 253.

4. Giller, Robert M., M.D., and Kathy Matthews. *Natural Prescriptions.* New York: Carol Southern Books, 1994, pp. 206ff.

5. Wei, Ming, et al. "Total Cholesterol and High Density Lipoprotein Cholesterol As important Predictors of Erectile Dysfunction," *American Journal of Epidemiology* 140(10): 930–937, 1994.

6. Kahn, Jason. "Smoking May Increase Risk of Impotence," *Medical Tribune,* Jan. 19, 1995, p. 5.

7. Jain, P., et al. "Testosterone Supplementation for Erectile Dysfunction: Results of a Meta-Analysis," *Journal of Urology* 164: 371–375, 2000.

8. Raifer, Jacob, M.D., et al. "Nitric Oxide Deficiency Causes Most Impotence," *Medical Aspects of Human Sexuality* 26(2): 7, 1992.

9. Raifer, Jacob, M.D., et al. "Nitric Oxide As a Mediator of Relaxation of the Corpus Cavernosum In Response to Nonadrenergic, Noncholinergic Neurotransmission," *New England Journal of Medicine* 326(2): 90–94, Jan. 9, 1992.

10. Mindell, Earl, R.Ph., Ph.D. *Earl Mindell's Vitamin Bible for the 21st Century.* New York: Warner Books, 1999, p. 281.

11. Pfeiffer, Carl C., Ph.D., M.D. *Mental and Elemental Nutrients.* New Canaan, Conn.: Keats Publishing, 1975, pp. 469ff.

12. Ito, T., et al. "The Effects of ArginMax, a Natural Dietary Supplement for Enhancement of Male Sexual Function," *Hawaii Medical Journal* 57: 741–744, Dec. 1998.

13. Kronhausen, Eberhard, Ed.D., et al. *Formula for Life.* New York: William Morrow and Co., 1989, pp. 552–553.

14. Rowland, David L., Ph.D., et al. "Yohimbine, Erectile Capacity, and Sexual Response in Men," *Archives of Sexual Behavior* 26(1): 49–62, 1997.

15. Teloken, Claudio, et al. "Therapeutic Effects of High Dose Yohimbine Hydrochloride on Organic Erectile Dysfunction," *Journal of Urology* 159: 122–124, Jan. 1998.

16. Whitaker, Julian, M.D. *Dr. Whitaker's Guide to Natural Healing.* Rocklin, Calif.: Prima Publishing, 1995, pp. 284ff.

17. Murray, Frank. *100 Super Supplements for a Longer Life.* Los Angeles, Calif.: Keats Publishing, 2000, pp. 171ff.

22 Why You Need to Exercise to Reduce Your Diabetes Risk

A low-fat diet and a half hour of walking and other moderate exercise each day can reduce the risk of developing diabetes in 58% of those at high risk for developing the disease. In one study, the risk of Type 2 diabetes was reduced by 25% and heart disease risk by 50% in those who were moderately active. This regimen can also lower weight in some people.

Insulin resistance is associated with large amounts of abdominal body fat, which may cause 25% of cardiovascular disease in men and 60% in women. Diabetics should have their health care provider tailor an exercise program especially for them, since a too-stressful program can cause undue oxidative stress in untrained exercisers.

Low-fat diets and a half hour of walking and other exercise daily can reduce the risk of developing diabetes by 58% among those at high risk for developing the disease, according to a national survey by the National Institutes of Health in Bethesda, Maryland. All of the 3,234 volunteers in the study were overweight and had trouble controlling the amount of sugar in their blood, a major contributor to Type 2 diabetes. Those who were counseled on lifestyle changes—such as diet and exercise—lost on average about 15 pounds during the 3-year study.[1]

"Diabetes is not inevitable," reported Robert E. Ratner of the MedStar Research Institute in Washington, D.C., one of the participants in the study. "Lifestyle modification is achievable and changes health outcomes. Those who can't sustain lifestyle modifications have a choice in taking metformin, a drug, that is significantly better than nothing."

Ratner went on to say that the study doesn't prove that these interventions will permanently prevent diabetes. However, even delaying the onset of the disease could prevent many costly complications, such as blindness and kidney failure.

In the study, one-third of the participants were given individualized counseling about diet, exercise, cooking, gym classes, et cetera. Another third took the diabetes drug metformin, while the remaining one-third were given placebos. In each year of the study, 11% getting a placebo developed diabetes, 7.8% getting the drug developed the disease, and only 4.8% in the counseling group developed diabetes.

Low-fat diets and a half hour of walking and other exercise daily can reduce the risk of developing diabetes by 58% among those at high risk for developing the disease, according to a national survey by the National Institutes of Health in Bethesda, Maryland. All of the 3,234 volunteers in the study were overweight and had trouble controlling the amount of sugar in their blood, a major contributor to Type 2 diabetes.

Researchers at the University of Ottawa and other Canadian facilities report that exercise training can reduce glycosylated hemoglobin (HBA1C) sufficiently to decrease the risk of diabetic complications. HBA1C is the substance formed when glucose is attached to hemoglobin molecules. This test determines the average blood sugar levels for the previous two months. Their conclusions came after reviewing a meta-analysis of controlled clinical trials (a compilation of data from various studies). Specifically, the analysis showed that exercise can reduce HBA1C by about 0.66%, an amount that could cut the risk of diabetic complications significantly, according to Normand G. Boule, M.A., and Elizabeth Haddad, M.D., lead authors of the report.[2]

The studies did not find significant weight loss in the exercise group when compared to other groups, but exercise should be thought of as beneficial on its own and not merely as an avenue for losing weight.

"Two of the major goals of diabetes therapy are to reduce hyperglycemia (abnormal amounts of glucose in the blood) and body fat," the researchers said. "Chronic hyperglycemia is associated with significant long-term complications, particularly damage to the kidneys, eyes, nerves, heart and blood vessels. Obesity, especially abdominal obesity, is associated with insulin resistance, hyperinsulinemia, hyperglycemia, dyslipidemia and hypertension. These abnormalities tend to cluster and are often referred to as the 'metabolic syndrome.'"

They added that elements of the metabolic syndrome are strong risk factors for cardiovascular disease, and that regular exercise in nondiabetic subjects has beneficial effects on virtually all aspects of the syndrome.

At Ohio State University College of Medicine at Columbus, a research team concluded that exercise is beneficial to Type 1 diabetics. They reported that exercise increases insulin sensitivity (the normal state in which the cells of the body are receptive to the action of insulin) and reduces blood glucose levels. They added that an appropriate diet and insulin monitoring enables Type 1 diabetics to exercise safely and regularly. To prevent hypoglycemia, the researchers suggested that the insulin dose may have to be reduced 30 to 50% before exercise begins. Avoiding taking regular insulin at bedtime and reducing the evening insulin dose may help to prevent nocturnal hypoglycemia after exercising.[3]

At Nagoya University in Japan, 10 Type 2 diabetics were managed by diet alone, and 14 other diabetics were placed on a diet and exercise program. The exercise group was required to walk at least 10,000 steps daily, which were monitored by a pedometer. The other group followed its usual daily routine. While the body weight of both groups went down significantly during the study, the exercisers lost the most weight. In addition, the glucose infusion rate and the metabolic clearance rate went up substantially in those who were exercising. The authors said that walking can be safely incorporated into a daily routine, and it can be recommended as an adjunctive therapy in the treatment of obese, Type 2 diabetes.[4]

Researchers at the University of Texas at Austin reported that epidemiological studies reveal that those who have a physically active lifestyle are less likely to develop Type 2 diabetes or impaired glucose tolerance. The protective effect of exercise is strongest for those who are at the highest risk of developing Type 2 diabetes. Older people who have vigorously exercised on a regular basis have a greater glucose tolerance and lower insulin response to glucose than sedentary elderly people of similar height and weight.[5]

Exercise results in loss of fat from the central regions of the body, and this should significantly prevent or alleviate insulin resistance. The researchers added that exercise training can prevent muscle atrophy and stimulate muscle development. As an example, several months of weight training can significantly lower the insulin response to a glucose challenge (consuming glucose in the diet) without affecting glucose tolerance. Exercise should be done on a regular basis, and exercising with a variety of different exercises and using different large muscle groups helps to prevent and treat insulin resistance, the researchers explained.

Writing in *Sports Medicine,* Johan G. Ericksson, M.D., reported that Type 2 diabetes increases with age, partly due to a reduction in muscle mass associated with aging. However, muscle mass can be enhanced with resistance training. An optimal exercise program consists of aerobic training, and a combination of aerobic endurance training and circuit-type resistance training.[6]

At the Foundation for Optimal Health and Longevity, Harold Elrick, M.D., said that the daily participation in a prescribed exercise program is highly beneficial to patients with diabetes, cardiovascular disease, arthritis, hyperlipidemia, depression, cancer, and chronic obstructive pulmonary disease. This is beneficial because it: a) increases blood supply to all organs and tissues; b) improves muscle/tendon/ligament strength, mobility and flexibility; c) releases endorphins, the feel-good hormones; d) enhances bone formation; and e) stimulates creativity.[7]

"Daily exercise is one of the four living habit patterns that are essential for optimal health/fitness, disease management and disease prevention," Elrick said. "Its physiological and psychological benefits cannot be provided by medication or surgery. This observation is based on 53 years of medical practice and experience with thousands of patients, as well as family and friends."

In a study of 1,263 Type 2 diabetics, 50 years of age, they were given a thorough physical between 1970 and 1993. During an average follow-up of 12 years, 18 had died. After adjusting for variables, the researchers found that those in the low-fitness group had an adjusted risk for all-cause mortality of 2.1, compared with the men who were fit. The diabetics who said they were physically inactive had an adjusted risk of death that was 7.7-fold higher than in the men who were physically active.[8]

Researchers at the University of Miami School of Medicine in Florida evaluated 10 male adolescents with Type 1 diabetes and 10 youngsters who were not diabetic, to see the effect of an aerobic, strength, and calisthenic circuit training type program. Mean age of the diabetics was 17.2 years. For 12 weeks the volunteers underwent a 45-minute exercise program three times weekly to exercise all the major muscle groups. The researchers reported that the diabetics improved their cardiorespiratory endurance, muscle strength, lipid profile, and glucose regulation with the exercise, and that such a program is safe for properly trained and monitored adolescent diabetics, the researchers said.[9]

Insulin resistance is associated with large amounts of abdominal body fat and may cause 25% of cardiovascular disease in men and 60% of that found in women. However, low-intensity exercise, including walking briskly for 45 minutes on a treadmill or outdoors, can lower a diabetic's insulin resistance and need for insulin. As an example, the risk of Type 2 diabetes was reduced by 25%, and heart disease risk by 50% in those who were moderately active.[10]

Researchers have found that insulin resistance is not associated with the total amount of excess fat on a person, but rather on how much fat is found in the abdominal cavity. In fact, one out of every four men, age 40 and over, has excess abdominal fat and insulin resistance. Researchers have further found that abdominal fat is associated with a 20 to 25% increase in apolipoprotein-B levels, which is a reliable predictor of ischemic heart disease.

Elevated insulin levels raise triglycerides and reduce high-density lipoprotein cholesterol (the beneficial kind), which increases the risk of hardening of the arteries. Raised levels of insulin and apo-B, which are found in insulin resistance syndrome, are said to bring an 11-fold increase in heart disease risk.

While exercise is an important therapeutic tool for diabetic patients, it also produces oxidative stress which, theoretically, can increase the risk of blood vessel complications in diabetics. Oxidative stress is associated with an increase in free radicals, since oxygen molecules are usually involved in the creation of these destructive elements. For example, hyperglycemia (too much glucose in the blood) can stimulate the production of oxidative free radicals in the blood of diabetics. Also, exercise results in a significant increase in oxygen uptake at the whole-body level and in skeletal muscle.[11]

In addition, exercise increases the activity of catalase, superoxide dismutase, and glutathione in skeletal muscle and the heart and liver. Catalase is an enzyme that aids in the decomposing of hydrogen peroxide into water, superoxide dismutase is an enzyme that helps to deactivate harmful free radicals, and glutathione is an antioxidant that protects against free radicals. It is also suggested that a lot of exercise in a Type 2 diabetic, who is untrained, would result in more sustained oxidative stress. A trained diabetic would sustain less oxidative stress, presumably due to the induction of certain antioxidant enzyme systems.

A research team studied 85 pairs of nondiabetic patients with ischemic heart disease and controls for the risk of ischemic heart disease. They found that the risk was significantly increased in men who had elevated fasting plasma insulin and apoprotein-B levels, as well as small, dense LDL particles, when compared to those who had normal levels for two of these three factors.[12]

Researchers have long known that exercise increases cardiac output, redistributes blood flow, and increases blood flow to the muscles. For most people, exercising at 65 to 75% of their VO2 maximum is a suggested goal. VO2 measures oxygen consumption. For a 40-year-old, a safe pulse rate ranges between 117 and 135 beats per minute. For a 60-year-old, the safe range is between 104 and 120 beats per minute.[13]

Exercise is necessary for the prevention and treatment of high blood pressure. As an example, a meta-analysis of 13 controlled studies on exercise showed a mean reduction of 11.3 mmHg in systolic blood pressure and 7.5 mmHg in diastolic pressure. In diabetics, exercise can reduce insulin resistance by 40%, according to an article in *Consultant.*

Obese children tend to have elevated insulin levels, which can normalize with exercise. Exercise can also benefit osteoarthritis and reduce LDL-cholesterol and increase HDL-cholesterol. Exercise can also help to prevent bone loss, reduce anxiety and stress, and elevate mood.

References

1. Christensen, Damaris. "Walking and Eating for Better Health," *Science News* 160(10): 159, Sept. 8, 2001.

2. Boule, Normand G., M.A., et al. "Effects of Exercise on Glycemia Control and Body Mass in Type 2 Diabetes Mellitus: A Meta-Analysis of Controlled Clinical Trials," *Journal of the American Medical Association* 286(10): 1218–1227, Sept. 12, 2001.

3. Fahey, Patrick J., M.D., et al. "The Athlete with Type 1 Diabetes: Managing Insulin, Diet and Exercise," *American Family Physician,* April 1996, pp. 1611ff.

4. Yamanouchi, Kunio, M.D., Ph.D. "Daily Walking Combined with Diet Therapy as a Useful Means for Obese, Non-Insulin Dependent Diabetes Mellitus Patients Not Only to Reduce Body Weight But Also to Improve Insulin Sensitivity," *Diabetes Care* 18(6): 775–778, June 1995.

5. Ivy, John L. "Role of Exercise Training in the Prevention and Treatment of Insulin Resistance and Non-Insulin-Dependent Diabetes Mellitus," *Sports Medicine* 24(5): 321–336, Nov. 1997.

6. Eriksson, J. G. "Exercise and the Treatment of Type 2 Diabetes Mellitus," *Sports Medicine* 27(6): 381–391, June 1999.

7. Hamilton, Kirk. "Exercise Is Medicine," *The Experts Speak.* Sacramento, Calif.: I.T. Services, 1997, p. 70. Also, Elrick, Harold, M.D. "Exercise Is Medicine," *The Physician and Sports Medicine* 24(2): 72–78, Feb. 1996.

8. Wei, M., et al. "Low Cardiorespiratory Fitness and Physical Inactivity as Predictors

of Mortality in Men with Type 2 Diabetes," *Annals of Internal Medicine* 132(8): 605–611, April 2000.

9. Mosher, Patricia E., Ed.D., et al. "Aerobic Circuit Exercise Training: Effect on Adolescents with Well-Controlled Insulin-Dependent Diabetes Mellitus," *Archives of Physical Medicine and Rehabilitation* 79: 652–657, June 1998.

10. Pramik, Mary Jean. "Exercise May Improve Insulin Sensitivity," *Medical Tribune,* June 18, 1996, p. 7.

11. Villa-Caballero, L., et al. "Oxidative Stress, Acute and Regular Exercise: Are They Really Harmful in the Diabetic Patient?" *Medical Hypotheses* 55(1): 43–46, 2000.

12. Lamarche, B., et al. "Fasting Insulin and Apoprotein-B Levels and Low-Density Lipoprotein Particle Sizes Risk Factors for Ischemic Heart Disease," *Journal of the American Medical Association* 279(24): 1955–1961, June 24, 1998.

13. Shahady, E. J. "Exercise As Medication: How to Motivate Your Patients," *Consultant,* Nov. 2000, pp. 2174–2178.

23 Don't Smoke! And Eliminate a Prime Diabetes Risk

There is convincing evidence that cigarette smoking is a risk factor for Type 2 diabetes, in both men and women. There is also a relationship between cigarette smoking and insulin levels, as well as lipoprotein levels. A lipoprotein is a combination of fats and protein in blood, and is responsible for the transport of fats through the system. In addition, smoking is related to elevated triglyceride and cholesterol concentrations. Since smokers metabolize vitamin C more rapidly than nonsmokers, smokers are often deficient in the vitamin.

Smoking is also associated with a 50% increase in the progression of hardening of the arteries, another complication of diabetes. Vitamin C, vitamin E, selenium, and other antioxidants can inactivate the dangerous oxygen free radicals that damage blood vessels and contribute to atherosclerosis.

More than 80% of diabetics die from some form of blood vessel or heart disease, according to the *Men's Health and Wellness Encyclopedia*. However, studies show that women with heart disease and diabetes are more likely to die than men with the same conditions. On average, smokers die at a 70% greater rate than nonsmokers.[1]

A debate as to whether or not there is an association between diabetes and smoking evolved in *The New England Journal of Medicine*, when Paul J. West, M.D., asked this question in the January 24, 2002, issue.[2,3] Responding to West's letter, Frank B. Hu, M.D., said that 60% of the patients they had studied were overweight and obese, and that a poor diet, lack of exercise, and smoking were associated with a significant elevated risk of diabetes. He added that there is convincing evidence that cigarette smoking is a risk factor for Type 2 diabetes, in both men and women.

A research team at the Veterans Affairs Medical Center at Palo Alto, California, reported that cigarette smoking is associated with elevated plasma triglycerides and decreases in plasma HDL-cholesterol concentrations. In addition to increasing the risk of coronary artery disease, smoking increases glucose and fats in the blood.[4]

The study evaluated the relationship between cigarette smoking and insulin mediated glucose uptake and lipoprotein levels. The researchers found that smokers had significantly higher very-low-density lipoprotein cholesterol (VLDL), triglycerides, and concentrations of cholesterol and lower HDL-cholesterol than nonsmokers.

While blood sugar levels in response to the rate of oral glucose intake were similar in both groups, blood insulin response in smokers was significantly higher. In addition, smokers had higher blood glucose levels in response to continuous infusion of glucose, insulin, and somatostatin, in spite of similar blood insulin levels. Somatostatin is a polypeptide that reduces the secretion of insulin and other hormones. The researchers added that chronic cigarette smokers have high insulin levels in the blood, as well as abnormal levels of fats in the blood, when compared with matched nonsmokers. This explains why smokers have an increased risk of cardiovascular disease or coronary artery heart disease, the researchers added.

At Sahlgrenka University Hospital in Goteborg, Sweden, a research team studied 36 smokers who smoked more than 10 cigarettes per day for 20 years along with 25 controls. It was found that smokers had lower HDL-cholesterol (the beneficial kind) and lipoprotein-A. In addition, smokers were both insulin resistant and lipid intolerant with impaired triglyceride clearance.[5] People with Type 2 diabetes are often insulin resistant. They produce enough insulin, but their bodies cannot respond to the action of the hormone. Similar to LDL-cholesterol, lipoprotein-A is a fairly newly defined risk factor for hardening of the arteries, including coronary and cerebrovascular vessels.

The *Journal of the American Medical Association* published two studies involving 18 U. S. cities, involving 72,144 men between the ages of 33 and 39, and 270,671 men between 37 and 40 (Study 1); and 10,025 men who were 18 or 19, 7,490 men between 40 and 59, and 6,229 women who were between 40 and 59 (Study 2). The researchers found that those who had lower cholesterol and blood pressure, and who did not smoke or have diabetes, heart attack, or electrocardiogram abnormalities, have a much longer life span.[6]

In another study, researchers evaluated 10,914 people between 1987 and 1989 from the Atherosclerosis Risk in Communities study and found that cigarette smoking was associated with a 50% increase in the progression of hardening of the arteries; past smoking was associated with a 25% increase. Exposure to environmental tobacco smoke was associated with 20% increase in atherosclerosis when compared to those not exposed to tobacco smoke. In addition, the adverse consequences of smoking on hardening of the arteries progression was greater in those with diabetes and high blood pressure.[7]

Ralph Golan, M.D., reported in *Optimal Wellness* that cigarette smoking, high blood pressure, and diabetes injure arteries, as does excessive vitamin D, iron, lead, and sugar, even in nondiabetics.[8]

Cigarette smoking impairs coronary microcirculation and interferes with the regulation of myocardial blood flow, according to an article in *Lancet*. In addition, smoking may cause oxidative damage to vascular cells. In studying 11 healthy smokers and 8 nonsmokers, it was found that blood flow in the heart muscle was 21% lower in smokers at the beginning of the study. The researchers also found that smokers have reduced blood and tissue concentrations of vitamin C. An infusion of 3 g of vitamin C normalized myocardial blood flow and coronary flow reserve in smokers, but there was no effect in nonsmokers.[9]

Since smokers apparently use up vitamin C more rapidly, low levels of the vitamin are the most frequent nutritional deficiency among smokers, according to *Family Practice News*. In fact, the suggested dose of 100 mg/day of vitamin C for smokers may be too low. A review of more than 12,000 adults showed that at the 100 mg/day level of dietary intake, more than twice as many smokers as nonsmokers had low levels of vitamin C (hypovitaminosis C). In the study, 34% of smokers and only 12% of nonsmokers had hypovitaminosis C, which was defined as blood levels of 0.4 mg/dl. When the vitamin was taken at 200 mg/day, the difference between smokers and nonsmokers evened out. The researchers added that in smokers who are not willing to stop smoking, vitamin C supplements at 200 mg/day may benefit them.[10]

At the University of Toronto in Canada, a research team said that normal blood levels of vitamin E do not prevent lipid peroxidation (the oxidizing of fats) in smokers, and an increase in vitamin E intake is needed to reduce lipid peroxidation. The recommended dietary allowance of vitamin E (15 IU/day) may not be sufficient for cigarette smokers to prevent lipid peroxidation to tissues, the researchers said.[11] Fats (lipids) and cholesterol are vulnerable to free-radical damage (oxidation), from causes such as cigarette smoke. These damaged substances form toxic elements called lipid peroxides, which can damage artery walls and aid in the progression of hardening of the arteries.

In the Canadian study, which involved 13 healthy smokers, researchers found increased levels of breath pentane output, a sign of increased lipid peroxidation. Cigarette smoking increases the production of oxidants and free radicals that accelerate lipid peroxidation, as mentioned. After supplementing the smokers with 800 mg/day of vitamin E for 2 weeks, the research team reported decreased levels of pentane in their breath, and the plasma (selenium-dependent) glutathione peroxidase level was restored to normal in 5 of the 13 volunteers in which it was initially low. Glutathione peroxidase is an antioxidant, and it requires the mineral selenium as a cofactor.

Researchers at the Rowett Research Institute, Aberdeen, Scotland, evaluated 50 men who smoked more than 15 cigarettes daily for 10 years and a similar number of people who never smoked, and studied them for vitamin E stores and lipid peroxidation products. They found that the red blood cells of male smokers with a habitually low vitamin E intake were more susceptible to the breakdown of hydrogen peroxide into free radicals than those from nonsmokers. Blood levels of lipid peroxides and other harmful substances were also elevated in smokers.

These indicators of oxidative stress were considerably decreased in smokers and nonsmokers who took 280 mg/dl of vitamin E for 10 weeks. The authors suggest that vitamin E intakes may benefit both smokers and nonsmokers, since elevated levels of lipid peroxidation are associated with the risk of hardening of the arteries.[12]

References

1. Inlander, Charles B., et al. *Men's Health and Wellness Encyclopedia.* New York: Macmillan/People's Medical Society, 1998, p. 293.

2. West, Paul J., M.D. "Diet and Risk of Type 2 Diabetes," *New England Journal of Medicine* 346(4): 297, Jan. 24, 2002.

3. Hu, F. B., et al. "Diet, Lifestyle and the Risk of Type 2 Diabetes in Women," *New England Journal of Medicine* 345: 790–797, Sept. 13, 2001.

4. Facchini, Francesco, et al. "Insulin Resistance and Cigarette Smoking," *Lancet* 339: 1128–1138, May 9, 1992. (Erratum, *Lancet* 339: 1492, 1992).

5. Eliasson, Bjorn, et al. "Insulin Resistance Syndrome and Postprandial Lipid Intolerance in Smokers," *Atherosclerosis* 129: 79–88, 1997.

6. Stamler, J., et al. "Low Risk-Factor Profile and Long-Term Cardiovascular and Noncardiovascular Mortality and Life Expectancy: Findings for Five Large Cohorts of Young Adult and Middle-Aged Men and Women," *Journal of the American Medical Association* 282(21): 2012–2018, Dec. 1, 1999.

7. Howard, George, Dr.P.H., et al. "Cigarette Smoking and Progression of Atherosclerosis," *Journal of the American Medical Association* 279(2): 119–124, Jan. 14, 1998.

8. Golan, Ralph, M.D. *Optimal Wellness.* New York: Ballantine Books, 1995, p. 332.

9. Morris, K. "Vitamin C Restores Early Coronary Impairments in Smokers," *Lancet* 356: 1007, Sept. 16, 2000.

10. "Increased RDA for Vitamin C for Smokers May Still Be Too Low," *Family Practice News* 20(15); 29, Aug. 1–14, 1990.

11. Hoshino, Etsto, M.D., et al. "Vitamin E Suppresses Increased Lipid Peroxidation in Cigarette Smokers," *Journal of Parenteral and Enteral Nutrition* 14(3): 300–305, May/June 1990.

12. Brown, Katrina M., et al. "Vitamin E Supplementation Suppresses Indexes of Lipid Peroxidation and Platelet Counts in Blood of Smokers and Nonsmokers but Plasma Lipoprotein Concentrations Remain Unchanged," *American Journal of Clinical Nutrition* 60: 383–387, 1994.

24 What Is Syndrome X?

Syndrome X is a combination of health conditions that place a person at high risk for heart disease. These conditions include Type 2 diabetes, high blood pressure, high insulin levels, and high levels of fat in the blood. The main elements that make up the syndrome include a waistline that measures 39 inches or more, a ratio of total cholesterol to HDL-cholesterol greater than 5, and triglyceride levels above 150 mg/dl. Smoking and alcohol intake are also contributing factors. Diet and exercise are the keys to controlling Syndrome X, and the nutrients listed in this chapter are beneficial in alleviating the problem.

Syndrome X involves a group of symptoms, including abnormal lipids in the blood, resistance to insulin, obesity, and elevated blood pressure, reported *Nutrition Reviews*. This syndrome is thought to increase degenerative changes in arterial walls, thereby contributing to coronary artery disease. The so-called typical Western diet, which is high in fat and refined carbohydrates and low in fiber, can induce insulin resistance and contribute to other aspects of Syndrome X.[1]

Syndrome X is a condition involving elevated triglycerides, glucose intolerance, high blood pressure, excessive abdominal fat, insulin resistance, and coronary artery disease, according to Seymour L. Alterman, M.D., and Donald A. Kullman, M.D. In addition to putting a person at risk for developing diabetes, Syndrome X also predisposes a person to hardening of the arteries and related cardiovascular disease problems.[2]

After the cluster of symptoms constituting Syndrome X is recognized, measures can be taken to control or eliminate the problem, the authors continued. The main elements that make up the syndrome include:

1. A waistline measurement greater than 39 inches in either men or women.

2. A ratio of total cholesterol to HDL-cholesterol greater than 5.

3. Elevated triglyceride levels—usually above 150 mg/dl—associated with normal total cholesterol and high LDL-cholesterol levels, along with low HDL-cholesterol.

The authors went on to say that the key to preventing or reversing Syndrome X is diet and exercise. With weight loss and less abdominal fat, there is improvement in insulin sensitivity. In addition, certain high blood pressure medications, beta-blockers, diuretics, tobacco, and a diet high in saturated fat may increase the risk of developing the syndrome.

The *Nutrition Review* authors recommend consuming a diet low in refined carbohydrates and high in fiber to offset this syndrome. In addition, regular physical activity can prevent insulin resistance and provide protection against Syndrome X.

They went on to say that consuming alcohol in large quantities suppresses fat oxidation, and elevates insulin and free fatty acids, as well as increasing concentrations of such things as lactate, which can influence kidney glucose production. Cigarette smoking reduces insulin sensitivity and contributes to Syndrome X.

Some of the nutrients that may be beneficial for addressing Syndrome X include:

1. alpha-lipoic acid, which improves blood glucose control

2. arginine, which promotes blood vessel health and improves insulin action

3. chromium, which improves blood glucose control and insulin action

4. coenzyme Q10, which reduces elevated blood pressure, improves blood glucose control and enhances insulin action, as well as improving blood lipid profiles and reducing oxidative stress

5. magnesium, which reduces blood pressure, improves blood glucose control, and improves insulin action

6. omega-3 fatty acids, which can improve insulin action and improve blood lipid profiles

7. selenium, which can improve blood glucose control, improve insulin action and reduce oxidative stress

8. vanadium, which can improve blood glucose control and improve insulin action

9. vitamin C, which promotes blood vessel health, reduces elevated blood pressure, improves blood glucose control, and improves insulin action

10. vitamin E, which promotes blood vessel health, improves insulin action, and reduces oxidative stress

As for dosages of the supplements, the authors recommend these amounts: 1) vitamin C, 500 to 1,000 mg/day; 2) vitamin E, between 100 and 1,200 IU/day; 3) coenzyme Q10, between 100 and 120 mg/day; 4) magnesium, 480 mg/day; 5) vanadium salt, 100 mg/day, with an upper limit not to exceed 1,000 mg/day; 6) chromium, 200 mcg/day. They added that arginine may be beneficial as a stimulator of nitric oxide, which is known to mediate insulin's vasodilating effects on the endothelium. Arginine-derived nitric oxide has been shown to enhance nutrient-stimulating insulin secretion, they added.

Even if you are not diabetic, there are several reasons you should be concerned about diabetes or at the very least, about pre-diabetic symptoms, according to Jack Challem, Burton Berkson, M.D., and Melissa Diane Smith in *Syndrome X*. For example, diabetes and all other degenerative diseases develop slowly, over years, meaning that various degrees of pre-diabetes may exist for years. Diabetes is not an all-or-nothing disease, and insulin resistance and Syndrome X are common forms of pre-diabetes, they added.[3]

"The early signs of diabetes are easy to overlook because the symptoms are often vague, and ambiguous symptoms can indicate almost any disorder," the authors continued. "Most doctors are taught that diseases have well-defined causes that respond to well-defined treatments. While this idea seems straightforward enough, it has a built-in defect.

"Diseases are most easily diagnosed in their later stages, not in their earlier stages. Unfortunately, treating diseases in their later stages is often a difficult, uphill battle. It is much easier to prevent disease or to change the course of the illness before the damage becomes entrenched and irreversible. If you know that glucose intolerance and insulin resistance are potentially early signs of diabetes or heart disease, you can correct them before you become diabetic or have a heart attack."

Exercise reduces the risk of developing insulin resistance (e.g., Type 2 diabetes) and associated conditions, such as cardiovascular disease and blood lipid abnormalities, the researchers added. Studies have shown that physical activity can reduce the risk of diabetes by 50%. Further, every 500 kcal increase in leisure time physical activity is associated with a 6% reduction in the risk of developing diabetes.

Diet and lifestyle play a significant role in the development of Syndrome X, according to Karen Roberts, M.S., and Kathleen Dunn, M.P.H., R.D. The typical American diet, high in fat and refined carbohydrates, and low in dietary fiber and nutrients, is a major factor in increasing the risk of insulin resistance, they said. Smoking, lack of exercise, and excessive alcohol intake also contribute to the risk of Syndrome X.[4]

Exercise reduces the risk of developing insulin resistance (e.g., Type 2 diabetes) and associated conditions, such as cardiovascular disease and blood lipid abnormalities, the researchers added. Studies have shown that physical activity can reduce the risk of diabetes by 50%. Further, every 500 kcal increase in leisure time physical activity is associated with a 6% reduction in the risk of developing diabetes. Roberts and Dunn report that cigarette smoking appears to be a strong contributor to Syndrome X, since smoking increases insulin resistance, elevates triglyceride concentrations, and lowers HDL-cholesterol (the good kind), which are classic signs of Syndrome X.

Studies show that especially risky for the development of Type 2 diabetes is what's known as visceral or truncal obesity, in which excess fat is carried mainly in the area of the abdomen, and around the hips and thighs, reported Porter Shimer in *New Hope for People with Diabetes*. Since more fat is near the liver, the fat has a tendency to find its way into the liver's blood supply, thereby interfering with sensitive hormonal processes required for proper glucose regulation. Studies also show that people who gain weight later in life—such as when we adopt our lounge-chair lifestyles—

are more apt to accumulate the weight in the area of the abdomen and thus increase the risk for diabetes, than those who have been overweight since childhood, Shimer said.[5]

The link between diabetes and abdominal obesity brought on by the quintessential couch potato lifestyle is now so well established that the term "diabesity" has been coined, Shimer continued. He quotes Gerald Bernstein, M.D., an endocrinologist at the Beth Israel Medical Center in New York, as saying, "These people frequently have high blood pressure and high blood fats, thus constituting a very risky situation—referred to as Syndrome X—which increases the risk of developing heart disease."

References

1. Roberts, K., et al. "Syndrome X: Medical Nutrition Therapy," *Nutrition Reviews* 58(5): 154–160, 2000.

2. Alterman, Seymour L., M.D., and Donald A. Kullman, M.D. *How to Prevent, Control and Cure Diabetes*. Hollywood, Fla.: Frederick Fell Publishers, 2000, pp. 183–184.

3. Challem, Jack, Burton Berkson, M.D., and Melissa Diane Smith. *Syndrome X*. New York: John Wiley & Sons, 2000, pp. 32ff.

4. Hamilton, Kirk. "Syndrome X, Diet and Exercise." *Clinical Pearls*. Sacramento, Calif.: I.T. Services, 2001, pp. 131–132. Also, Roberts, Karen, M.S., and Kathleen Dunn, M.P.H., R.D. "Syndrome X: Medical Nutrition Therapy," *Nutrition Reviews,* May 2000, pp. 154–160.

5. Shimer, Porter. *New Hope for People with Diabetes*. Roseville, Calif.: Prima Publishing/Random House, 2001, pp. 4ff.

25 You Probably Already Eat Too Much Sugar

Since its use in India around 400 B.C., sugar has become one of our most pervasive substances. In the United States alone, the average person consumes more than 150 pounds of sugar annually. Unfortunately, it is almost impossible to tell how much sugar we are consuming, since it is used in so many foods and products.

Prominent nutritionists such as John Yudkin, M.D., have said that the body reacts to the metabolizing of sugar in a number of different ways. If its effects were produced by a food additive, he said, sugar would undoubtedly be banned from the marketplace. He and other experts have agreed that sugar plays a significant role in several diseases of civilization, such as diabetes. Those insisting on having sugar should consider stevia, an herb that is said to improve glucose utilization.[1]

American consumption of sugar in 1996 and 1997 rose to 9.8 million short tons from the previous year, reported Nutrition Week. U.S. sugar consumption rose by about 1 million tons in six years, or by 2.5 pounds per person.[2]

Table sugar is obtained mostly from sugar cane and sugar beets, but various types of sugar are available in the marketplace, such as molasses, raw sugar, brown sugar, turbinado sugar, and others.

Sugary foods have lots of calories but are lacking in any kind of nutrition. While some nutritionists recommend small amounts of sugar for diabetics, the sugar recommendations are at the tip of the Food Pyramid. Diabetics should review their sugar intake with their health care provider.

Excess sugar intake can increase triglyceride levels in diabetics, contributing to the risk of heart disease. High sugar intake can also lead to overweight, another major problem for diabetics.

Stevia (Stevia rebaudiana*), an herb in the* Chrysanthemum *genus, can be used as a sugar substitute by some diabetics, since it contains virtually no calories and is said to not raise blood sugar levels. Its use by diabetics should, however, be reviewed by their doctor.*[3]

The definitive essay on the case against sugar is Surgeon-Captain T. L. Cleave's book, *The Saccharine Disease*, reports Robert C. Atkins, M.D. Cleave shows example after example of societies in which the addition of sugar to the diet was the obvious starting point for the development of diabetes and of hardening of the arteries in the epidemic proportions now typical of a Western nation. Two striking examples in Cleave's global studies were Iceland, beginning in 1920, and among the nomadic Yemenite Jews. Before sugar was introduced into these cultures, there was no diabetes or atherosclerosis. Two decades after their diets became similar to ours, because sugar was added, they began to develop nearly as high an incidence of these illnesses as we have today.[4]

"Another of Cleave's great contributions was the discovery of the Law of Twenty Years," Atkins said. "In every culture he studied, it took exactly 20 years after the dietary change for the first cases of diabetes and atherosclerosis to appear. In American terms this means that the increase in consumption of sugar and of highly refined flour between 1895 and 1910 could easily be invoked to explain the beginning of the heart attack era and the increase in diabetes prevalence noted between 1915 and 1930. This increase has continued—in the years between 1935 and 1968, for example, the prevalence increased by 600%."

In 1972, A. M. Cohen, a leading Israeli scientist, published a paper in *Metabolism* called "Genetics and Diet as Factors in the Development of Diabetes Mellitus: An Experimental Model." Cohen described how he and his associates were able to create a strain of diabetic rats by feeding them sugar and selectively breeding the most sugar-susceptible rats. This process took just six generations. This work was confirmed with striking similarity by H. Laube and R. Pfeiffer, of the University of Ulm in Germany, who were contributing editors to the book *Diabetes, Obesity and Vascular Disease.*

"Now, I won't bog you down with all the evidence implicating sugar as a contributing cause of diabetes—along with hereditary predisposition—as laid out in Dr. Cohen's rat model," Atkins continued. "But it seems to be proven that sugar raises insulin and triglyceride levels and has been used to create diabetes. Insulin and triglycerides, in turn, have been shown to help cause atherosclerosis. I hope you can see the connection."

In reading books and magazines devoted to diabetes, I am always astonished at how many recipes call for sugar or sugar substitutes. The fact remains that the body is perfectly capable of converting meat, cheese, fruits, vegetables, and other foods into glucose, so that sugar is not really necessary, except as an occasional treat.

The consumption of sugar varies from year to year, but it is estimated that the average American consumes more than 154 pounds of sugar annually. And you nearly have to be a Ph.D. to ascertain the sugar content on typical labels, since sweeteners can be listed as sucrose, fructose, maltose, honey, dextrose, corn syrup, fruit juices, et cetera.

A label is *supposed* to list the largest amount of sugar in the most prominent place, but when you add up the various sugars scattered throughout the label, some of the products, such as breakfast cereals, rightfully belong on the candy counter. When children are sent off to school each morning having eaten sugar-coated cereals, doughnuts, and other sweet foods, is it any wonder that their hyperactivity begins to surface about mid-morning? Candy bars, soft drinks, and other sweets taken later in the day ensure further unruly behavior.

In my book, *Program Your Heart for Health,* I quoted John Pekkanen and Mathea Falco, in an article in *Atlantic,* as saying that sugar, called "white gold," is said to be addictive and that many doctors and researchers believe that it poses a dire threat to our national health. At the time of the article, in 1975, the authors said that the average American consumed nearly 2 pounds of sugar a week, or some 130 pounds a year. When you consider that many people consume little or no sugar, such as infants, that raises the per capita amount of the sweetener even higher for those who do.[5]

Pekkanen and Falco quoted Abraham Nizel, Ph.D., professor of nutrition and dentistry at Tufts University in Boston, Massachusetts, as saying that one widely accepted and advertised value of sugar is as a supplier of quick energy, but energy can be obtained from many other foods that also supply minerals and vitamins at the same time.

"Refined sugar is an additive, a sweetener, a filler, a texturizer and a preservative, but it does not make us stronger or give us the sole source of quick energy," said Pekkanen and Falco. "In fact, because of its effect on blood sugar levels, some researchers believe it may do quite the reverse."

The myth that we need sugar to survive has been discounted by many knowledgeable scientists and nutritionists. The late Roger J. Williams, Ph.D., of the University of Texas at Austin, who discovered the B vitamin, pantothenic acid, told me that it is generally accepted that sugar is not itself a nutritional requirement for the body. Various amino acids (proteins) and the glycerol from fats can be converted in the body to glucose. Glucose, of course, is the main fuel used by the brain and other tissues, and it is regularly supplied in the blood for this purpose. If glucose is not supplied in the food, it is derived from the other sources and released continuously by the liver into the blood.

A fact sheet from The Sugar Association, Inc., in New York, said that chemists recognize more than 100 sweet substances that are described as "sugars," but only one is commonly called "sugar." It is sucrose ($C_{12}H_{22}O_{11}$), which is usually obtained in crystalline form from sugarcane or sugar beets. It is defined as a disaccharide of the carbohydrate family—disaccharide because it is a chemical union of two monosaccharides: glucose (dextrose) and fructose (levulose), and carbohydrate because it is a chemical compound in which hydrogen and oxygen in the proportion of 2:1, as in water, are combined with carbon.

In addition to levulose and dextrose (corn sugar), other types of sugars include:

1. Lactose or milk sugar, found in milk. It is usually made from whey and skim milk and is used mostly in pharmaceuticals.

2. Maltose, or malt sugar, which is made from starch and yeast. It is often mixed with dextrose for infant foods, in bread-making, and for other foods.

3. Corn syrup, a viscous liquid consisting of maltose, dextrin, dextrose, and other polysaccharides. It is often produced by heating corn starch with a dilute acid or by enzymatic action.

4. Molasses, which consists of concentrates extracted from sugar plants, usually the thick liquid produced when the sugar is being refined. It also contains other substances that occur naturally in sugarcane and sugar beets. The highest grade, called edible molasses, is used as table syrup or in such applications as spice and fruit cakes, rye and whole wheat breads, cookies, baked beans, gingerbread, candies, and others. It

contains some minerals, primarily iron. Blackstrap molasses is produced in the final step in the manufacture of sugar, and it contains no nutrients that are not already present in molasses.

5. Honey is an invert sugar with a small excess of levulose. It is made by an enzyme (honey invertase) from the nectar brought back to the hive by worker bees. The flavor and composition of honey depend on the type of nectar (orange blossom, sage, clover, tupelo, etc.). Its constituents include levulose (27 to 44%); dextrose (22 to 41%); maltose (6 to 16%); sucrose (0.25 to 7.5%); higher sugars (0.13 to 13%); water (13 to 23%); and other substances (0.13%).

6. Maple sugar and syrup come from the sap of the maple tree. The sugar contains approximately 93% of solids, and the syrup, 66%. Maple sugar is 90.69% sugar, 6.19% invert sugar, and 0.98% ash. Maple syrup is 95.12% sugar, 2.24% invert sugar, and 1% ash.

The late Jean Mayer, M.D., of Tufts University in Boston, once said, "Today, although it is a major component of the American diet, practicing nutritionists, especially those who work with children and the poor, consider sugar a menace to good nutrition. After reviewing the evidence, I believe it is adequate to show that the habitual consumption of large amounts of sugar is highly undesirable from the viewpoint of health and that sugar consumption should be reduced."

Mayer said that we have more or less conquered most of the infectious diseases and nutritional deficiencies (scurvy, beriberi, etc.) only to fall prey to another set of ills, such as atherosclerotic diseases of the heart and blood vessels, cancer, diabetes, high blood pressure, obesity, and tooth decay. He quoted a survey in 1974 as saying that of 78 cereals tabulated, only 26 contained less than 10% sugar. He stated that some cereal manufacturers have been known to combine the various grains and separate the sugars on the list of ingredients. Only thus can they keep cereal first on the list.

Mayer added that, whether sugar calories are called "empty," "naked," or "frivolous," they are unaccompanied by nutrients. Moreover, they increase the requirement for certain vitamins, such as thiamine (B_1), which are needed to metabolize carbohydrates. They may increase the need for the trace mineral chromium as well. Thus, a greater burden is placed on the other components of the diet to contribute all the necessary nutrients, in other words, other foods need to show extraordinary "nutrient density" to compensate for the emptiness of the sugar calories.

A large sugar intake means that huge amounts of rapidly digested and absorbed simple sugars (glucose and fructose) flood the body at intervals. This sudden glucose influx may represent a stress on the body such that the insulin-secreting islets of the pancreas of individuals genetically prone to diabetes cannot cope. A number of studies, while not totally conclusive, support the view that a large sugar intake promotes diabetes in susceptible people, Mayer said.

He added that preadolescent and adolescent boys are the nation's highest consumers of sugars and sweets, at a time when, to lower triglyceride and blood cholesterol, sugar intake should be cut along with a considerable decrease in saturated fat and cholesterol. Unfortunately, some children find sugar as addictive as tobacco or alcohol, and many of them get used to sweet desserts and snacks and feel deprived if these are not available. Clearly, he said, it is better to restrict sugar use from birth than to try to cut down later.

Appearing before the Select Committee on Nutrition and Human Needs of the United States Senate in Washington, D.C., John Yudkin, M.D., the eminent English nutritionist, said that there is no physiological need for sucrose. In fact, there is reason to believe that sugar, sucrose, plays a part in several diseases of civilization, such as dental caries, obesity, coronary thrombosis, and diabetes.

Yudkin said that these diseases have more than one cause. For example, in coronary heart disease, it is widely agreed that reduced physical activity, cigarette smoking, and obesity are among the causes. Thus, the most that can be expected from epidemiological studies in diseases of multiple causes is that they can provide a clue to the causes.

Yudkin said that, in the whole organism, sugar reduces the growth rate of animals in spite of them taking the same number of calories. It shortens

What Foods and Products Contain Sugar?

This pervasive substance is everywhere. Here are some of the applications.

Alcohol, alcoholic beverages, vitamin C, baby foods, bacon curing, baked beans, bakery products, bee feeding, beverage concentrates and bases, beverages, bread, candy, canning (fruits, fruit juices, vegetables, meats, soups, baby foods), catsup, cereal products (breakfast cereals, dry-mixed foods), chewing gum, chili sauce, chocolate, cider, citric acid, cocoa, condensed milk, condiments, confectionery (rock candy, candied peels, etc.) conserves, cordials, curing (fish, meat, and poultry), dairy products (ice cream, ice cream mix, ices, sherbet, milk drinks, frozen custards, frozen eggs, sugar egg yolks, yogurt).

Desserts, dried fruits, drink mixes, drugs, edible dyestuffs, elixirs, emulsifiers, flavorings, flavoring extracts, flavoring syrups, folic acid, fountain syrups, freezing (eggs, fruits, vegetables), fruit butters, fruit nectars, gelatin desserts, glace fruits, grain mill products, ham curing, jams, jellies, liqueurs, lozenges, macaroni, malted milk mix, maraschino cherries, marmalades, mayonnaise, meat products, mince meat, noodles.

Penicillin, pharmaceuticals, pickled fruits and vegetables, pickles, preserved fruits, puddings, preserved nuts, relishes, salad dressings, soft drinks, spaghetti, syrups, table syrups, tobacco products (including cigarettes), tomato sauces, water softeners, wieners, wines, and yeast culture.

Source: Frank Murray. *Program Your Heart for Health.* New York, Larchmont Books, 1977, pp. 185–186.

the lifespan, and it accelerates the production of protein deficiency, since it interferes with protein utilization. In addition, sugar increases the deposition of fat; it increases the concentration of cholesterol and triglycerides in the blood, and it reduces glucose tolerance and, therefore, produces the diabetic condition. Sugar sometimes increases and sometimes decreases the blood concentration of insulin; and it increases the blood concentration of another potent hormone of the adrenal cortex–corticosteroid, he continued.

"On the organs of the body, sugar increases the size of the liver, not simply by expanding each of the cells of the liver but actually by making the liver cells divide," Yudkin said. "It increases the amount of liver fat, kidney size and it produces pathological changes in the kidneys, as Aharon M. Cohen, M.D., has pointed out. In the laboratory, one finds that human volunteers and experimental animals that have been fed with sugar show a disturbed behavior of the blood platelets that are concerned with blood clotting. And it changes considerably the activity of many enzymes in the liver and in fat tissue."

The effects of sugar on disease can occur in three ways, he added: 1) by pushing out other foods from the diet; 2) by being taken in addition to other foods; and 3) by the particular properties of sucrose. Actually, sugar is the only common food that provides calories free from any trace of nutrients, he said.

At the end of World War I, statistics clearly showed that from 1914 to 1918, the mortality rates for diabetes had fallen sharply in Germany and only slightly less in England, the countries most affected by food rationing, according to Eberhard Kronhausen, Ed.D., et al., in *Formula for Life*. The most pronounced food shortages were of fats, meats, and sugars, all known today to contribute to diabetes. The same thing happened during World War II, but still nobody made the connection.[6]

The authors said that most people did not note the significance of another wartime dietary change, the milling of flour. In Denmark, they reported, high-fiber barley meal and rye meal further raised the fiber content of flour products during the Second World War. Consequently, the diet of some European countries during the war years was considerably lower in fats and much higher than usual in fiber. Both fat and fiber content in the diet are crucial factors in the cause and control of diabetes, the authors added.

At the University of Michigan, Jerome W. Conn and L. E. Newburgh found that sugar levels were most balanced when blood sugar was produced from protein and not refined carbohydrates, reported R. O. Brennan, D.O., in *Nutrigenetics*. That's because protein takes longer to be digested, absorbed, and metabolized in the blood. He noted that the U.S. Department of Agriculture had found that, because protein takes longer, the bloodstream receives a greater supply of glucose.[7]

> ## What Are the Nutrients in Sugar?
>
> One tablespoon of granulated cane or beet sugar contains calories (50), protein (0), fat (0), total carbohydrate (12), calcium (0), iron (0), vitamin A (0), vitamin B_1 (0), vitamin B_2 (0), vitamin B_3 (0), and vitamin C (0).[8]

"If Americans were getting enough protein and other nutrients, eating sugar (which lacks nutrients), would not cause as much damage as it does," Brennan said. "A Mysore, India, experiment showed that the sugar level remained relatively healthy and steady when glucose was eaten with high amounts of protein. Only alone, in snacks and desserts, do carbohydrates cause the large peaks and valleys in the blood-sugar level."

Writing in *Tired–So Tired*, William G. Crook, M.D., said that sugars derived from cane, beet, or corn are "bad" carbohydrates, because they have been stripped of minerals, vitamins, and other nutrients. He added that a USDA report stated that the average American is consuming an estimated 154-plus pounds of caloric sugars each year, and the calories replace those that could and should be obtained from the good carbohydrates.[9]

"Digestion of these simple sugars stimulates insulin release from the pancreas," Crook added. "Insulin lowers the blood sugar and makes people irritable, hungry and jittery and causes them to eat more sweets. One of the results is that more Americans are becoming obese. Simple sugars encourage multiplication of the yeast *Candida albicans* in the digestive tract. A research study in the early 1900s at St. Jude Hospital in Memphis, showed that mice receiving dextrose in their diet–as compared to controls–had a 200-fold increase in *Candida albicans* proliferation."

Researchers at San Diego State University in California evaluated 24 San Diego County public middle schools, grades 6 through 8, with children who were between 11 and 13 years of age. Snacks purchased from student stores averaged 8.7 g of fat and 23 g of sugar. Overall, 88.5% of store inventory was high in fat and/or sugar. Sugar candy accounted for one-third of the sales.[10]

A study by the NASA Langley Research Center reported that sugar is the most important dietary factor related to heart disease in women, according to the *Journal of Orthomolecular Medicine*. Heart disease mortality in men is related to animal fat. The researchers added that simple sugars raise triglyceride levels and lower the density of lipoproteins, which are risk factors for cardiovascular disease. They said that sugar intake accounts for more than 150,000 premature deaths from heart disease in the United States annually. There would be a reduction in heart failure and related conditions from reducing simple sugars in the diet, they added.[11]

In his book, *Intelligent Medicine*, Ronald L. Hoffman, M.D., said that one of the most common abuses, or perhaps *the* most common abuse of the body in America today, is the high-carbohydrate, sugar-laden diet that leads ultimately to some form of sugar disease, or—in its most damaging form—to diabetes. He added that you can get away with this kind of diet for 20 or 30 years, or maybe even longer, but it will damage the system, whether or not the damage shows up right away.[12]

"If you've never paid attention to your sugar consumption, perhaps now is the time to begin," Hoffman said. "Remember that sugar in its refined form, sucrose (table sugar), is not a naturally occurring food. It has to be refined through a chemical process from plant material, much as cocaine is refined from cocoa leaves, or medicinal drugs are extracted from rain-forest plants. In fact, sugar is more potent in the body than many drugs."

An individual may succumb to sugar cravings a million times in a lifetime, Hoffman said, generating a staggering overproduction of insulin and leading to Syndrome X, which is a precursor of heart disease and diabetes, as explained in the previous chapter. In fact, he added, the term "sugar disease" is a catch-all for a host of modern conditions that result from unbridled intake of sugar or refined carbohydrates. We can look at sugar disease as passing through three stages, from a milder form to more advanced and destructive forms; that is: 1) hypoglycemia; 2) Syndrome X; and 3) diabetes.

References

1. Mozersky, R. P. "Herbal Products and Supplements Used in the Management of Diabetes," *Journal of the American Osteopathic Association* 99 (Suppl. 12): S4–S9, Dec. 1999.

2. "Sugar and American Consumption," *Nutrition Week* 27(11):7, March 21, 1997.

3. Richard, David. *Stevia Rebaudiana: Nature's Sweet Secret*. Bloomingdale, Ill.: Vital Health Publishing, 1999, pp. 62ff.

4. Atkins, Robert C., M.D. *Dr. Atkins' Health Revolution*. Boston: Houghton Mifflin Co., 1988, pp. 85–86.

5. Murray, Frank. *Program Your Heart for Health*. New York: Larchmont Books, 1978, pp. 184ff.

6. Kronhausen, Eberhard, Ed.D., et al. *Formula for Life*. New York: William Morrow and Co., 1989, pp. 259–260.

7. Brennan, R. O., D.O. *Nutrigenetics*. New York: M. Evans and Co., 1975, p. 35.

8. *Food, The Yearbook of Agriculture.* Washington, D.C.: U.S. Department of Agriculture, 1959, p. 264.

9. Crook, William G., M.D. *Tired—So Tired—and the "Yeast Connection."* Jackson, Tenn.: Professional Books, 2001, pp. 138–139.

10. Wildey, M. B., et al. "Fat and Sugar Levels Are High in Snacks Purchased from Student Stores in Middle Schools," *Journal of the American Diabetes Association* 100(3): 319–322, March 2000.

11. "Heart Disease and Sugar," *Journal of Orthomolecular Medicine* 13:95–104, 1998.

12. Hoffman, Ronald L., M.D. *Intelligent Medicine.* New York: Simon & Schuster, 1997, pp. 102–103.

26 The Importance of Fiber

Dietary fiber consists of insoluble fiber, which helps to prevent constipation, colonic inflammation, and hemorrhoids, and soluble fiber, which slows starch digestion and glucose uptake, thus lowering the amount of insulin needed to process blood glucose after a meal. Fiber can also lower blood cholesterol and triglyceride levels, which are associated with coronary artery disease.

Sources of insoluble fiber include the skins of fruits and vegetables, whole grains, high-fiber cereals, dried beans, bran, and others. Soluble fiber includes cooked dried beans, chickpeas, barley, lentils, oat bran, rice bran, guar gum, pectin, psyllium, and others.

The high-complex carbohydrate, high-fiber diet advocated by James W. Anderson, M.D., can significantly lower blood fats; reduce fasting blood sugar, glycosylated hemoglobin, and blood lipids; help to maintain a desirable body weight; reduce insulin and oral hypoglycemic medications; and eliminate them entirely. In one study, the recommended diet improved glycemic control and reduced insulin requirements by 30 to 40% for Type 1 diabetics, and 75 to 100% for Type 2 diabetics. In most cases, insulin has been discounted after 10 to 21 days in Type 2 diabetics.

Neil Stamford Painter, M.D., and his colleagues in Great Britain were among the first to explain that low-fiber diets and too much white sugar and refined carbohydrates in the diet were responsible for increases in diabetes, heart disease, appendicitis, obesity, and other common health problems.

For example, Surgeon Captain T. L. Cleave of the Royal Navy, author of the landmark book, *The Saccharine Disease,* spent a lifetime collecting evidence showing that the refining of carbohydrates, and in particular the eating of purified sugar, was responsible for diabetes, coronary thrombosis, and other disorders. He explained that the removal of fiber from sugarcane and sugar beets concentrates sugar in a form that fools the appetite, so that the mechanism that regulates our intake of calories is bypassed. Cleave added that refined sugar is the cause of diabetes, because of the unnatural strain imposed on the pancreas, and this is the cause of coronary heart disease because of the striking association of diabetes to that disorder.[1]

Denis P. Burkitt, M.D., another British researcher, wrote as early as the 1960s and early 1970s that highly refined starches and sugars are responsible for diabetes, coronary heart disease, varicose veins, gallstones, ulcerative colitis, colon cancer, and other health problems. He added, "Appendicitis always begins at least a generation before the other diseases, but they all go together."

Fiber, also called roughage or bulk, consists of a mixture of various nonstarch complex carbohydrate and noncarbohydrate materials. This breaks down to cellulose, hemicellulose, pectin, muculage, gums, algal materials, and lignin, according to Robert A. Ronzio, Ph.D. Insoluble fiber, which includes cellulose and lignin, swell in water, increasing stool weight and stool frequency. These substances help to prevent constipation, colonic inflammation, and hemorrhoids by softening stools and speeding up transit time of waste through the intestine. While cellulose is not digested, colon bacteria break down 40 to 80% of it. Lignin, which may lower cholesterol levels, is not degraded and passes through the system unchanged.[2] Dietary fiber reduces the speed at which carbohydrates are converted into glucose, and it can reduce cholesterol and triglyceride levels, which contribute to heart attacks and strokes.

Bran, which is derived from the outer husk of wheat and other grains, is the most common insoluble fiber. Bran contains cellulose and other materials, which slows the rise of blood sugar following a meal and may help to prevent precancerous polyps in the colon.

Soluble fiber swells in water and forms a glue-like gel. It consists of noncellulose carbohydrates, such as pectins, gums, algalpolysaccharides, and some types of hemicellulose. Soluble fiber slows starch digestion and glucose uptake, thus lowering the amount of insulin needed to process blood glucose after a meal. This, of course, may help those with diabetes. Oat bran is thought to effectively lower blood sugar levels.

Good sources of insoluble fiber include the skins of vegetables and fruits, whole grains (excluding white flour), high-fiber cereals, dried beans, broccoli, bulgar wheat, and bran. Reliable sources of soluble fiber include fruits, cooked dried beans, chickpeas, barley, lentils, navy beans, squash, carrots, barley, oat bran, rice bran, guar gum, glucomannan, and pectin. Note: Patients with diverticulitis, ulcerative colitis, and Crohn's disease should not take fiber supplements without medical supervision. High levels of fiber can impede the absorption of iron, calcium, zinc, copper, and other minerals.

Whole grain foods are a rich source of antioxidants, such as vitamin E and selenium, as well as other vitamins, trace minerals, phenolic acids, lignins, and phytoestrogens, according to James W. Anderson, M.D., of the Veterans Affairs Medical Center at Lexington, Kentucky. Other trace minerals such as copper, zinc, and manganese are found in the outer layer of grains. Also, phytic acid, considered an antinutrient, may also function as an antioxidant. Whole grains are a potent source of numerous antioxidant compounds, which may help to inhibit oxidative damage.[3]

The effects of whole grain foods on insulin resistance are of great importance in reducing the risk of coronary heart disease, Anderson said. As an example, the insulin resistance syndrome affects as many as 80 million people in the United States, and it is an important forerunner of Type 2 diabetes. He added that the dietary glycemic index has been shown to be positively associated with the risk of both diabetes and coronary heart disease.

According to studies by S. Liu, et al., and previous publications, it seems that the consumption of two to three servings of whole grains daily has significant benefit in the prevention of cardiovascular disease. Recommending that an individual incorporate moderate amounts of whole grains, including dark bread, whole grain breakfast cereals, popcorn, cooked oatmeal, or brown rice in their diet may have important implications in the prevention of Western disease.

In a study involving 13 Type 2 diabetics, the volunteers were given two diets, each for 6 weeks. One of the diets, recommended by the American Diabetes Association (ADA), contained 24 g of total fiber (8 g were soluble fiber and 16 g were insoluble fiber); and the other was a high-fiber diet containing 50 g of total fiber (25 g were soluble fiber and 25 g were insoluble fiber). In week 6 of the high-fiber diet, as compared to week 6 of the ADA diet, mean after-eating blood glucose levels were 13 mg/dl lower and mean daily urinary glucose excretion was 1.3 g lower. In all, the high-fiber diet reduced total blood cholesterol concentrations by 6.7%, triglycerides by 10.2%, and very low-density lipoprotein cholesterol by 12.5%.[4]

Oats: Oat gum is as effective, if not better, than guar gum in lowering after-meal glucose and insulin levels in human beings, reported a research team from the University of Ottawa in Canada. In the study, glucose and insulin response to consuming 14.5 g of oat gum with 50 g of a glucose drink were compared to responses from consuming guar gum with glucose or glucose alone. Healthy volunteers were given test meals after a 12-hour fast, while blood samples were recorded at minus-15 and 0 minutes, each 10 minutes after the test meal up to 100 minutes, and then at 120, 150, and 180 minutes.[5]

Each of the volunteers consumed three different test meals at least 3 days apart. The test glucose drink brought a greater risk in after-eating blood glucose concentrations after 20 and 60 minutes than either the oat gum or guar gum. Reductions in after-eating glucose and insulin levels were similar for both guar gum and oat gum.

Oat gum is a soluble fiber from oats, of which about 80% of the gum is beta-D-glucan or beta-glucan. This sticky fiber consists of about 4% of rolled oats and 7% to 10% of oat bran. The researchers said that, based on their study, oat gum is potentially helpful in stabilizing after-meal glucose and insulin levels.

At the Beltsville Human Nutrition Research Center in Maryland, researchers evaluated the effect of beta-glucan in oats on 23 volunteers between the ages of 38 and 61, who had moderately high cholesterol levels. The participants consumed oat extract with either 1 or 10% soluble beta-glucans added. The extracts comprised 10% of energy and were consumed in a 5-week crossover study. There were 16 females and 7 males in the study.

The reactions of glucose were reduced by both extracts in both men and women. The reactions of insulin did not vary between men and women, but were lower after oat extracts were eaten. The authors said that oat extract can be substituted for fat energy with minimal changes in over-all food selection to improve the diets of those at risk for heart disease and diabetes. The extracts can have a beneficial effect on high blood sugar factors, they added.[6]

In another study by James W. Anderson, M.D., and his colleagues at the University of Kentucky College of Medicine and the HCF Diabetes Foundation at Lexington, they concluded that a ready-to-eat cereal containing oat bran, if consumed in ample amounts, can be an effective way of incorporating oat bran into the diet to lower blood lipid levels.

In the study, men with high cholesterol levels were given a diet containing either corn flakes (the controls) or oat bran cereal, which provided 25 g/day of oat bran. Other macronutrients in the diet resembled a typical American diet; that is, 16% protein, 41% fat, and 43% carbohydrate. The results showed that the oat bran cereal lowered serum cholesterol and LDL-cholesterol levels by up to 8.5% when compared to the controls.[7]

At the University of Alberta in Canada, researchers studied 8 Type 2 diabetics, with a mean age of 45, during a 24-week crossover study. Four of the men ate high-fiber, oat bran concentrate bread at the beginning, while 4 others were given white bread. After 12 weeks, the volunteers switched diets. Mean dietary fiber intake was 19 g/day in the white bread group, compared with 34 g/day in the oat bran group.[8]

The researchers found that mean glycemic and insulin response areas were lower for the oat bran group than for the white bread group. It was also found that the oat bran group had a lower total cholesterol and LDL-cholesterol.

Swedish researchers studied 42 heart attack survivors with Type 2 diabetes, who consumed either oat husk at 5 g/day for 6 weeks or 10 g/day for 4 weeks. It was reported that plasminogen inhibitory activity was reduced with 10 g/day of oat husks, although this was not significant. Plasminogen is a precursor of plasmin, an enzyme that dissolves fibrin in blood clots, thus protecting against heart attacks and strokes.[9] LDL-cholesterol went down on average by 18.2% in the study group and 7.4% in the controls. HDL-cholesterol rose in both groups by about 30%.

Psyllium: The addition of psyllium (*Plantago psyllium*) to a traditional diet for those with diabetes is safe and well tolerated, and improves glycemic and lipid control in men with Type 2 diabetes and moderate cholesterol levels, according to James W. Anderson, M.D., mentioned earlier. After 2 weeks of dietary stabilization, 34 men with Type 2 diabetes and mild-to-moderate cholesterol levels were randomly assigned to receive 5.1 g of psyllium or a cellulose placebo twice daily for 8 weeks. In analyzing the results, the research team reported that there were significant improvements in glucose and lipid values compared to the volunteers getting a look-alike or placebo substance. For example, serum total and LDL-cholesterol (the bad kind) concentrations were 8.9 and 13%, respectively, in the psyllium group compared to controls.[10]

In a study at the Medical College in Lucknow, India, 24 patients with Type 2 diabetes were given 3.5 g of psyllium husk twice daily for 90 days. The researchers reported that psyllium significantly decreased total cholesterol by 19.7%, LDL-cholesterol by 23.7%, and triglycerides by 27.2%, as well as the LDL-HDL cholesterol ratio by 24.1%. HDL-cholesterol (the beneficial kind) went up by 15.8% during the study but did not continue after the treatment was stopped. There were no adverse side effects.[11]

According to researchers at the University of Virginia and Diabetes Associates, Inc., psyllium reduces after-meal glucose and insulin levels in Type 2 diabetics, regardless of whether or not their disease is controlled by diet or requires oral hypoglycemic drugs. In the study, 18 Type 2 diabetics consumed psyllium or placebos twice during each 15-hour crossover phase, in other words before breakfast and dinner. Fasting glucose levels were recorded prior to the morning supplement and meal. Psyllium was not consumed during the lunch meal, so that residual or second-meal effects could be measured.[12]

The research team reported that maximum after-eating glucose elevation decreased 14% at breakfast and 20% at dinner in the fiber-supplemented group compared to controls. In addition, after-meal blood insulin levels after breakfast dropped 12%. Second-meal effects after lunch brought a 31% reduction in glucose in the psyllium volunteers compared to controls.

Psyllium can lower blood cholesterol levels by increasing fecal excretion of bile acids and preventing their normal reabsorption, according to researchers at the University of Minnesota, the Department of Medicine at Hennepin County Medical Center in Minneapolis, and Procter and Gamble Company in Cincinnati, Ohio. The study involved 75 male and female patients with slightly elevated cholesterol, who followed the American Heart Association Step 1 low-fat, low-cholesterol diet for 12 weeks before adding 1 teaspoon (3.4 g) of psyllium or a placebo to the diet three times daily for 8 weeks.[13]

The fiber brought a 4.8% reduction in total cholesterol when compared to placebo. LDL-cholesterol came down 8.2%, and apolipoprotein-B levels were reduced 8.8%. In all, 78% of the volunteers experienced a significant lowering of their total and LDL-cholesterol. No changes were recorded for blood pressure, HDL, triglycerides, serum glucose, or iron. No adverse effects were recorded. (In studying 1,045 patients who had recently suffered a heart attack, those who had high levels of apolipoprotein-B were eight times more likely to have a second heart attack than those with low levels of the protein.)[14]

Barley: In Iraq, barley bread is a common treatment for diabetes, since it modulates the glycemic response to carbohydrate ingestion, slow weight loss, and excessive water consumption. One of the advantages of barley is that it contains about 5.69 mcg of chromium per gram.[15]

Grapefruit: Grapefruit pectin decreased blood levels of cholesterol an average of 7.6% and LDL-cholesterol went down 10.8%, according to researchers at the University of Florida College of Medicine. In addition, the ratio of LDL-cholesterol and HDL-cholesterol decreased 9.8%. In the study, 27 volunteers at medium to high risk of developing coronary heart disease consumed 15 g/day of grapefruit pectin supplements or a placebo. There were no changes in diet or lifestyle during the 16-week study.

The researchers concluded that a prudent diet aimed at preventing hardening of the arteries should include pectin-rich foods such as grapefruit. Pectins are water-soluble substances in plants that yield a gel that is the basis of fruit jellies.[16]

Guar Gum: Guar gum reduced after-meal blood glucose, insulin requirements, and total blood cholesterol in Type 1 diabetics, according to a research team at Helsinki Hospital and the National Public Health Institution in Finland. During the study, 9 Type 1 diabetics ate a regular diet plus a 5 g placebo four times a day before meals for 4 weeks. The volunteers were then given a guar gum supplement diet for 4 weeks. Granulated guar gum was taken in 5 g doses four times daily before eating. Following 4 weeks of guar gum therapy, blood glucose response to a test meal was significantly reduced when compared to the placebo diet.[17]

Insulin sensitivity was unchanged, but the average daily insulin dose was slightly lower by 5% after the guar gum supplementation. This was attributed to the smaller after-meal glucose rise. Blood levels of total cholesterol fell 21% following the guar gum period, with a similar reduction in LDL-cholesterol. There was no change in HDL-cholesterol. The researchers said that, because diabetics have an increased risk for heart disease, the cholesterol-lowering effect of guar gum can contribute to long-term positive prognosis in Type 1 diabetics.

Guar gum can be consumed for an extended period by Type 2 diabetics without compromising mineral balance, according to researchers at the USDA Beltsville Human Nutrition Research Center and Sinai Hospital in Baltimore, Maryland. They added that guar gum is an effective aid to glycemic control and its use might have a role in the treatment of Type 2 diabetes.

In the study, 16 volunteers were given either granola bars containing 6.6 g of guar gum or a look-alike bar without the gum. Average granola bar consumption at the end of the 6-month study was 4.8 bars/day. This provided an average of 31.7 g/day of guar gum.[18]

The researchers examined feces and urine for iron, zinc, copper, calcium, magnesium, and manganese, and no differences in mineral content were recorded between the two groups. Also, there were no differences found in hemoglobin, serum iron, and other parameters.

However, guar gum seems to interfere with selenium utilization, according to researchers at the University of Nebraska at Lincoln. Guar gum is a vegetable gum derived from the Indian cluster bean. The researchers found that selenium excretion in urine and feces increased when the volunteers were given selenium supplements; however, fecal secretion of the mineral increased even more when guar gum was consumed with the supplement. Also, overall selenium balance and glutathione peroxidase activity decreased when guar gum was eaten. Glutathione peroxide is an antioxidant that inactivates oxidized fats and hydrogen peroxide, which are converted to dangerous free radicals.

These effects were found regardless of how much selenium was in the diet.[19] Glutathione peroxidase, which requires selenium as a co-factor, is an antioxidant that inactivates oxidized lipids (lipid peroxides) and hydrogen peroxide, which break down to free radicals, the wayward chemicals that can damage cells.

At the Helsinki University Hospital in Finland, 17 Type 1 diabetics were randomly assigned 5 g of granulated guar gum or a placebo four times daily before meals and in the evening snack for 6 weeks. Patients getting the guar gum had a significant reduction in glucose, hemoglobin A1C, LDL-cholesterol and the LDL:HDL ratio. The reductions were 20% in the LDL-cholesterol and 28% in the LDL:HDL cholesterol ratios. The placebo group recorded no changes.[20]

Carbohydrate Diet: The high-complex carbohydrate, high-fiber diet advocated by James W. Anderson, M.D., can significantly lower blood fats; reduce the risk of cardiovascular disease; reduce fasting blood sugar, glycosylated hemoglobin, and blood lipids; help maintain desirable body weight; reduce insulin and oral hypoglycemic medications; and eliminate them entirely.[21]

This diet includes 70% calories as complex carbohydrates with 35 g of dietary fiber per 1,000 kcal. The diet has been shown to improve glycemic control and reduce insulin requirements by 30 to 40% for Type 1 diabetics, and 75 to 100% for Type 2 diabetics. In most cases, Anderson has reported that insulin has been discontinued after 10 to 21 days of dietary treatment in Type 2 diabetics. In addition, serum cholesterol levels are reduced 30% for Type 1 diabetics and 24% for Type 2 diabetics. He has found water-soluble fibers are especially effective, such as those from oat bran and dried beans.

For those pursuing the high-carbohydrate, high-fiber diet at home, this includes 50 to 60% calories from carbohydrates (two-thirds of which are complex carbohydrates), 15 to 20% protein (minimum of 45 g/day), 20 to 25% fat (less than 10% saturated fat), 200 mg or less of cholesterol daily, 40 to 50 g total dietary fiber (25 g/1,000 kcal), and 10 to 15 g of soluble fiber daily. Anderson added that excellent water-soluble fiber sources include oat bran, oatmeal, oat bran muffins, beans, psyllium, and soy fiber.

Fiber Supplements: In a study at the University of Minnesota at Minneapolis, researchers evaluated the effects of 10 or 20 g/day of a fiber supplement, compared to a look-alike supplement, and found that total cholesterol, LDL-cholesterol, and the ratio of LDL:HDL were significantly reduced in those in the 10-g fiber group and the 39 in the 20-g group, compared to 48 volunteers who took a placebo. However, the fiber supplement had no effect on HDL-cholesterol or triglycerides. The fiber supplement contained guar gum, pectin, soy, pea, and corn bran.[22]

In a study involving niacin (vitamin B₃) and oat bran, the niacin therapy brought a 10% reduction in total cholesterol and a 16% drop in LDL-cholesterol, according to researchers at the University of Minnesota at Minneapolis. Some 10% of the volunteers experienced even more dramatic lipid-lowering effects when they combined niacin and oat bran.

Insoluble Fiber: Over the years, several researchers have suggested that an increase in dietary fiber might inhibit the absorption of minerals and contribute to the development of mineral deficiencies. This concern is unfounded, according to a study at the USDA Beltsville Human Nutrition Research Center and the University of Maryland. Volunteers were given a basic diet alone or one supplemented with the insoluble fiber cellulose (Nacarboxymethylcellulose) or one of the soluble fibers—locust bean gum or karaya gum at a concentration of 7.5 g fiber/1,000 calories. Urine and fecal samples were collected during the final 8 days of the 1-month study and analyzed for weight and mineral content.

The insoluble fiber had an adverse effect on manganese absorption, but it did not affect the absorption of calcium, magnesium, iron, copper, or zinc. The soluble gum fibers did not affect mineral absorption, while karaya gum improved the absorption of all of the minerals.[23]

Niacin: In a study involving niacin (vitamin B₃) and oat bran, the niacin therapy brought a 10% reduction in total cholesterol and a 16% drop in LDL-cholesterol, according to researchers at the University of Minnesota at Minneapolis. Some 10% of the volunteers experienced even more dramatic lipid-lowering effects when they combined niacin and oat bran.

In the study, the volunteers consumed oat bran alone (2 oz./day) for 6 weeks, then oat bran plus niacin (1,500 mg/day) for 6 weeks, followed by a 32-week period of niacin alone. Seventy percent of the people completed the study, while 11 discontinued the study because of adverse side effects or liver enzyme abnormalities.[24]

Popcorn: While popcorn is considered a good source of fiber, a large order of popcorn at some of the large theater chains has more than a day's worth of fat and two-day's worth of "artery-clogging fat," according to the Center for Science in the Public Interest in Washington, D.C. And this is without butter. With the butter-flavored topping, the heart-unhealthy fat is equal to nine McDonald's Quarter Pounders, the Center said.

It is said that 7 out of 10 movie theaters use coconut oil, which is about 80% saturated fat. Some of the nonbutterless products are partially hydrogenated soybean oil, which contributes both saturated and trans fatty acids. Trans fats are thought to elevate cholesterol levels. If the theaters use partially hydrogenated canola shortening, not canola oil, this can also be unhealthy. However, oils do not contain trans fatty acids.[25]

A Review of Part 1 and a Look Forward to Part 2

In part 1, I have reviewed the causes of diabetes and the life-threatening consequences of having the disease for an extended period. Admittedly, there are technical and semi-technical terms that may not be familiar (see glossary), but in a disease as complex as diabetes, this terminology is to be expected.

The chapter on obesity is especially cogent because, for those who are overweight, diabetes is waiting in the wings. Unfortunately, many people have the disease and don't know it, so it is important for everyone to review the typical signs. But diabetes can often be prevented by losing weight and engaging in an unstressful exercise program.

In the middle section of part 1, there are useful chapters on how to protect the eyes, feet, kidneys, and thyroid gland. Otherwise, diabetics may develop cataracts, lose their eyesight, have a foot or leg amputated, or find that their kidneys are not functioning properly.

While cholesterol is necessary for remaining healthy, too much of this waxy substance can clog arteries and lead to heart attacks and stroke. Triglycerides, another fat, can also damage the body. Homocysteine, a normally benign amino acid, can build up in the body and lead to cardio-vascular problems, especially in diabetics.

Hypertension, or high blood pressure, is a problem for both Type 1 and Type 2 diabetics. It is called a "silent killer" because there are no symptoms, and it often goes undetected until a physical exam is given. High blood pressure, brought on by overweight, severely damages arteries, thus causing the heart to work harder. It also contributes to hardening of the arteries, a prelude to heart attack and stroke. Hypertension also damages the kidneys, eyes, and nerves, possibly leading to erectile dysfunction in men and circulatory problems.

While I leave diets and menus to physicians—to be tailored to individual needs—I do explain the importance of a healthful diet. In planning diets, it is necessary to keep in mind the glycemic index, which indicates which foods are more likely to affect blood sugar levels. A high-fiber diet is also important in preventing and controlling diabetes. While many diabetes experts say that diabetics can eat sugar, I find this counterproductive, since a high-sugar diet may be responsible for their illness in the first place. It is amazing how pervasive this non-nutritive substance is in the marketplace. While sugar tickles the taste buds, it is not necessary to remain healthy. Meat, cheese, fruits, vegetables, and other foods can provide the glucose that is necessary as the body's source of energy. Needless to say, a no-smoking policy is recommended for anyone wishing to avoid diabetes and other potentially life-threatening conditions.

As we have seen in part 1, diabetes is a national problem that may be spiraling out of control. As more Americans become overweight or obese, diabetes and its accompanying problems soon follow: high blood pressure, heart disease, stroke, blindness, impotence, and the amputation of limbs.

In part 2, we change pace and show which natural vitamins, minerals, herbs, and other supplements can provide help for many diabetics. Since many diabetics may not be eating a nutritious diet, they may be lacking important nutrients. That's where supplements can provide necessary support. For example, in one study vitamin C lowered blood sugar levels on average by 30% and daily insulin requirements by 27%, and sugar excretion in the urine could almost be eliminated.

Low levels of the mineral chromium in the blood are associated with diabetes, cataracts, and cardiovascular disease. Selenium, another mineral, and vitamin E have overlapping functions, so that each nutrient may replace the other in helping to prevent cataract, heart disease, cancer, diseases of the liver, cardiovascular or muscular disease, and aging.

Vanadium, another mineral, is being used to treat both Type 1 and Type 2 diabetes.

Alpha-lipoic acid, a vitamin-like substance found in beef and spinach, is needed in supplement form to provide protection. The supplement prevents beta-cell destruction leading to Type 1 diabetes, and it enhances glucose uptake in Type 2 diabetes. It is the number one treatment for diabetes in Germany.

Other chapters detail how various supplements can prevent or control diabetes. These chapters should be shown to doctors treating diabetics, so that many medications may not be needed. While diabetes is a complex disease, many natural approaches offer many possible answers.

References

1. Adams, Ruth, and Frank Murray. *The Good Seeds, The Rich Grains, The Hardy Nuts for a Healthier, Happier Life.* New York: Larchmont Books, 1973, pp. 7ff., 24ff., 33ff.

2. Ronzio, Robert A., Ph.D. *The Encyclopedia of Nutrition and Good Health.* New York: Facts on File, Inc., 1997, pp. 175ff.

3. Anderson, James W., and Tammy J. Hanna. "Whole Grains and Protection Against Coronary Heart Disease: What Are the Active Components and Mechanisms," *American Journal of Clinical Nutrition* 70: 307–308, 1999.

4. Chandalia, M., et al. "Beneficial Effects of High Dietary Fiber Intake in Patients with Type 2 Diabetes Mellitus," *New England Journal of Medicine* 342(19): 1392–1398, May 11, 2000.

5. Braten, J., et al. "Oat Gum Lowers Glucose and Insulin After an Oral Glucose Load," *American Journal of Clinical Nutrition* 53: 1425–1430, 1991.

6. Hallfrisch, Judith, et al. "Diets Containing Soluble Oat Extracts Improve Glucose and Insulin Responses of Moderately Hypercholesterolemic Men and Women," *American Journal of Clinical Nutrition* 61: 379–384, 1995.

7. Anderson, James W., et al. "Oat-Bran Cereal Lowers Serum Total and LDL-Cholesterol in Hypercholesterolemic Men," *American Journal of Clinical Nutrition* 52: 495–499, 1990.

8. Pick, Mary E., M.Sc., R.D., et al. "Oat Bran Concentrate Bread Products Improve Long-Term Control of Diabetes: A Pilot Study," *Journal of the American Dietetic Association* 96(12): 1254–1261, Dec. 1996.

9. Guzie, B., et al. "The Effect of Oat Husk Supplementation in Diet on Plasminogen Activator Inhibitor Type 1 and Diabetic Survivors of Myocardial Infarction," *Fibrinolysis* (Suppl. II): 444–446, 1994.

10. Anderson, James W., et al. "Effects of Psyllium and Glucose and Serum Lipid Responses in Men and Type 2 Diabetes and Hypercholesterolemia," *American Journal of Clinical Nutrition* 70: 466–473, 1999.

11. Gupta, R. R., et al. "Lipid-Lowering Efficacy of Psyllium Phydrophilic Muciloid in Non-Insulin-Dependent Diabetes Mellitus with Hyperlipidemia," *Indian Journal of Medical Research,* Nov. 1994, pp. 237–241.

12. Pastors, J., et al. "Psyllium Fiber Reduces Rise in Postprandial Glucose and Insulin Concentrations in Patients with Non-Insulin-Dependent Diabetes," *American Journal of Clinical Nutrition* 53: 1431–1435, 1991.

13. Bell, L., et al. "Cholesterol-Lowering Effects of Psyllium Hydrophilic Mucillido," *Journal of the American Medical Association* 261: 3419–3423, 1989.

14. "Heart Attack," *Nutrition Week,* July 16, 1999, p. 29.

15. Mahdi, G., et al. "Role of Chromium in Barley in Modulating the Symptoms of Diabetes," *Annals of Nutrition and Metabolism* 35: 65–70, 1991.

16. Cerda, J., et al. "The Effects of Grapefruit Pectin on Patients At Risk for Coronary Heart Disease Without Altering Diet or Lifestyle," *Clinical Cardiology* 11: 589–594, 1988.

17. Ebeling, P., et al. "Glucose and Lipid Metabolism and Insulin Sensitivity in Type 1 Diabetics: The Effect of Guar Gum," *American Journal of Clinical Nutrition* 43: 98–103, 1988.

18. Behall, K., et al. "Effect of Guar Gum on Mineral Balances in NIDDM Adults," *Diabetes Care* 12: 357–364, 1989.

19. Choe, M., and C. Kies. "Selenium Bioavailability: The Effect of Guar Gum Supplementation on Selenium Utilization in Human Subjects," *Nutr. Rep. Int.* 39: 557-563, 1989.

20. Vuorinen-Markkola, Helena, et al. "Guar Gum and Insulin-Dependent Diabetes: Effects on Glycemic Control and Serum Lipoproteins," *American Journal of Clinical Nutrition* 56: 1056–1060, 1992.

21. Anderson, James W., M.D. "High Fiber Diet for Diabetes: Safe and Effective Treatment," *Postgraduate Medicine* 88(2): 157–168, Aug. 1990.

22. Hunninghake, Donald B., et al. "Hypocholesterolemic Effects of a Dietary Fiber Supplement," *American Journal of Clinical Nutrition* 59: 1050–1054, 1994.

23. Behall, K., et al. "Mineral Balance in Adult Men: Effect of Four Refined Fibers," *American Journal of Clinical Nutrition* 46: 304–314, 1987.

24. Keenan, J., et al. "A Clinical Trial of Oat Bran and Niacin in the Treatment of Hyperlipidemia," *Journal of Family Practice* 34: 313–319, 1992.

25. Hurley, Jayne, and Stephen Schmidt. "Movie Theater Snacks," *Nutrition Action,* May 1994, pp. 1, 9.

Part Two

Reducing Your Insulin Dependency if You Have Diabetes or a Risk of Diabetic Complications

27 Vitamin A

Vitamin A is a fat-soluble vitamin that is available in milk, butter, eggs, liver, and fish-liver oils, and it is formed in the liver from beta-carotene (provitamin A). Since it is stored in the liver and not excreted as the water-soluble vitamins are (C and B-complex), excessive amounts can be toxic. Beta-carotene is found in green and yellow fruits and vegetables. Vitamin A is essential for the health of eyes, skin, teeth, gums, and mucous membranes.

Vitamin A is useful in treating macular degeneration, retinitis pigmentosa, cataract, and other eye disorders. A deficiency is related to "night blindness," in which it is difficult to see in a darkened theater, in the glare from car headlights at night, or in bright sunlight. The recommended daily requirement is around 5,000 IU/day for most adults.

Also known as retinol, axerophthol, biosterol, anti-infective vitamin, and other names, vitamin A was discovered in 1912 by Elmer V. McCollum and Marguerite Davis at the University of Wisconsin. They had determined that something in butterfat or egg yolk fat made the difference between moderate success in the nutrition of young rats on certain diets and prompt nutritive failure.

This something turned out to be vitamin A, and this theory was confirmed several months later by Thomas Burr Osborne and Lafayette Benedict Mendel at Yale University. Incidentally, the first vitamin (thiamine, B_1) had been isolated in 1911 by Dr. Casimir Funk, a Polish scientist working at the Lister Institute in London, England, who had isolated what became B_1 from rice polishings that prevented beriberi.[1]

Vitamin A is available from such animal sources as milk, butter, eggs, liver, and fish-liver oils. However, it can be formed in the liver of humans and animals from beta-carotene (provitamin A). Experiments show that carotene—found in green- and yellow-colored fruits and vegetables—is utilized less effectively than vitamin A; however, individuals differ in their ability to convert carotene into vitamin A.

Vitamin A is essential for the health of eyes, skin, teeth, gums, and mucous membranes. Those who have difficulty seeing at night or when they enter a darkened theater, or are bothered by an oncoming car at night, are said to have "night blindness" and are probably deficient in vitamin A. This is also true for those who are bothered by the glare of sunlight during the day.

The daily requirement for vitamin A, a fat-soluble vitamin, is given in retinol equivalents (RE), reported Robert A. Ronzio, Ph.D. One RE is defined as 1 mcg of retinol or 6 mcg of beta-carotene. The vitamin is also listed in international units (IU), with 1 IU of vitamin A activity equal to 0.3 mcg of retinol or 0.6 mcg of beta-carotene.

The Recommended Daily Allowance (RDA) of vitamin A for men, ages 25 to 50, is 1,000 mcg of retinol or retinol equivalents, and 800 mcg (RE) for nonpregnant women. Pregnant women should not take vitamin A without a doctor's recommendation, since amounts above 10,000 IU (3,000 RE) are thought to cause birth defects.[2] Prior to the RE designation by the National Research Council, the RDA for vitamin A for most adults was 5,000 IU.

Researchers reported that 4,500 RE—that is, 15,000 IU—per day of vitamin A caused no toxic manifestations of too much vitamin A in young and middle-aged adults with retinitis pigmentosa during a 12-year follow-up.[3]

At the Massachusetts Eye and Ear Infirmary in Boston, researchers said that 15,000 IU/day of vitamin A had a beneficial effect in dealing with retinitis pigmentosa, while 400 IU/day of vitamin E had an adverse effect. The study involved 601 patients, ranging in age from 18 to 49, who were diagnosed with the eye disorder.[4]

In the first National Health and Nutrition Examination Survey, which collected data between 1971 and 1972, the frequency of consumption of fruits and vegetables rich in vitamin A, in those 45 years of age or older, was inversely related to age-related macular degeneration.[5]

In studying 2,900 people between the ages of 49 and 97, higher intakes of vitamin A, protein, vitamin B_3, vitamin B_1, and vitamin B_2 were associated with a reduced risk for nuclear cataract. The researchers also found that polyunsaturated fatty acid intake was also associated with a reduced risk for cortical cataract.[6]

Since free-radical formation is a common biological occurrence, an organism must be able to defend itself against this form of cellular damage, reported Medical and Health Annual 1995. Vitamins play a significant role in these defenses. For example, vitamins A and E have been shown to absorb free radicals, and vitamin C, which is present in circulating blood, is part of the first line of defense against free radicals. In fact, vitamin C has been shown to regenerate the electron-absorbing capacity of vitamin E. Because of their capacity to defend the body against the oxygen free radicals, vitamins A, E, and C have been termed antioxidants.[7]

Vitamin A, along with beta-carotene, is of particular importance to diabetics, since they not only pick up infections easily but also have very poor wound-healing abilities, according to Eberhard Kronhausen, Ed.D., et al., in *Formula for Life*.[8]

"Vitamin A has definitely been shown by researchers at Albert Einstein College of Medicine in New York to be of help with regard to diabetic animals," the authors said. "It is not yet known whether these benefits also apply to humans, but indications are that they may."

References

1. Murray, Frank. *Program Your Heart for Health*. New York: Larchmont Books, 1997, pp. 291ff.

2. Ronzio, Robert A., Ph.D. *The Encyclopedia of Nutrition and Good Health*. New York: Facts on File, Inc., 1997, p. 444.

3. Sibulesky, L., et al. "Safety of 7500 RE (25,000 IU) Vitamin A Daily in Adults with Retinitis Pigmentosa," *American Journal of Clinical Nutrition* 69: 656–663, 1999.

4. Berson, Eliot L., M.D. "A Randomized Trial of Vitamin A and Vitamin E Supplementation for Retinitis Pigmentosa," *Archives of Ophthalmology* 111: 761–772, June 1993.

5. Goldberg, J., et al. "Factors Associated with Age-Related Macular Degeneration: An Analysis of Data from the First National Health and Nutrition Examination Survey," *American Journal of Epidemiology* 128(4): 700–710, 1988.

6. Cumming, R. G., et al. "Diet and Cataract: The Blue Mountain Eye Study," *Ophthalmology* 107(3): 450–456, March 2000.

7. Denke, Margo A., M.D. "Diet and Nutrition," *Medical and Health Annual*. Chicago: Encyclopedia Britannica, 1995, p. 268.

8. Kronhausen, Eberhard, Ed.D., et al. *Formula for Life*. New York: William Morrow and Co., 1989, p. 257.

28 Beta-Carotene and the Carotenoids

Carotenoids are naturally occurring compounds that are abundant in fruits and vegetables. However, only a few of the 600 or so carotenoids are found in human blood and tissues. These include alpha-carotene, beta-carotene (provitamin A), lutein, zeaxanthin, cryptoxanthin, and lycopene. In spite of their similarities in structure, the carotenoids play a variety of roles in the human body. For example, they function as chain-breaking antioxidants, thus protecting the cells and other body components against dangerous free radicals.

Oxidative damage resulting from free-radical attacks are related to premature aging, cancer, high blood pressure, cataracts, age-related macular degeneration, and a variety of degenerative diseases, such as heart attack and stroke. Antioxidants, such as beta-carotene, vitamin E, and others, protect against insulin-damaging free radicals, thus reducing the risk of developing diabetes.

Carotenoids are naturally occurring compounds that are abundant in plants, according to Sharon Landvik, M.S., R.D. While 500 to 600 carotenoids have been identified, only a small number of them are found in appreciable quantities in human blood and tissues. The major carotenoids are alpha-carotene, beta-carotene, lutein, zeaxanthin, cryptoxanthine, and lycopene.[1]

Carotenoids have diverse biological functions, and despite their similarities in structure, they play different roles, Landvik continued. Certain carotenoids are precursors of vitamin A and can be metabolically converted into the vitamin; however, beta-carotene has the highest potential vitamin A activity. Other provitamin A carotenoids are alpha-carotene and cryptoxanthin.

"Carotenoids are effective quenchers of singlet oxygen, with lycopene exhibiting the highest singlet oxygen quenching activity," Landvik continued. "Carotenoids function as chain-breaking antioxidants, protecting cells and other body components from free radical attack. Oxidative damage resulting from free radical attack has been linked to the onset of premature aging, cancer, atherosclerosis, cataracts, age-related macular degeneration and an array of degenerative diseases." (Free radicals, which are dangerous molecules that sometimes contain oxygen, can multiply by chain reactions, making them even more devious. Singlet oxygen, a higher energy form of oxygen, can react with atmospheric pollutants to cause smog formation, thus providing harmful biological effects.)

Lutein and zeaxanthin are the only carotenoids found in the macular region of the retina. They are linked to normal function of the macula, which is responsible for sharp and detailed vision. The two carotenoids are thought to serve as filters for harmful blue light in the macula and as scavengers of singlet oxygen in retinal tissues. (For more information on these two carotenoids, see the chapter on eye health.)

As indicated, free radicals are by-products of metabolic processes and originate from environmental pollutants—nitrogen dioxide and ozone in polluted air, heavy metals, halogenated hydrocarbons, ionizing radiation, and cigarette smoke, Landvik said. If they are unchecked by an antioxidant, the highly reactive free radicals attack the cell walls and cell constituents, including DNA and other opportune targets, especially those containing polyunsaturated fatty acids (PUFAs).

Currently, there is no officially recommended dietary intake for carotenoids. Based on dietary guidelines of governmental agencies for optimal intake of fruits and vegetables to help prevent chronic disease, it appears that a daily intake of 6 mg of beta-carotene could be recommended. The Alliance for Aging Research has recommended 10 to 30 mg/day of beta-carotene for optimal health, especially in older people. In

Food Sources of Carotenoids

The richest dietary sources of carotenoids are fruits and vegetables. Apricots, cantaloupe, carrots, leafy green vegetables, pumpkin, sweet potato, and winter squash are good sources of beta-carotene.

Carrots and pumpkin are good sources of alpha-carotene.

Lutein and zeaxanthin are found in leafy green vegetables, pumpkin, and red pepper.

Guava, pink grapefruit, tomatoes and tomato products, and watermelon are rich in lycopene.

Cryptoxanthin is found in mangoes, nectarines, oranges, papaya, peaches, and tangerines.

Source: Sharon Landvik, M.S., R.D. "VERIS Research Summary," LaGrange, Ill., Aug. 1997.

the United States, the amount of carotenoids supplied by the average diet is estimated at 1.5 mg/day of beta-carotene.

Carotene supplements are available over the counter in 6 and 15 mg soft gelatin capsules, 2-piece capsules, and/or powdered tablets. Some of the vitamin A supplements available in stores contain beta-carotene. The only common side effect associated with high intakes of carotenoids (30 mg/day or more) from supplements or carotenoid-rich foods is yellowing of the skin, which is harmless, and goes away when the amount of carotenoid is reduced, Landvik said.

Beta-carotene, as an antioxidant, may reduce the risk of certain diseases, such as heart disease and cancer. Researchers studied disease and dietary patterns in 12,733 men and women who participated in the ongoing Atherosclerosis Risk in Communities Study. It was found that, in both men and women, carotenoid-rich foods were associated with a substantially lower prevalence of cholesterol deposits in the carotid artery, which is a major blood vessel. Women eating beta-carotene-rich diets benefited more than men.[2]

It was also found that women eating diets rich in beta-carotene had a 16% lower risk of developing cholesterol deposits in the carotid artery. Also, women smokers gained the most benefits with high-carotenoid diets, with a 33% reduction in risk when compared with smokers eating a low-carotenoid diet.

In a study involving 106 Type 2 diabetics and 201 matched controls, those with diabetes had lower serum levels of beta-carotene and vitamin E. High levels of the two nutrients were associated with a reduced risk for Type 2 diabetes, but this association disappeared after adjusting for cardiovascular risk factors.[3]

Physicians have long suggested that diet is a principal risk factor for Type 2 diabetes, and that a high intake of refined carbohydrates and sugar is associated with an increased risk of getting the disease. In a study published in the *American Journal of Epidemiology*, a research team studied blood levels of various carotenoids in 1,665 volunteers, ranging in age from 40 to 74.[4]

It was found that the highest beta-carotene levels were in those with normal glucose tolerance; however, levels declined progressively among those with impaired glucose tolerance and diabetes. Further, people with impaired glucose tolerance had beta-carotene levels 13% below normal, and those with newly diagnosed diabetes had beta-carotene levels 20% below normal.

While the study did not demonstrate a protective effect of beta-carotene, the findings were consistent with existing research which shows that antioxidants may protect against insulin-damaging free radicals and, therefore, reduce the risk of developing diabetes.

In a study reported in the *American Journal of Clinical Nutrition*, it was found that in studying 56 men with cardiovascular disease, between the ages of 30 and 69, the visceral fat at the vertebra was not significantly greater in cardiovascular disease patients without diabetes than in the controls. However, the visceral fat area was much greater in cardiovascular disease patients with diabetes than in the controls at both the L1 and L4 vertebra.[5]

It was also reported that the cardiovascular disease patients had higher blood levels of homocysteine and lower blood levels of superoxide dismutase than controls. Superoxide dismutase is an antioxidant that destroys harmful free radicals. Blood levels of lycopene and beta-carotene were lowest in the cardiovascular patients with diabetes. Superoxide dismutase (SOD) is an enzyme that extinguishes the harmful free radicals. Homocysteine may be more dangerous than cholesterol in some patients.

Beta-carotene and other carotenoids, which are fat-soluble antioxidants, prevent free-radical damage to fats, a process called lipid peroxidation, which contributes to cell damage leading to heart disease. In a study reported in the *Journal of the American College of Nutrition*, 9 women were fed a very low-carotenoid diet and/or given beta-carotene and mixed carotenoid supplements.[6]

It was found that women consuming low levels of carotenoids had high blood levels of malondialhyde-thiobarbituric acid (MDA-TBA), which is an established signal for lipid peroxidation. When the women were given supplements of beta-carotene and mixed carotenoids, the MDA-TBA levels went down.

It is believed that free-radical damage (oxidation) to low-density lipoprotein cholesterol (LDL, the harmful kind) is a major cause of coronary heart disease. Researchers asked 22 healthy smokers and nonsmokers to eat fruits and vegetables rich in carotenoids. The foods were carrots (beta-carotene); pear tomatoes (lycopene); and French beans, cabbage, and spinach (lutein). The foods added about 30 mg of mixed carotenoids to the daily diet. The researchers then tested the blood levels of carotenoids in the volunteers and whether or not their LDL resisted oxidation.[7]

After eating a high-carotenoid diet for 2 weeks, blood levels of carotenoids increased 23% in the smokers and 11% in the nonsmokers.

This was considered significant, since smokers tend to have lower cholesterol levels. Also, the ability of LDL to resist oxidation increased by 14% in smokers and 28% in nonsmokers. The researchers concluded that a mix of dietary carotenoids can help to resist the oxidation of LDL cholesterol and probably lower the risk of coronary heart disease.

After eating a high-carotenoid diet for 2 weeks, blood levels of carotenoids increased 23% in the smokers and 11% in the non-smokers. Also, the ability of LDL to resist oxidation increased by 14% in smokers and 28% in non-smokers. The researchers concluded that a mix of dietary carotenoids can help to resist the oxidation of LDL cholesterol and probably lower the risk of coronary heart disease.

A research team at Erasmus University Medical School in Rotterdam, the Netherlands, and other facilities in the Netherlands and Germany, reviewed evidence that antioxidants provide protection against ischemic heart disease, and decided to test this suggestion on a group of elderly volunteers, ranging in age from 55 to 95.[8] The researchers reported that high dietary intakes of beta-carotene provided protection against heart disease.

The preferred form of carotenoid supplements are those derived from algae, such as *Dunaliella salina*, or whole-food concentrates, according to Robert C. Atkins, M.D. An average adult may opt to take 10,000 to 25,000 IU/day for preventive care, he said. For those with cancer, he often prescribes 75,000 IU/day, and many German oncologists use considerably more. For protection against cancer and macular degeneration, Atkins bolsters *D. salina*'s carotenoids with additional lycopene, lutein, and zeaxanthin.[9]

References

1. Landvik, Sharon, M.S., R.D. *Carotenoids Fact Book*. LaGrange, Ill.: VERIS Research Information Service, 1996.

2. Kritchevsky, S. B., et al. "Provitamin A Carotenoid Intake and Carotid Artery Plaques: The Atherosclerosis Risk in Communities Study," *American Journal of Clinical Nutrition* 68: 726–733, 1998.

3. Reunanen, A., et al. "Serum Antioxidants and Risk of Non-Insulin Dependent Diabetes Mellitus," *European Journal of Clinical Nutrition* 52: 89–93, 1998.

4. Ford, E. S., et al. "Diabetes Mellitus and Serum Carotenoids: Findings from the Third National Health and Nutrition Examination Survey," *American Journal of Epidemiology* 149: 168–176, 1999.

5. Jang, Y., et al. "Differences in Body Fat Distribution and Antioxidant Status in Korean Men With Cardiovascular Disease With or Without Diabetes," *American Journal of Clinical Nutrition* 73: 68–74, 2001.

6. Dixon, Z. R., et al. "The Effect of a Low Carotenoid Diet on Malondialdehyde-Thiobarbituric Acid (MDA-TBA) Concentrations in Women: A Placebo-Controlled Double-Blind Study," *Journal of the American College of Nutrition* 17: 54–58, 1998.

7. Hininger, I., et al. "Effect of Increased Fruit and Vegetable Intake on the Susceptibility of Lipoprotein to Oxidation in Smokers," *European Journal of Clinical Nutrition* 51: 601-606, 1997.

8. Klipstein-Grobush, Kerstin, et al. "Dietary Antioxidants and Risk of Myocardial Infarction in the Elderly: the Rotterdam Study," *American Journal of Clinical Nutrition* 69(2): 261–266, Feb. 1999.

9. Atkins, Robert C., M.D. *Dr. Atkins' Vita-Nutrient Solution.* New York: Simon & Schuster, 1998, p. 52.

29 The B-Complex Vitamins

The eight members of the B-complex play significant roles in preventing or treating diabetes. Some work directly to help Type 1 and Type 2 diabetics, while others deal with life-threatening problems for diabetics, such as heart attack and stroke. Since the members of this complex are water-soluble, they should be taken in supplement form in divided doses during the day, since large amounts pass out of the body via urine and feces.

- Vitamin B_1 (thiamine) is a co-factor in many enzyme systems and plays an active role in carbohydrate metabolism.

- Vitamin B_2 (riboflavin) is also necessary for carbohydrate metabolism, and it becomes deficient when patients are under severe stress.

- Vitamin B_6 (pyridoxine) is needed for amino acid (protein) metabolism, hemoglobin formation, and hormone synthesis. It is being used to treat high homocysteine levels and neuropathy.

- Vitamin B_{12} (cobalamin) plays an important role in hemoglobin synthesis and lowering of homocysteine levels, and a deficiency may result in altered glycosylated hemoglobin.

- Vitamin B_3 (niacin) helps to lower cholesterol levels and protect against hardening of the arteries.

- Another form of B_3, inositol hexaniacinate, is even more effective in many applications and it doesn't cause flushing.

- Folic acid is instrumental in lowering homocysteine levels and in preventing cardiovascular disease.

- Biotin may help to prevent diabetic neuropathy, and it is used to treat low blood sugar.

- Pantothenic acid aids in the production of energy from fat, protein, and carbohydrates, and a form of the vitamin—pantethine—helps to lower cholesterol and triglyceride levels.

- Choline and inositol, two B-complex cousins, are also useful to diabetics.

The eight members of the B-complex work individually and in unison to keep us healthy. Some of them work directly to protect diabetics, while others are necessary for protecting against heart disease, stroke, and other disorders affecting diabetics.

The eight members are thiamine (B_1), riboflavin (B_2), niacin (B_3), pyridoxine (B_6), cyanocobalamin (B_{12}), folic acid, pantothenic acid, and biotin. Three vitamin B-like substances—choline, PABA, and inositol—have not officially been declared B vitamins. The B vitamins are water-soluble, so vitamin B supplements should be taken in divided doses, since they pass out of the body in urine and feces during the day.

In *The Diabetes Educator*, Daniel E. Baker, Pharm.D., and R. Keith Campbell report concerning the B-complex that many of these vitamins and minerals as well are important for diabetics. For example, vitamin B_1 is a co-factor in many enzymes and plays an active role in carbohydrate metabolism and the transmission of nervous system impulses. Vitamin B_2 is also necessary for carbohydrate metabolism, and it can become deficient under severe stress.[1]

Vitamin B_6 is important in amino acid metabolism, hemoglobin formation, nerve impulses, and hormone synthesis. In a double-blind trial using vitamin B_6 at 200 mg/day in 8 patients with diabetic mononeuropathy (nerve damage), it was found that the vitamin is associated with improvements in motor and sensory activity in the median nerve and sensory activity in the ulnar nerve (in the upper arm). In addition, vitamin B_6 may be considered an alternative form of therapy with diabetics who have failed to respond to other forms of traditional therapy for carpal tunnel syndrome (a painful nerve in the wrist).

Vitamin B_{12} plays a significant role in hemoglobin synthesis, and it helps to maintain a normal, healthy nervous system. A deficiency in the vitamin may result in altered glycosylated hemoglobin (amount of glucose in the blood). When vitamin B_{12} therapy is given along with iron, hemoglobin A1C levels have been shown to decrease after three weeks. The authors said that it does not appear that this reduction in hemoglobin A1C improves glycemic control, but instead, improved glycemic control indicates an increase in the erythrocyte (red blood cell) population. Most of the hemoglobin—the oxygen-carrying component in red blood cells—exists in a form known as hemoglobin A. A small amount is converted into hemoglobin A1C or glycosylated hemoglobin. A glycosylated hemoglobin test indicates a person's average blood glucose level for the previous two or three months.

Vitamin B_3 is necessary for energy, growth, nerve function, healthy skin, and gastrointestinal function. The vitamin should be used with caution by diabetics, since it can deteriorate glycemic control, the authors added. Most diabetics using niacin experience an increase in blood glucose and glycosylated hemoglobin levels; therefore, diabetics using the vitamin should be monitored for glucose levels.

Biotin is needed for the production of fatty acids and the conversion of food into energy. Pantothenic acid is important in the production of steroid hormones and in obtaining energy from carbohydrates and fat. Folic acid is needed in amino acid metabolism and nucleic acid synthesis. A deficiency in folic acid can result in anemia, gastrointestinal lesions, poor growth, and glossitis (inflammation of the tongue).

Swiss researchers evaluated the vitamin status in 6 patients, ranging in age from 45 to 66, and 4 men between the ages of 28 and 40 who, due to kidney disease caused by analgesics or diabetes, underwent Continuous Ambulatory Peritoneal Dialysis (CAPD). When compared to healthy controls, B_1, B_6, C, and folic acid in the blood were in the lower range of normal, and vitamin A and B_{12} concentrations were elevated.[2]

After supplementing with 8 mg of B_1, 8 mg of B_{12}, 10 mg of B_6, 50 mg of B_3, 10.9 mg of pantothenic acid, 30 mcg of biotin, 2 mg of folic acid, and 100 mg of vitamin C, given twice daily for 7 weeks, levels of B_6 and C were normalized, while folic acid levels in the blood increased. B_1 and B_2 levels remained unchanged. After 13 weeks, levels of vitamin A and B_{12} following supplementation tended to normalize.

The researchers said that improved methods of dialysis lead to an ever growing loss of essential nutrients, and even those regarded as insoluble in water are eliminated. This can lead to depleted body stores and malfunction, especially in long-term dialysis patients.

For these patients, the researchers recommend 30 mg of B_1, 10 to 50 mg of B_6, 0.5 to 1 mg of folic acid, and 100 to 200 mg of vitamin C, all twice daily. They question whether one can ensure an adequate supply of vitamins by choosing marginal values in healthy people as a reference for patients undergoing chronic dialysis.

Now let's look at the individual B vitamins in detail.

Vitamin B_1: At the University of Pavia in Italy, in a 9-year vitamin B_1 metabolism study, researchers evaluated 2 patients with megaloblastic anemia that was associated with diabetes and deafness caused by nerve damage. Megaloblastic anemia is a blood condition in which red blood cells have a reduced oxygen-carrying capacity. It was reported that the content of B_1 and that of its red blood cell constituents were within the normal range, but amounts of B_1 and B_1 compounds were reduced by 40% when compared to controls.[3]

The 2 patients were given 50 mg/day of vitamin B_1 for 9 years. The authors concluded by saying that the cells from patients with megaloblastic anemia contain low levels of B_1 compounds, probably because they cannot properly metabolize the vitamin. Patients with this type of anemia are unable to properly transport the vitamin to red blood cells.

In *Body, Mind and the B Vitamins*, Ruth Adams and I reported on the case of a 3-year-old girl who suffered from diabetes and deafness, who later developed pernicious anemia. Doctors at Duke University in North Carolina gave her vitamin B_{12} and folic acid, the usual treatment for this anemia, but it did not help. She began to improve after they gave her a high-potency multi-vitamin supplement.[4]

She returned home without any supplements, and her condition worsened, and her insulin requirements also went up. Again admitted to the hospital, the girl was given large amounts of each of the vitamins in the multi-vitamin tablet. Her insulin requirements lessened with large amounts of vitamin B_1. She was sent home once gain without supplements, and again she relapsed. Finally, the doctors gave her 20 mg/day of vitamin B_1 and sent her home with instructions for her family to continue this treatment. The child had no more relapses.

Why did B_1 make the difference? The doctors concluded that the child had a defect in a single B_1-dependent enzyme which made the difference,

Food Sources of B₁

Brazil nuts, enriched bread, soybeans, brewer's yeast, dried whey, wheat germ, turkey, broccoli, cabbage, kidney, salmon, brown rice, cashews, sunflower seeds, chicken, liver, peas, lentils, mushrooms, eggs, flounder, chickpeas, and cauliflower.

and that dietary amounts were insufficient to keep her from developing anemia. The doctors could not tell whether or not B_1 affected her diabetes, deafness, or other health problems, but they feared that their treatment came too late to reverse the damage that had already been done.

A research team from the University of Michigan at Ann Arbor, and other locations, reported in the *Journal of the American Dietetic Association* that a B_1 deficiency may occur in a large number of patients with congestive heart failure, and that a dietary deficiency in the vitamin may contribute to an increased risk.[5]

They found a B_1 deficiency in 8 of 38 patients, and a risk for dietary thiamine deficiency in 10 of 38 patients. Those with congestive heart failure frequently experience cardiac cachexia, which is a type of malnutrition. Previous studies have shown that a B_1 deficiency may be the result of increased urinary losses in association with loop therapy for congestive heart failure, they said.

How safe is vitamin B_1? According to the Council for Responsible Nutrition, thiamine is very nontoxic and has a long history as an oral supplement without adverse effects. It is safe at intakes up to 50 mg and perhaps as high as 200 mg/day. There are no reports of adverse effects by taking B_1 supplements, even at dosages of several hundred milligrams.[6]

Vitamin B₂: Formerly known as vitamin G, riboflavin is widely distributed in foods of plant and animal origin. Some of the best food sources are milk, meat, liver, heart, kidney, cheese, eggs, leafy green vegetables, and whole-grain cereals and bread. Chemical research on B_2 started in 1879, but its function and importance in nutrition were not realized until the 1930s, when Otto Warburg and W. Christian in Germany in 1932 studied a yellow enzyme in yeast and were able to split it into a protein and a pigment (flavin).[7]

Deficiency in B_2 and B_3 may result in soreness and redness of the tongue and lips, atrophy of papillae (small bumps) on the surface of the tongue, and cracks at the corners of the mouth. In B_2 deficiency, dermatitis of the scrotum may also spread to other areas of the body. Another complication is disturbances in the blood vessels in the eye.

Riboflavin is excreted when protein in the body is broken down, and it is retained when protein is being accumulated. Thus, in acute starvation, uncontrolled diabetes, and other conditions associated with negative nitrogen balance, excretion in the urine does not adequately reflect body stores of the vitamin, the publication said.

In 1941, government statistics showed that many Americans were not getting sufficient amounts of B_1, B_2, B_3, and iron, so the Food and Nutrition Board—to build strong bodies during World War II—proposed that the four nutrients be added to flour and bread. The government then ruled that this "enrichment" program should be utilized by the Army and Navy, as well as the general public. However, B_2 was not available in adequate amounts until the end of 1943.[8]

When researchers evaluated 368 gluten-free products, they found that many do not provide the same levels of B_1, B_2, and B_3 as enriched wheat flour products. Those who consume a gluten-free diet could be deficient in one or more of the three vitamins. Celiac disease patients on a gluten-free diet should be checked for B vitamin deficiencies.[9]

Fiber products, such as Metamucil, are used as bulk laxatives to lower cholesterol, to improve blood sugar in diabetics, and for weight reducing, according to Sheldon Saul Hendler, M.D., Ph.D. However, long-term use of these products can negatively affect vitamin B_2, zinc, iron, manganese, copper, and beta-carotene, he said.[10]

Is vitamin B_2 safe? There are no reports of adverse effects from orally consumed riboflavin, according to the Council for Responsible Nutrition. Although the data are sparse at very high intakes, there is sufficient evidence to suggest that oral intakes of 200 mg/day are perfectly safe, the Council added.[11]

Vitamin B_3: The importance of niacin surfaced when researchers found that it was a cure for pellagra (a disorder marked by skin lesions and digestive and nervous disturbances), which spread around the world with the cultivation of corn, which is a poor source of vitamin B_3. This vitamin is a "cluster" that includes nicotinic acid and nicotinamide, both of which are natural forms of the vitamin with equal niacin activity. In the body, both forms are active as nicotinamide adenine dinucleotide (NAD) and nicotinamide adenine dinucleotide phosphate (NADP); they serve as coenzymes, often in conjunction with B_1 and B_2 coenzymes to produce energy within cells, according to *Food & Nutrition Encyclopedia.*[12]

NAD and NADP function in many important enzyme systems which are necessary for cell respiration, and they are involved in the release of energy from carbohydrates, proteins, and fats. In addition, the two coenzymes are involved in the synthesis of fatty acids, protein, and DNA. However, for these processes to occur, they require three B vitamins—B_6, pantothenic acid, and biotin.

The Top Food Sources of Vitamin B₃

Liver and kidney, lean meat, poultry, fish, rabbit, mushrooms, nuts, milk and cheese, eggs, and enriched cereals.

Nicotinic acid—but not nicotinamide—reduces the levels of cholesterol, and niacin in large amounts is beneficial in protecting against recurrent nonfatal myocardial infarction (heart attack). Niacin is closely associated with tryptophan, the amino acid, and the amino acid can be converted to niacin in the body. In effect, 60 mg of tryptophan is equivalent to 1 mg of niacin, the publication added.

According to researchers at the University of Bristol in England, nicotinamide is being used as a potential way of preventing Type 1 diabetes in high-risk, first-degree relatives. In a review of the literature, it was found that at very high doses there is reversible hepatoxicity (toxic damage to the liver) in both animal and human studies. Minor abnormalities of liver enzymes have surfaced with dosages used for diabetes prevention. The research team added that long-term nicotinamide use appears to be highly favorable, and this may be an excellent treatment for diabetes prevention.[13]

Further, high-dose nicotinamide can protect beta cells in response to a range of toxic and immune stimuli in animal and test-tube models, suggesting that the vitamin may react as a free-radical scavenger. High-dose nicotinamide or niacin has been recommended for schizophrenia at doses between 1.5 and 6 g/day for 3 months to 5 years' duration. For skin conditions such as pemphigoid (large blisters), nicotinamide has been used at doses between 1.5 and 3 g/day for from 2 weeks to 6 months. In radiotherapy, the vitamin has been used at doses up to 6 g/day, the researchers continued.

For Type 1 diabetes, doses have ranged from 200 mg/day to 30 mg/kg—equivalent to 3.5 g/day—for 12 months. To prevent Type 1 diabetes in high-risk groups, doses have ranged from 1 to 3 g/day for from 4 months to 4 years. The researchers added that the vitamin has been used at pharmacological doses for many years with a low incidence of side effects or toxicity. Most maximum doses are about 3.5 g/day, but some researchers have used doses as high as 6 g/day.

Nicotinic acid has been known as a cholesterol-lowing agent since 1955, according to Jeffrey L. Probstfield, M.D., of the Fred Hutchinson Cancer Research Center in Seattle, Washington. Daily doses between 2 and 12 grams can have a major effect in lowering LDL-cholesterol (the bad kind), he said. Dosage is generally 3 g/day or less, since larger doses can cause flushing and itching in susceptible people. Excess amounts can also cause gastrointestinal complaints, high amounts of glucose in the blood, injury to the liver, a buildup of uric acid, and gout. Some of these side effects can be minimized by taking the supplement with food, gradually increasing or decreasing the dose. Sustain-release dosages, which are also available over the counter, have been shown to reduce symptoms, but they are also related to liver damage and reduced efficiency in increasing HDL-cholesterol levels (the good kind).[14]

While there is a recorded 26% reduction in LDL-cholesterol with 20 mg of lovastatin per day, LDL can also be reduced by 5%, 16%, and 23% with 1.5, 3, and 4.5 g/day of nicotinic acid, respectively. The vitamin was more effective than the drug in increasing HDL-cholesterol and apolipoprotein-A1 levels, as well as decreasing triglycerides and lipoprotein-A levels. A 1 mg increase in HDL-cholesterol could decrease coronary heart disease risk by 2 to 3%, Probstfield said.

He also said that nicotinic acid would be useful for Type 2 diabetics with cholesterol, triglyceride, and other fat abnormalities, except that it must be used with caution because it can affect blood glucose control. It may be useful to start with a low dose of 100 to 125 mg three times daily, which may produce fewer symptoms and better patient compliance with a slow buildup to gram doses. The flushing can be reduced by giving the vitamin during or after meals.

By keeping lipid levels normal, vitamin B_3 should protect diabetics against the most dangerous chronic side effect—hardening of the arteries—according to Abram Hoffer, M.D., Ph.D., in *Orthomolecular Medicine for Physicians*. The vitamin may also have an effect on glucose levels in the blood, on the glucose tolerance curve, and on insulin requirements. Insulin requirements may be increased or decreased, he added.[15]

Hoffer said that some researchers (Vague, et. al) concluded that niacinamide given to young Type 1 diabetics produced a remission of the disease. Their double-blind experiment involved 16 newly diagnosed Type 1 diabetics, ranging in age from 10 to 35. After 1 week of intensive insulin, the volunteers were started on 3 g/day of niacinamide or a placebo. If insulin was needed after 6 months, the vitamin was discontinued.

"Our results and those found from animal experiments indicate that, in Type 1 diabetes, niacinamide slows down destruction of B-cells and enhances their regeneration, thus extending remission time," the researchers said. Of the 16 treated volunteers, 3 reached 2-year remissions.

Researchers at the University of Massachusetts at Amherst reported that niacinamide may prevent the onset of Type 1 diabetes. Doses of up to 3,000 mg/day were said to be non-toxic. The vitamin's role is thought to be involved in DNA damage/repair processes, or in providing protection against free-radical damage.[16]

The researchers added that both vitamin C and vitamin E may prevent high blood sugar levels, and that vitamin E, given at 100 IU/day, can greatly lower glycosylated hemoglobin levels (amount of glucose in the blood). Further, red blood cell lipid peroxidation is associated with glycosylated hemoglobin levels, and 100 IU/day of vitamin E can correct this abnormality. Lipid peroxides are dangerous molecules that can harm the body. Also, 126 mg/day of sodium vanadate (vanadium) has been shown to lower insulin requirements and plasma cholesterol levels in Type 1 diabetics, the researchers said.

At the Center for Human Nutrition in Dallas, Texas, 13 Type 2 diabetics were given 1.5 g of nicotinic acid three times daily or a placebo for 8 weeks. The researchers found that the niacin supplement reduced cholesterol by 24%, triglycerides by 45%, very low-density lipoprotein (VLDLs) by 58%, and low-density lipoprotein cholesterol by 15%, with a 34% increase in high-density lipoprotein cholesterol.[17]

The vitamin therapy altered blood sugar control with a 16% increase in plasma glucose, 21% increase in glycosylated hemoglobin levels, and increased glycosuria (glucose in urine). There was also an increase in uric acid, which is a potent antioxidant. However, the researchers did not recommend this therapy for first-time Type 2 diabetics with elevated cholesterol.

Researchers have concluded that nicotinamide may protect beta-cells in Type 1 diabetes, while nicotinic acid may help with insulin resistance in Type 2 diabetes. Type 2 diabetics often produce sufficient insulin, but their bodies do not regulate the insulin, hence insulin resistance, a major cause of Type 2 diabetes. In studying 4 case studies, it was reported that 250 to 750 mg/day of niacin were shown to benefit patients with diabetes, high blood pressure, congestive heart failure, and circulatory problems. Beta-cell injury is thought to be associated with low nicotinamide adenine dinucleotide (NAD) and adenosine triphosphate (ATP) levels, which results in oxidative injury and organ failure. Antioxidants, plus vitamin B_3, which is an NAD precursor, may prevent this condition, and NAD levels are known to be low in diabetics.[18]

John P. Cleary, M.D., of Madison, Wisconsin, said that in the early 1940s, nicotinamide was used to reduce insulin requirements in treating diabetes, but following World War II, vitamin B_3 was not of much interest in treating the disease. However, he said, low NAD may impair NaK-ATPase, which can cause impaired glucose transport, and insulin may not be able to correct this defect. Type 1 diabetics utilize nicotinamide, which inhibits the poly (ADP-ribose) synthetase enzyme leading to a loss of NAD in the beta-cells and subsequent loss of insulin production. But 25 mg/kg of body weight per day of nicotinamide is recommended to correct the problem.

Cleary added that 100 to 200 mg/day of nicotinamide in the early onset of diabetes may be useful. For Type 2 diabetics, 500 mg/day of nicotinic acid is recommended. Larger amounts are not recommended, since some patients can experience liver dysfunction, glucose intolerance, hyperuricemia (large amounts of uric acid in the blood), and flushing.

At the University of Rome and the University Cattolica in Rome, Italy, researchers reported that Type 1 diabetics might benefit from taking nicotinamide. This therapy brought a partial remission of diabetes, indicated by reduced insulin need in 32% of 22 volunteers given 200 mg/day of the B vitamin for 1 year. A control group of 13 patients who were given only insulin had a 7.5% partial remission rate. Total remission, or no insulin, was reported in 3 patients getting the vitamin but not in the controls.[19]

Researchers in California gave 56 Type 1 diabetics 25 mg/kg of nicotinamide or a placebo for 12 months. Their data showed that the vitamin can be added to insulin in these patients to prevent beta-cell destruction. Beta-cells in the pancreas make and release insulin.[20]

A combination of niacinamide and vitamin E may be beneficial in future trials of insulin-dependent diabetes (Type 1) at the beginning of the disease, according to a research team at St. Bartholomew's Hospital Medical College in London, England. These observations were made following a study of 84 Type 1 diabetics, ranging in age from 5 to 35. Forty-two of the volunteers were given 15 mg/kg body weight per day of vitamin E for 1 year, and the other 42 received niacinamide for 1 year at 25 mg/kg of body weight per day.

All of the diabetics were getting 3 or 4 insulin injections daily. Glycosylated hemoglobin and insulin were similar in both groups. In patients under the age of 15 who were getting vitamin E, there was an increased need for insulin compared to the niacin-treated patients 1 year after diagnosis. The researchers added that the two vitamins have similar effects in protecting beta-cell function in patients recently diagnosed with Type 1 diabetes.[21]

In spite of current recommendations against the use of niacin in treating diabetes, lipid modifying doses of timed-release vitamin B_3 can be used safely in patients with stable, controlled Type 2 diabetes, according to Marshall B. Elam, Ph.D., M.D., et al., of the University of Tennessee at

Memphis. They added that niacin may be considered an alternative to statin drugs or fibrates in those with diabetes in whom these drugs are not tolerated, or in whom they fail to sufficiently correct high levels of triglycerides or low levels of HDL-cholesterol.[22]

The study was conducted at 6 clinical centers from August 1993 to December 1995, and involved 468 participants, including 125 with diabetes, who had diagnosed peripheral arterial disease. The volunteers were selected to receive either 3,000 mg/day of niacin (64 with diabetes and 173 without the disease) or placebo (61 with diabetes and 170 without diabetes) for up to 60 weeks. Niacin significantly increased HDL-cholesterol (the good kind) 29% in both groups, and decreased triglycerides by 23% and 28%; low-density lipoprotein cholesterol (LDL, the bad kind) dropped as well, 8% and 9%, respectively. Statins and fibrates are two of the most common lipid-lowering drugs.

The optimum dose of niacin varies from 3 g/day (3,000 mg) to 6 g/day (6,000 mg) in 3 divided doses, according to Abram Hoffer, M.D., Ph.D. This can begin suddenly, or by starting with smaller doses and gradually increasing them. Few people will not have pronounced vasodilation (flush) beginning in the forehead and extending downward. Most will flush very little after a period of days or weeks.[23]

If the flush remains a problem, Hoffer added, the niacin may need to be discontinued. It may then be replaced by a niacin derivative such as Linodil (inositol niacinate) if the beneficial vascular effect is essential, or by niacinamide if it is not. Or the flush can be moderated by using aspirin, 1 tablet before each dose of niacin for a few days, or by using antihistamines. Also, tranquilizers can decrease the intensity of the flush. Few people will flush with niacinamide, he said.

Writing in *Psychodietetics*, E. Cheraskin, M.D., D.M.D., et al., reported that nicotinic acid, lecithin, vitamin C, and grain and vegetable fiber help the body to regulate cholesterol levels. They added that megadoses of vitamin B_3 help to stabilize blood glucose levels. They also said that vitamin B_6 can help the niacin to work more effectively and that hypoglycemics who are continually troubled by excess fatigue may benefit from a wheat germ oil supplement at mealtime.[24]

Vitamin B_6: Found in foods in three forms—pyridoxine, pyridoxal, and pyridoxamine—this B vitamin is rapidly absorbed from the upper part of the small intestine, thence it enters the body by the portal vein, according to *Foods & Nutrition Encyclopedia*. It is present in many body tissues, with high concentrations in the liver.[25]

Vitamin B_6 in its coenzyme forms, usually as pyridoxal phosphate but sometimes as pyridoxamine phosphate, is involved in a large number of physiologic functions, especially in protein (nitrogen) metabolism and to a lesser extent in carbohydrate and fat metabolism. It is an essential part of phosphorylase, the enzyme that brings about the conversion of glycogen to glucose-1-phosphate in muscle and liver. It also takes part in fat metabolism, and is believed to be involved in the metabolism of the unsaturated fatty acid, linoleic acid, into another fatty acid, arachidonic acid.

> **Top Food Sources of Vitamin B_6**
>
> Liver and kidney, fish, soybeans, poultry, brown rice, nuts, bananas, lean meat, avocados, and whole grains.

Writing in *Vitamin B_6 Therapy*, John M. Ellis, M.D., reported that a vitamin B_6 deficiency is common in both Type 1 and Type 2 diabetes. In Type 1, the pancreas does not produce enough insulin, and in the later stages, it does not produce any insulin. In Type 2, the pancreas produces some insulin, but it is ineffective. In 1989, Ellis and colleagues began an intensive study of 21 diabetics, all but 1 taking 100 to 300 mg/day of vitamin B_6.[26]

"We can conclude from our studies that every diabetic at every stage should be given a therapeutic dose of 100 to 300 mg/day of B_6," Ellis said. "A quick response to vitamin B_6 is not so evident in the late stages of diabetic retinopathy and nephropathy. However, it is in the prevention of these catastrophic conditions the vitamin becomes important. The rheumatic improvements seen within three months of beginning treatment with vitamin B_6 signal the long-term prevention of diabetic retinopathy and nephropathy."

Ellis went on to say that the biochemistries and cellular activities in the different bodily tissues, including those of the eye, are responsive for a number of enzymatic activities, many of which require vitamin B_6, and affect the collagen in the vitreous and retina, and the matrix of the retina. This explains why one result of a long-term vitamin B_6 deficiency is the leakage of serum and lipids, including cholesterol, into the vitreous and retina. Detailed reports from Ellis's study reveal the beneficial effects of vitamin B_6 in treating diabetes and its complications.

Diabetes is a condition in which blood glucose levels are high and vitamin B_6 levels are low in the body, according to Chandra Mohan, Ph.D. If vitamin B_6 levels are low, the insulin response is reduced and the circulating levels of insulin are lower, which leads to further increases in blood glucose levels. When there is a B_6 deficiency, storage of glycogen in the liver is impaired, leading possibly to hypoglycemia (low blood sugar).[27]

For diabetics, Mohan recommends a well-balanced meal, as recommended by the American Diabetes Association, which consists of 20% protein, about 50 to 55% carbohydrate, and 30% fat, along with fiber from food sources.

Vitamin B$_6$ has been used with some success in treating gestational diabetes, the type of the disease that sometimes accompanies pregnancy, reported Alan Gaby, M.D. In addition, B$_6$ can improve the abnormal glucose tolerance that develops in some women who take birth control pills.

There is a reduced level of B$_6$ and an increased amount of blood glucose and uncontrolled hyperglycemia (high levels of glucose in the blood), Mohan said. In time this can lead to damage to the eyes, kidneys, and nervous and vascular systems. Also, reduced amounts of B$_6$ can cause problems with amino acid (protein) transport and perhaps protein synthesis. Inefficient protein synthesis is a major problem with diabetics, since they need insulin for protein synthesis. In addition, she continued, diabetics have a high rate of protein breakdown due to the needs of amino acids for gluconeogenesis processing (the synthesis of glucose from noncarbohydrates, such as protein or fat).

Tissues cannot detect the high glucose levels and uncontrolled glucose production that occur via gluconeogenesis, Mohan said. A person needs at least 120 grams of glucose for the brain daily. When you estimate the amount of glucose needed (120 g), and the amount of protein needed to produce 120 grams of glucose, that breaks down to about 200 grams of protein. However, this process is not exactly efficient, since some amino acids (proteins) are oxidized and some are ketogenic amino acids and do not produce glucose. Ketones are breakdown products of fat, and they can build up in the body and cause dehydration.

As for dosages, Mohan recommends about 2 g/day of vitamin B$_6$, which is the so-called Recommended Daily Allowance. For someone taking two to three times the RDA, that is not going to cause complications, Mohan said.

Vitamin B$_6$ has been used with some success in treating gestational diabetes, the type of the disease that sometimes accompanies pregnancy, reported Alan Gaby, M.D. In addition, B$_6$ can improve the abnormal glucose tolerance that develops in some women who take birth control pills. It seems that B$_6$ is related to xanthurenic acid (XA), a by-product of tryptophan (amino acid) metabolism. B$_6$-deficient patients have abnormalities in their tryptophan metabolism that leads to the production of excess XA. This by-product possesses a dangerous property of being able to bind into insulin and inactivate it, Gaby said.[28]

He discussed the work of Charles L. Jones, D.P.M., a podiatrist, and Virgilio Gonzalez, M.D., who studied 10 Type 1 diabetics who had symptoms of peripheral neuropathy. The patients excreted more XA than did other diabetics without neuropathy, suggesting that a B_6 deficiency was more pronounced in the patients with neuropathy. When the researchers gave each patient 50 mg of B_6 three times daily for 6 weeks, XA excretion became normal, suggesting that B_6 deficiency had been corrected. Symptoms of neuropathy disappeared in all 10 patients. Most of the patients noticed some relief of pain and paresthesia (tickling sensation) in about 10 days. The diabetics also reported that their eyes "felt better."

"Seven of the patients continued on B_6 supplements and did well," Gaby added. "The other three stopped taking the vitamin and noticed a recurrence of their symptoms about three weeks later. When they resumed taking B_6, their symptoms again disappeared. Two patients also had a marked improvement in their blood sugar measurements, which had been chronically elevated (275 and 315 mg/100 ml), respectively, and difficult to control. After B_6 therapy, their glucose levels fell to 195 and 200, respectively, and remained there as long as they continued taking B_6."

Vitamin B_6 may be an effective therapy in the treatment of diabetic neuropathies, according to researchers at Kaiser Permanente Medical Center in Hayward, California. Volunteers who reported chronic, painful diabetic neuropathies were given 160 mg/day of B_6, and then monitored monthly for 4 months and 2 months afterward.

Results were assessed by a pain questionnaire, electrophysiologic testing of motor and sensory nerves and clinical evaluations. The researchers said that pain consistently decreased and activity increased with B_6 supplements. Also, complaints of pain decreased and mood increased. The researchers also found that hypoglycemic drugs, such as insulin or oral medications, were reduced with the supplement. No adverse side effects were recorded.[29]

How safe is vitamin B_6? Pyridoxine produces no reliably identified adverse effects at intakes up to 200 mg/day, reported the Council for Responsible Nutrition. Daily intakes of 2,000 to 6,000 mg have caused a distinct pattern of sensory neuropathy, which slowly and perhaps incompletely regresses after the megadoses are stopped. An intake of 500 mg/day carries some risk of neurotoxicity. The validity of the single report in the literature of adverse effects at daily intakes near 100 mg remains controversial.[30]

Vitamin B$_{12}$: Like other members of the B-complex, vitamin B$_{12}$ is not a single substance but consists of a number of closely related compounds with similar activity. The term *cobalamin* is applied to these substances since they contain the mineral cobalt. The vitamin is called cyanocobalamin and is named for the cyanide ion in the molecule. Other compounds include hydroxocobalamin and nitrocobalamin.[31]

Vitamin B$_{12}$ is involved in the synthesis of nucleoproteins, and it has a close association with folic acid in stimulating blood regeneration. Pernicious anemia is the most important disease due to B$_{12}$ deficiency. The deficiency is due not necessarily to a dietary deficiency, but to failure of absorption of the vitamin from the intestinal tract in the absence of intrinsic factor in the gastric juice. Intrinsic factor is a substance produced by gastrointestinal mucosa that facilitates the absorption of B$_{12}$.

The vitamin is available in animal foods such as liver and kidney. Other sources include muscle meats, milk, cheese, fish, and eggs. There is no known B$_{12}$ in fruits and vegetables.

A research team at the Tokyo Metropolitan Geriatric Hospital in Japan evaluated homocysteine plasma levels in 52 Type 2 diabetic patients with microangiopathy, 84 diabetic patients without the condition, and 57 nondiabetic controls. *Microangiopathy* refers to blood clots in small blood vessels. It was found that total plasma homocysteine levels were higher in the patients who had microangiopathy than in those who did not.[32]

Further, high levels of homocysteine were clearly associated with the presence of diabetic microangiopathy. However, when the patients were given 1,000 mcg/day of methylcobalamin (B$_{12}$) for 3 weeks, plasma levels of homocysteine in 10 diabetics were significantly reduced.

A panel of experts met at the U.S. Institute of Medicine and reported that vitamin B$_{12}$ should probably be added to any folic acid supplement to avoid masking of a B$_{12}$ deficiency, according to an article in *Lancet*. They added that B$_{12}$ is apparently nontoxic even at high doses of 1 mg/day. B$_{12}$ is usually prescribed in micrograms. Homocysteine levels indicate a folic acid, B$_{12}$, and B$_{6}$ deficiency, and screening for homocysteine levels is beneficial for cardiovascular disease. Also, methylmalonic acid excess is considered a more reliable indicator of a B$_{12}$ deficiency. Methylmalonic acid is an important intermediate in fatty acid metabolism.[33]

It was also reported that 1 to 3 g/day of choline, a vitamin B-like substance, can reverse steatosis when given intravenously. *Steatosis* is a somewhat obsolete term for abnormal fatty deposits.

Vitamin B_{12} supplements have been used with some success in treating diabetic neuropathy, according to Michael T. Murray, N.D., in *Diabetes and Hypoglycemia*. It is not apparent that the success is due to the correction of a deficiency or the normalization of the deranged B_{12} metabolism seen in diabetics. Clinically, he added, diabetic neuropathy is very similar to that of classical B_{12} deficiency. A typical symptom of B_{12} deficiency is megaloblastic anemia, which is characterized by abnormal red blood cells in the bone marrow.[34]

A researcher in Louisiana reported on an elderly man with mild diabetes who was unable to open his right eyelid and was diagnosed with peripheral neuropathy. Following vitamin B_{12} therapy for 6 weeks, the eyelid became perfectly normal. The researcher, Vincent F. Chicola, M.D., began adding one-fourth cc of B_{12} to the protocol for patients on insulin, and he has found no problem with peripheral neuropathy.[35]

How effective is a vegetarian diet in alleviating diabetes? Since 1980, Milton Crane, M.D., of Weimar Institute in California, has been using the lacto-ovo-vegetarian diet in his practice. He initially began prescribing the diet in 1946, realizing that a more restrictive diet excluding milk, meat, eggs, and refined foods (sugars, refined cereals, free fats, shortening or margarine) was very effective in alleviating diabetes, high blood pressure, and coronary artery disease. He said that 80% of the patients with systemic, distal diabetic neuropathy have relief of pain in 4 to 17 days.

In addition, one-third of the Type 2 diabetics and 10% of those with Type 1 diabetes can be maintained with a fasting glucose level below 120 mg/dl with this therapy. In addition, 80% of male hypertensives and 50% of female hypertensives (those with blood pressure of 160/90 or above) can be maintained with normal blood pressure below 140/90 without medication after 1 month on this program.[36]

Diabetic neuropathy, a common factor in the disease, has an unknown etiology, Crane continued. It is most likely related to a combination of factors related to faulty diet and inadequate exercise. It is theorized that the changes in the nerve bundles, as a result of faulty metabolism of carbohydrates, cause tissue swelling, and therefore pain. The two pathologic changes seem to be ischemia to the nerve and/or accumulation of certain metabolites of sugar within the cells that result from inadequate insulin.

Since many vegetarians are deficient in vitamin B_{12}, Crane recommended a B_{12} supplement. He went on to say that all total vegetarians (vegans) are at risk of becoming B_{12} deficient unless they allow beneficial germs to grow in their food or on their eating utensils on a routine basis.

Chief Food Sources of Folic Acid

Beef liver, lima beans, spinach, cottage cheese, kidney, peanuts, filberts, walnuts, potatoes, endive, asparagus, turnip greens, lentils, cowpeas, collards, cabbage, sweet corn, lettuce, chard, beet greens, and whole-grain bread.

However, it may take a year or up to 10 years for evidence of a B_{12} deficiency to become symptomatically evident.

"There are no foods that are consistently eaten that contain B_{12} naturally or which have been supplemented by B_{12}," Crane continued. "The increasing concern over cleanliness in our society to avoid infectious diseases decrease the number of bacteria that would produce B_{12} in foods. I believe strongly that it does not make sense to wait for vitamin B_{12} levels to go down before taking a supplement."

He added that when B_{12} is taken orally in adequate amounts, the intrinsic factor is the initial limiting factor and the intestinal wall is the second limiting factor. If excess B_{12} is absorbed, the excess is readily disposed in the urine. He said that three sea vegetables—arame, wakame, and kombu—may be sources of B_{12} for the strict vegetarian, but studies indicate that this needs to be confirmed.

How safe is vitamin B_{12}? No toxic effects of vitamin B_{12} have been reported in man or animals at any level of oral intake, according to the Council for Responsible Nutrition. There is a case of cobalamin-induced acne in association with an unspecified dosage given by injection twice weekly, and a single case of contact dermatitis has been found in the literature. There is sufficient experience with intakes up to 3,000 mcg (3 mg) to establish the safety of this amount.[37]

Folic Acid: This B vitamin is sometimes referred to as folacin, pteroylmoboglutamic acid, and antianemia factor. The importance of folacin for the manufacture of blood cells in man apparently resides in its function in the formation of purines and pyrimidines.[38]

Folic acid stimulates the formation of blood cells in certain anemias (megaloblastic anemia, for example), which are characterized by oversized red blood cells and the accumulation in the bone marrow of immature red blood cells called megaloblasts. Bone marrow is the organ that manufactures blood cells, but it can't complete the process without folic acid. Vitamin B_{12} is also required for the formation of blood cells and is effective in the treatment of a number of anemias (specifically pernicious anemia).

Folic acid is also related to vitamin C and tyrosine, the amino acid. In addition to the anemias, folic acid deficiency causes diarrhea, inflammation of the tongue, and sprue (celiac disease and the malabsorption of nutrients).

In addition to its various human needs, folic acid is instrumental in decreasing plasma concentrations of homocysteine. An amino acid, homocysteine is a natural product of the synthesis and breakdown of protein. While it is normally processed by the body, it can build up in the bloodstream and increase the risk of stroke, heart attack, and blood clots in the legs and lungs, according to researchers at Wageningen Agricultural University in the Netherlands. A dose of 250 mg/day of the vitamin decreased homocysteine levels significantly in an 8-week, placebo-controlled study involving 144 healthy women, ranging in age from 18 to 40.[39]

Since the causes of abnormal homocysteine levels are multi-faceted and vitamin supplements can lower homocysteine, it would be prudent to include folic acid, B_6, and B_{12} in a supplement intended to lower homocysteine in those with abnormal levels of the amino acid, according to a team of researchers in Belfast, Northern Ireland, the University of Berne in Switzerland, and the University of Pennsylvania. They added that the possibility of increasing the intake of the three B vitamins through dietary means, either through public health recommendations or food fortification, should be investigated.[40]

The researchers found that supplementing a group of volunteers with folic acid, B_6, and B_{12}—in doses 2.5 to 10 times the Recommended Daily Allowance—lowered homocysteine levels by about 32%. The reduction in the amino acid occurred whether or not vitamin E, vitamin C, and beta-carotene were included in the protocol.

At the General Clinical Research Center in Portland, Oregon, a research team found that African-American women had higher blood levels of homocysteine and lower amounts of folic acid in their blood than did white women. This was apparently due to lifestyle factors, which may contribute to the greater rate of coronary artery disease in premenopausal black women than premenopausal white women.[41]

Researchers in Canada evaluated 5,506 men and women, ranging in age from 35 to 79, and found 165 coronary heart disease deaths among the group. They reported that there was a statistically significant association between the blood levels of folic acid and the risk of coronary heart disease. The lower the folate levels, the higher the risk.[42]

Writing in the *Netherlands Journal of Medicine,* a research team reviewed the role of high amounts of homocysteine in the development of hardening of the arteries in renal failure patients. For patients with chronic renal failure, homocysteine levels are significantly higher at an early stage. They reported that 5 mg/day of folic acid significantly lowers homocysteine levels in chronic renal failure patients.

They added that cardiovascular disease is a major cause of death in patients on maintenance dialysis. The deaths from cardiovascular disease of those on dialysis are only partially accounted for by the high prevalence of high blood pressure, smoking, excess fat in the blood, and diabetes, they said.[43]

The risk of heart attack in smokers may be partially attributed to high homocysteine levels and low amounts of folic acid in the blood. Smoking seems to affect folate status and total homocysteine levels adversely, according to an article in *Atherosclerosis*.[44]

Researchers at the University of Pretoria in South Africa evaluated folic acid, B_{12}, and B_6 levels in 44 healthy men with moderate elevated levels of homocysteine, and compared them with 274 controls without elevated levels. The research team found lower levels of folic acid, B_{12}, and B_6 in the group with high homocysteine. In fact, the prevalence of suboptimal levels of B_6, B_{12}, and folic acid in the men with raised homocysteine was 25%, 56.8% and 59.1%, respectively. In a placebo-controlled follow-up study, a daily vitamin containing 10 mg of B_6, 1 mg of folic acid, and 400 mcg of B_{12} normalized homocysteine levels within 6 weeks. The authors said that an increased risk of premature hardening of the arteries due to raised homocysteine levels should be easy to prevent with the B vitamins.[45]

Folic acid appears to be an effective treatment for the reduction of both normal and increased plasma homocysteine concentrations in patients who have had a heart attack, according to researchers at County Hospital in Kalmar, Sweden. They suggest that folic acid should be used when studying the effect of homocysteine and its relation to a heart attack. The typical dosage was 2.5 to 10 mg/day of folic acid.[46]

At the Cleveland Clinic Foundation in Ohio, Killian Robinson, M.D., and colleagues, evaluated the B_6, B_{12}, and folic acid status of 176 dialysis patients with a mean age of 56 years. Abnormally high amounts of homocysteine were found in 149 patients (85%) with end-stage kidney disease. Vitamin B_6 deficiency was noted more frequently in dialysis patients than in normal populations (18% versus 2%).[47]

Robinson said that high blood levels of homocysteine are an independent risk factor for hardening of the arteries in kidney disease patients, and that those patients may benefit from higher doses of the three B vitamins. Folic acid doses of up to or even greater than 15 mg/day may be required to lower certain homocysteine levels, Robinson added.

Researchers at the University of Calgary in Alberta, Canada, evaluated 1,171 patients for blood levels of folic acid. Patients were 65 years of age or older. Those with the lowest amounts of the B vitamin in their blood were associated with an increased risk of stroke.[48]

Vitamin B_6 and folic acid may help to reduce the risk of cardiovascular disease in dialysis patients, according to *The Nutrition Report*. Patients undergoing hemodialysis were given 300 mg/day of B_6 and 5 mg/day of folic acid. The B_6 therapy brought a 7% reduction in cholesterol levels, and folic acid supplementation resulted in a reduction of blood levels of homocysteine by 30%.[49]

> ## Top Food Sources of Biotin
>
> Cheese, wheat germ, brewer's yeast, nuts and peanut butter, eggs, chocolate, sardines, salmon, cauliflower, mushrooms, and chicken.

Although congenital forms of elevated homocysteine levels are rare, it has been suggested that milder but prolonged elevations of homocysteine in the blood of otherwise normal people can slowly take their toll on the body's vascular system, according to Seymour L. Alterman, M.D., and Donald A. Kullman, M.D.[50]

Homocysteine levels, which can be measured by a lab test, are considered normal at levels of 12mM/1 or less. Levels between 12 and 15 mM/1 are considered borderline, while those greater than 15mM/1 are said to be associated with a high risk for cardiovascular disease, they said.

Biotin: Like vitamin B_1, biotin is a sulfur-containing vitamin. It is absorbed primarily from the upper part of the small intestine. However, avidin, a protein found in raw egg white, binds biotin and prevents its absorption. Cooking inactivates the protein. The vitamin plays a significant role in the metabolism of carbohydrates, fats, and proteins.[51]

A great deal of biotin is synthesized by intestinal bacteria, since three to six times more biotin is excreted in the urine and feces than is ingested. A number of variables affect the microbial synthesis of biotin in the intestines, including the carbohydrate sources of the diet (starch, glucose, sucrose, etc.), along with the presence of other B vitamins, and the presence or absence of antimicrobial drugs and antibiotics. The vitamin is closely related to folic acid, pantothenic acid, and B_{12}.

Diabetics tend to be low in B vitamins, perhaps because diabetes uses up B vitamins and because poorly controlled diabetes causes these water-soluble nutrients to be excreted in the urine, according to Mary Dan Eades, M.D., medical director of the Arkansas Center for Health and Weight Control at Little Rock. For example, some people may benefit from taking biotin in amounts up to 15 mg (15,000 mcg) a day, she said. A study by Japanese researchers reported that biotin helps cells in muscle tissue to use sugar more effectively.[52]

Biotin, at up to 2,000 mcg three times daily, may help neuropathy, especially if it is diabetes-related, reported Ralph Golan, M.D. And the vitamin has successfully reversed symptoms of peripheral neuropathy. The recommendation is 10 mg/day intramuscularly for 6 weeks, followed by 5 mg/day orally. The 10 mg/day dosage can be taken orally without injections, he said.[53]

To treat hypoglycemia (low blood sugar), Golan recommends chromium (200 to 300 mcg three times daily); biotin; B-complex (25 to 50 mg of each three times daily); pantothenic acid (500 mg one to three times daily); niacin (500 to 1,000 mg twice daily); vitamin C (up to 1,000 mg three times daily); brewer's yeast (1/2 tsp daily); calcium and magnesium (1,000 mg/day of calcium and 500 mg/day of magnesium); and an amino acid cocktail containing glutamine, 5-hydroxy tryptophan, and tyrosine.

"For hypoglycemia, approximately 1,000 mcg three times daily of biotin with meals will enhance glucose utilization, generally improve low blood sugar symptoms, as well as tend to reduce sugar cravings," Golan added. "Biotin is largely synthesized by friendly intestinal bacteria, and if you have used antibiotics (which kill these bacteria), this vitamin is particularly important to use. Once your condition has stabilized, 300 mcg/day should suffice."

Knowing that several of the B-complex vitamins are crucial to the utilization of carbohydrates and the release of energy, you can see how a deficiency of these vitamins could contribute to hypoglycemia, says Golan. For example, biotin is a critical co-factor for glucokinase, an enzyme that is involved in the initial step of glucose utilization by the cells.

Robert C. Atkins, M.D., commenting on the continuing use of complementary medicine, said, "We were particularly excited about the idea of using biotin in milligram doses, rather than the microgram doses we usually administer, and, after studying a report in the *Annals of the New York Academy of Sciences* showing a significant improvement in glucose readings, we incorporated mega-biotin therapy into our routine."[54]

Concerning other nutrients, he said that one of the most promising is pyridoxine alpha-ketoglutarate (PAK), which he began using in 1988. Studies in Italy showed that this compound of two nutrients significantly reduced the sugar elevations in both Type 1 and Type 2 diabetics, Atkins continued. Similarly, Japanese researchers demonstrated improvement in diabetic parameters using coenzyme Q10, although their first study involved Q7.

Pantothenic Acid: Present in all cells, pantothenic acid plays a significant role in energy production from fat, carbohydrate, and protein, according to Robert A. Ronzio, Ph.D. It forms the core of coenzyme A, the enzyme helper that carries fatty acids throughout metabolism, which includes fat synthesis and fat degradation.

Coenzyme A helps to synthesize compounds such as citric acid and most fats, including cholesterol, steroid hormones, and ketone bodies. Ketones are substances formed by the liver when the digestion of fats is compromised, which occurs in diabetes. CoA is also required for the synthesis of acetylcholine, a chemical needed for nerve transmission. It also is involved in the synthesis of heme for the formation of hemoglobin.[55]

> ## Food Sources of Pantothenic Acid
>
> Liver, beans, peas, whole grains, wheat germ, brewer's yeast, dark green leafy vegetables, nuts, peanuts, and eggs.

Pantethine, a molecule of pantothenic acid, may help to lower cholesterol and triglyceride levels. Ronzio states it may be easier to convert pantethine to coenzyme A than to convert pantothenic acid, thus, pantethine may be more effective therapeutically in certain instances.

For hypoglycemia, Ralph Golan, M.D., recommends pantothenic acid—or calcium pantothenate—to boost the adrenal glands. Extra amounts may be needed for those who have not responded to B-complex supplements for chronic fatigue and characteristic low blood sugar symptoms in 1 month. He recommends 500 mg one to three times daily with meals for 1 to 3 months, then gradually reduce the dosage.[56]

Reporting in *Nephrologia*, Francisco Coronel, M.D., of San Carlose University Hospital in Madrid, Spain, said that of 92 kidney transplant patients studied, 27, or 29.3%, suffered from excess fats in the blood. In the remaining 22 patients, pantethine was administered in doses of 900 mg/day. After 2 months of treatment, there was a significant decrease in total cholesterol, triglycerides, and very low-density lipoprotein cholesterol, LDL-cholesterol, and the total cholesterol/HDL ratio. These readings continued to be reduced at 4 and 6 months.[57]

Three of the transplant recipients stopped the pantothenic acid due to gastric irritation. These data suggest that pantethine may be an effective and well-tolerated lipid-lowering substance in hyperlipidemic renal transplant patients without affecting immunotherapy or kidney function.

The escalation of our two most dangerous blood fats—LDL cholesterol and triglycerides—stops dead in its tracks when confronted by pantethine, according to Robert C. Atkins, M.D. In one study, a daily dose of 900 mg of pantethine led to a 32% drop in triglycerides, a 19% drop in total cholesterol, and a 21% drop in LDL-cholesterol. At the same time, HDL-cholesterol rose by 23%, he said.[58]

Atkins found more than half a dozen similar accounts in the medical literature, and all of them documented dramatic improvements in supplement takers' blood fats, even when the lipid abnormality was due to other illnesses. The popular statin drugs create a shortage of the vital heart nutrient—coenzyme Q10—and all the other drugs were associated with death rates from noncardiac causes that were higher than the controls. Pantethine outperforms these two-edged swords every way, Atkins said.

Pantethine protects the heart and arteries in other ways, Atkins says. For example, it encourages the production of enzymes that help break down fats and helps vitamin E's action against cholesterol buildup. In addition, pantethine is one of the few nutrients that increase the amount of clot-busting omega-3 fatty acids and reduce clot-promoting fats in cell membranes, he said. By generating more coenzyme A, pantethine enhances metabolism in the heart muscle, strengthens the force of its contractions, and slows the rate at which it beats. In short, he continued, pantethine helps the heart in so many different ways, no heart patient should be without it.

Some research has indicated that pantethine helps in preventing the clumping of proteins in the eye that causes cataracts, according to Robert M. Giller, M.D.[59]

For some reason, pantethine has significant lipid-lowering characteristics, while pantothenic acid has little value in lowering cholesterol and triglyceride levels, according to Michael T. Murray, N.D. A dose of 900 mg/day of pantethine has reduced significantly serum triglyceride and cholesterol levels while increasing HDL-cholesterol (the beneficial kind).

These effects are especially impressive, since it has virtually no toxicity when compared to conventional lipid-lowering drugs, Murray said. Pantethine's mode of action is due to its ability to inhibit cholesterol synthesis and accelerate the utilization of fat as an energy source. There appears to be no toxicity or side effects from pantethine, he added.[60]

Pantothenic acid is closely related to lipid metabolism, and thus may be of help to obese patients, according to Li-Hung Leung, M.D., of Central Hospital, Hong Kong, Republic of China. The B vitamin may be beneficial in its ability to mobilize fatty acids and convert them to fully utilized energy.[61]

In the study, involving 60 Chinese males and 60 Chinese females, between the ages of 15 and 55, who were on a 1,000-calorie-a-day diet, 10 g of pantothenic acid was given in 4 divided doses. The average weight loss was 1.2 kg/week. Ketones in the urine were monitored and they were found absent in most instances. To maintain body weight after reaching a desired goal, Leung recommended 2 to 3 g/day, which allows the body to freely mobilize fat for energy. The study also used the B vitamin to treat acne vulgaris.

Choline: A constituent of lecithin, choline is necessary for the prevention of fatty livers, the transmitting of nerve impulses, and the metabolism of fat. Choline is a lipotropic agent, meaning that it has an affinity for fat. In this role, the substance prevents the abnormal accumulation of fat in the liver by promoting its transport as lecithin or by increasing the utilization of fatty acids in the liver.

> **Key Food Sources of Choline**
>
> Egg yolk, brewer's yeast, liver, soybeans, potatoes, cabbage, wheat germ, rice bran and polish, buttermilk and dried skimmed milk, hominy, turnips, wheat flour, whole grains, and blackstrap molasses.

Without choline, fatty deposits build up inside the liver, blocking its hundreds of functions and throwing the whole body into a state of ill health. Although associated with the B-complex, choline is not officially a B vitamin.[62]

Of the various related compounds that can replace choline, the primary one is betaine, which derives its name from the Latin word "beta" from the beet family, which is a rich source. Thus, choline can be replaced by betaine in preventing fatty liver in some species. Methionine, the amino acid, and vitamin B_{12} can also spare choline in certain species.

Patients who have induced choline deficiency have developed liver dysfunction, such as fatty liver, which is seen in choline-deficient animals, according to Steven H. Zeisel, M.D., Ph.D., of the University of North Carolina at Chapel Hill. The fatty liver occurs in choline deficiency because phosphatidylcholine (PC) synthesis is needed for the production of very-low-density lipoprotein cholesterol secretion. This could ultimately lead to liver cancer.[63]

"Fatty liver" is common in diabetes, according to Adelle Davis, probably because choline and inositol are so readily lost in urine. Biopsies of the livers of diabetic patients taken before and 6 weeks after they had adhered to a diet particularly high in protein and the B vitamins, and supplemented with choline, inositol, and vitamin B_{12}, showed that even the more serious cases were corrected in this period. Vitamin C and vitamin E and the sulfur-containing amino acids in eggs are also particularly valuable in correcting fatty liver.[64]

Fifty-one out of 102 people with fatty livers, recognized as a choline deficiency, had high blood urea and albumin in the urine, showing mild nephrosis (kidney disease), which quickly disappeared when choline was given with an adequate diet, Davis said. In a study involving 48 people, their blood pressure fell to normal and albumin cleared from the urine when choline was taken. Albumin, a protein, coagulates upon heating and provides the method by which albumin is usually detected in the urine to diagnose complications in the kidney.

A combination of choline-phosphatidylcholine and lecithin fights heart disease in a variety of ways, according to Robert C. Atkins, M.D. While PC brings only a modest reduction in total cholesterol, it improves the ratio between good and bad cholesterol. PC serves as the main source of choline, which is essential for the formation of acetylcholine, an important neurotransmitter. And choline is essential for our bodies to make lecithin, Atkins said.[65]

Researchers at Rush Medical College and Presbyterian-St. Luke's Medical Center, Chicago, reported that those with untreated high levels of homocysteine develop premature vascular disease, thrombosis, and thromboembolism, which bring on strokes and coronary occlusion.

As reported elsewhere in this book, B_6 and B_{12} are useful in lowering homocysteine levels. In addition, a restriction of choline in the diet along with folic acid deficiency increases the severity of high homocysteine levels. Betaine supplementation effectively corrects most types of high homocysteine, the researchers said.[66]

In a study of 14,916 male physicians between the ages of 40 and 84, with no prior history of myocardial infarction (heart attack) or stroke, 271 men who subsequently developed a heart attack were evaluated for homocysteine levels. The research team, headed by Meir J. Stampfer, M.D., reported that moderately high levels of homocysteine are associated with the subsequent risk of a heart attack. These high levels can be easily treated with B_6, B_{12}, folic acid, betaine, and choline, Stampfer added.[67]

Even though the mechanism of high homocysteine (hyperhomocysteinemia) is unknown, small amounts of folic acid and sometimes B_6, choline, or betaine, can return levels of homocysteine to normal, reported M. R. Malinow. These substances are innocuous in the absence of pernicious anemia. It might be prudent that those with hardening of the arteries or family members be screened for the presence of homocysteinemia and should be treated on an individual basis as is the case for other risk factors, Malinow said.[68]

Choline-free diets have induced nerve-muscle transmission problems, and increased liver transaminase enzyme levels, including liver damage, according to *Nutrition Action Health Letter.* Avoiding cholesterol often leads to avoiding choline. In evaluating 37 people who ran a Boston marathon, all but 1 had reduced choline levels. The stress of running may have made the deficiency worse in borderline deficient people.[69]

Inositol: Widely distributed in foods and closely related to glucose, inositol has been known as a chemical compound since 1850. It was initially referred to as "muscle sugar." In animal cells it occurs as a component of phospholipids, substances containing phosphorus, fatty acids, and nitrogenous bases. It is largely stored in brain, heart muscle, and skeletal muscle. Small amounts are normally excreted in the urine; however, diabetics excrete rather large amounts in urine. While associated with the B-complex, it has not been officially named a B vitamin.[70] Food sources include kidney, brain, brewer's yeast, liver, wheat germ, citrus fruits, and blackstrap molasses.

Inositol escapes freely from the nerve cells of diabetics, according to Robert C. Atkins, M.D. This loss may be partly responsible for diabetic neuropathy, the painful destruction of nerves in the arms and legs following years of poor blood sugar control. He added that he has been using inositol in his diabetes treatment protocol since reading an impressive study in 1978, in which 1 g/day eased pain and improved nerve function in a group of patients with neuropathy. Vitamin C may head off the loss of inositol, he added.[71]

Reduced magnesium in diabetic patients can reduce inositol transport by 50%, according to Robert Matz, M.D. Inositol and myoinositol deficiency can be important factors in some of the underlying complications of chronic diabetes.[72]

If either inositol or choline are undersupplied, lecithin cannot be produced in adequate amounts, reported Adelle Davis. When patients recovering from heart attacks receive daily 2,000 and 750 mg of choline and inositol, respectively, the size of the cholesterol particles and the amount of fat in the blood quickly decreases. Two months later, the blood cholesterols have dropped to normal, she said.

If either inositol or choline are undersupplied, lecithin cannot be produced in adequate amounts, reported Adelle Davis. When patients recovering from heart attacks receive daily 2,000 and 750 mg of choline and inositol, respectively, the size of the cholesterol particles and the amount of fat in the blood quickly decreases. Two months later, the blood cholesterols have dropped to normal, she said.[73]

Inositol has been shown in experiments to prevent the development of cataracts, according to Robert M. Giller, M.D. The recommended dosage is 500 to 1,000 mg/day.[74]

Researchers at the University of Birmingham in England reported that diabetes is associated with a reduction in serum magnesium levels. The magnesium ion is a positive effector of inositol transport and is capable of promoting a 2.5-fold increase in the affinity for the transporter for inositol. In fact, magnesium reduction in diabetes may cause reductions in inositol transport in diabetic patients by a factor of 1.5- to 2-fold.[75]

Writing in the *New England Journal of Medicine,* Bruce J. Holub, Ph.D., said that adults consume a total of about 1 g/day of inositol in animal products and from plant sources, especially inositol hexaphosphate or phytic acid. Inositol is in high amounts in breast milk. Clinical interest in inositol is focused on impairment of growth and development, nerve function, diabetes mellitus, renal disease, and respiratory distress syndrome, he said.[76]

With the milling of coarse cereal grains that has occurred in industrialized and developing countries, and the elimination of coarse cereals from the diet, there has been a substantial reduction in dietary phytic acid, with a concomitant reduction in urinary phosphorylated inositols, according to *Lancet.* This may be a key factor in the increased incidence of kidney stones in modern societies, the publication said.[77]

Phytic acid is a constituent of inositol found in various grains, nuts, and legumes. Phytic acid often combines with calcium and other minerals, which may also be related to kidney stones.

The safest form of niacin is inositol hexaniacinate, according to Michael T. Murray, N.D. This form of B_3 has been used in Europe to lower cholesterol levels and to improve blood flow. This form yields slightly better results than niacin and is better tolerated during long-term use, he said. In one study, 153 patients treated with inositol hexaniacinate at dosages ranging from 600 to 1,800 mg/day experienced no side effects.[78]

Patients who experience the niacin flush can take inositol hexaniacinate, a form of inositol nicotinate that is less likely to cause flushing. The suggested dosage is 500 to 1,000 mg three or four times daily, according to Mary Dan Eades, M.D., medical director of the Arkansas Center for Health and Weight control at Little Rock. The inositol combination seems to slow the release of niacin, she said.[79]

The antioxidant function of inositol hexaphosphate (IP-6) makes it ideal for controlling the damage done to the heart muscle (myocardium) during heart attacks, according to AbulKalam M. Shamsuddin, M.D., Ph.D. Following a heart attack, there is damage to ischemia or loss of the blood supply. Consequently, blood vessels may be locked by clots or temporarily constricted, thus stopping the flow of blood. However, the heart muscle cells can be saved if the area is successfully filled (reperfused) with oxygenated blood. If the lack of blood circulation to the area is cut off for an extended period, many heart muscle cells will die.[80]

Shamsuddin reported on experiments in which intravenous injections of IP-6 were given at 15 mg/kg of body weight, 75 mg/kg, and 150 mg/kg to rats 30 minutes before the experiment began (equal to 1 g for a 150-pound human). Ischemia was induced in the rats' hearts after 30 minutes, followed by 30 minutes of reperfusion. The animals getting 75 and 150 mg/kg of IP-6 showed protection of the heart muscle from reperfusion injury.

References

1. Baker, Daniel, Pharm.D., and R. Keith Campbell. "Vitamin and Mineral Supplementation in Patients with Diabetes Mellitus," *Diabetes Educator* 18(5): 420–427, Sept/Oct. 1992.

2. Hanck, A. "Vitamin Intake Under CAPD," *Nieren-Und Hochdruckkrankheimten* 21 (Suppl. 1): S64–S69, May 1992.

3. Rindi, C., et al. "Thiamine Transport by Erythrocytes and Ghosts in Thiamine-Responsive Megaloblastic Anemia," *Journal of Inherited Metabolism and Diseases* 15: 231–242, 1992.

4. Adams, Ruth, and Frank Murray. *Body, Mind and the B Vitamins.* New York: Larchmont Books, 1975, pp. 173–174.

5. Brady, Jennifer A., M.S., R.D., et al. "Thiamine Status, Diuretic Medications and the Management of Congestive Heart Failure," *Journal of the American Dietetic Association* 95: 541–544, 1995.

6. Hathcock, John N., Ph.D. *Vitamin and Mineral Safety.* Washington, D.C: Council for Responsible Nutrition, 1997, p. 7.

7. *Food, The Yearbook of Agriculture.* Washington, D.C.: U.S. Department of Agriculture, 1959, pp. 142–143.

8. Ibid., p. 21.

9. Thompson, T. "Thiamine, Riboflavin and Niacin Content of the Gluten-Free Diet: Is There Cause for Concern?" *Journal of the American Dietetic Association* 99(7): 858–862, July 1999.

10. Hendler, Sheldon Saul, M.D., Ph.D. *The Doctors' Vitamin and Mineral Encyclopedia.* New York: Simon and Schuster, 1990, p. 435.

11. Hathcock, John N., Ph.D. *Vitamin and Mineral Safety.* Washington, D.C.: Council for Responsible Nutrition, 1997, p. 7.

12. Ensminger, A., et al. *Foods and Nutrition Encyclopedia.* Clovis, Calif.: Pegus Press, 1983, pp. 1588ff.

13. Knip, M., et al. "Safety of High-Dose Nicotinamide: A Review," *Diabetologia* 43: 1337–1345, 2001.

14. Probstfield, Jeffrey L., M.D. "Nicotinic Acid As a Lipoprotein-Altering Agent: Therapy Directed by the Primary Physician," *Archives of Internal Medicine* 154: 1557–1559, July 25, 1994.

15. Hoffer, Abram, M.D., Ph.D. *Orthomolecular Medicine for Physicians*. New Canaan, Conn.: Keats Publishing, 1989, pp. 42–43.

16. Cunningham, J. J. "Micronutrients As Nutraceutical Interventions in Diabetes Mellitus," *Journal of the American College of Nutrition* 17(1): 7–10, 1998.

17. Garg, Abhimanyu, M.D., and Scott M. Grundy, M.D., Ph.D. "Nicotinic Acid As Therapy for Dyslipidemia in Non-Insulin-Dependent Diabetes Mellitus," *Journal of the American Medical Association* 264(6): 723–726, Aug. 8, 1990.

18. Cleary, John P., M.D. "Vitamin B_3 in the Treatment of Diabetes Mellitus: Case Reports and Review of the Literature," *Journal of Nutritional Medicine* 1: 217–225, 1990.

19. Pozzilli, P., et al. "Nicotinamide Therapy in Patients with Newly-Diagnosed Type 1 (Insulin-Dependent Diabetes)," *Diabetologia* 31: A533, 1988.

20. Pozzilli, P., et al. "Double Blind Trial of Nicotinamide in Recent-Onset Insulin-Dependent Diabetes Mellitus," *Diabetologia* 38(7): 848–852, 1988.

21. Pozzilli, P., et al. "Vitamin E and Nicotinamide Have Similar Effects in Maintaining Residual Beta Cell Function in Recent Onset Insulin-Dependent Diabetes (The IMDTAB IV Study)," *European Journal of Endocrinology* 137: 234–239, 1997.

22. Elam, Marshall B., Ph.D., M.D., et al. "Effect of Niacin on Lipid and Lipoprotein Levels and Glycemic Control in Patients with Diabetes and Peripheral Arterial Disease. The ADMIT Study: A Randomized Trial," *Journal of the American Medical Association* 284(10): 1263–1270, Sept. 13, 2000.

23. Hoffer, Abram, M.D., Ph.D., *Orthomolecular Medicine for Physicians*. New Canaan, Conn.: Keats Publishing, 1989, pp. 151–152.

24. Cheraskin, E., M.D., D.M.D., et al. *Psychodietetics*. New York: Stein and Day/Publishers, 1974, pp. 87, 165.

25. Ensminger, A., et al. *Foods and Nutrition Encyclopedia*. Clovis, Calif.: Pegus Press, 1983, pp. 2234ff.

26. Ellis, John M., M.D., and Jean Pamplin. *Vitamin B_6 Therapy*. New York: Avery Publishing Group, 1999, pp. 69ff.

27. Hamilton, Kirk. "Diabetes Mellitus and Vitamin B_6," *The Experts Speak*. Sacramento, Calif.: I.T. Services, 1996, pp. 102–103. Also, Mohan, Chandra, Ph.D. "Vitamin B6 Metabolism and Diabetes," *Biochemical and Metabolic Biology* 52: 10–17, 1994.

28. Gaby, Alan, M.D. *B_6: The Natural Healer*. New Canaan, Conn.: Keats Publishing, 1987, pp. 107ff.

29. Bernstein, A., et al. "Treatment of Painful Diabetic Neuropathies with Vitamin B_6: A Clinical and Electrophysiologic Study," *FASEB Journal* 2: A438, 1988.

30. Hathcock, John N., Ph.D. *Vitamin and Mineral Safety*. Washington, D.C.: Council for Responsible Nutrition, 1997, p. 8.

31. *Food, The Yearbook of Agriculture*. Washington, D.C.: U.S. Department of Agriculture, 1959, pp. 147–148.

32. Araki, Atsushi, et al. "Plasma Homocysteine Concentrations in Japanese Patients with Non-Insulin-Dependent Diabetes Mellitus: Effect of Parenteral Cobalamin Treatment," *Atherosclerosis* 103: 149–157, 1993.

33. Rowe, Paul M. "IOM (Institute of Medicine) Examines Folate, B_{12} and Choline Needs," *Lancet* 349: 780, March 15, 1997.

34. Murray, Michael T., N.D. *Diabetes and Hypoglycemia*. Rocklin, Calif.: Prima Publishing, 1994, pp. 99–100.

35. Chicola, Vincent F., M.D. "Vitamin B_{12} Bats An Eye," *Cortlandt Forum*, July 1996, p. 122.

36. Hamilton, Kirk. "Diabetic Neuropathy, Vegetarian Diets and Vitamin B_{12}," *The Experts Speak*. Sacramento, Calif.: I.T. Services, 1996, pp. 104-105. Also, Crane, Milton, M.D. "Vitamin B_{12} Studies in Total Nutrition," *Journal of Nutrition* 4: 419–430, 1994.

37. Hathcock, John N., Ph.D. *Vitamin and Mineral Safety*. Washington, D.C.: Council for Responsible Nutrition, 1997, p. 8.

38. *Food, The Yearbook of Agriculture*. Washington, D.C.: U.S. Department of Agriculture, 1959, pp. 146ff.

39. Brouwer, Ingeborg A., et al. "Low-Dose Folic Acid Supplementation Decreases Plasma Homocysteine Concentrations: A Randomized Trial," *American Journal of Clinical Nutrition* 69: 99–104, 1999.

40. Woodside, Jayne V., et al. "Effect of B-Group Vitamins and Antioxidant Vitamins on Hyperhomocysteinemia: A Double-Blind, Randomized, Factorial-Design, Controlled Trial," *American Journal of Clinical Nutrition* 67(5): 858–866, May 1998.

41. Gerhard, Glenn T., et al. "Higher Total Homocysteine Concentrations and Lower Folate Concentrations in Premenopausal Black Women Than in Premenopausal White Women," *American Journal of Clinical Nutrition* 70: 252–260, 1999.

42. Morrison, Howard I., Ph.D., et al. "Serum Folate and Risk of Fatal Coronary Heart Disease," *Journal of the American Medical Association* 275(24): 1893–1896, June 26, 1996.

43. Janssen, M. J. F. M., et al. "Hyperhomocysteinemia: A Role in the Accelerated Atherogenesis of Chronic Renal Failure," *Netherlands Journal of Medicine* 46: 244–251, 1995.

44. Christensen, B., et al. "Whole Blood Folate, Homocysteine in Serum and Risk of First Acute Myocardial Infarction," *Atherosclerosis* 147: 317–326, 1999.

45. Ubbink, Johan B., et al. "Vitamin B_{12}, Vitamin B6 and Folate Nutritional Status in Men With Hyper-homocysteinemia," *American Journal of Clinical Nutrition* 57: 47–53, 1993.

46. Landgren, F., et al. "Plasma Homocysteine in Acute Myocardial Infarction: Homocysteine-Lowering Effect of Folic Acid," *Journal of Internal Medicine* 237: 381–388, 1995.

47. Robinson, Killian, M.D., et al. "Hyper-homocysteinemia Confers an Independent Increased Risk of Atherosclerosis in End-Stage Renal Disease and Is Closely Linked to Plasma Folate and Pyridoxine Concentrations," *Circulation* 94(11): 2743–2748, Dec. 1, 1996.

48. Ebly, E. M., et al. "Folate Status, Vascular Disease and Cognition in Elderly Canadians," *Age and Aging* 27: 485–491, 1998.

49. "Vitamin B_6, Folic Acid Benefit Dialysis Patients," *The Nutrition Report*, March 1994, p. 21.

50. Alterman, Seymour, L., M.D., and Donald A. Kullman, M.D. *How to Prevent, Control and Cure Diabetes*. Hollywood, Fla.: Frederick Fell Publishers, 2000, p. 182.

51. Ensminger, A., et al. *Foods and Nutrition Encyclopedia*. Clovis, Calif.: Pegus Press, 1983, pp. 210ff.

52. *Prevention's Healing with Vitamins.* Emmaus, Penn.: Rodale Press, 1996, p. 220.

53. Golan, Ralph, M.D. *Optimum Wellness.* New York: Ballantine Books, 1995, pp. 188, 191–193, 360, 396.

54. Atkins, Robert C., M.D. *Dr. Atkins' Health Revolution.* Boston: Houghton Mifflin Co., 1988, pp. 102–103.

55. Ronzio, Robert A., Ph.D. *The Encyclopedia of Nutrition and Good Health.* New York: Facts on File, Inc., 1997, pp. 335–336.

56. Golan, Ralph, M.D., *Optimum Wellness.* New York: Ballantine Books, 1995, p. 192.

57. Coronel, F., et al. "Lipid-Lowering Treatment with Pantethine in Renal Transplant Patients," *Nephrologia* 15(1): 68–73, 1995.

58. Atkins, Robert C., M.D. *Dr. Atkins' Vita-Nutrient Solution.* New York: Simon and Schuster, 1998, pp. 84–85.

59. Giller, Robert M., M.D., and Kathy Matthews. *Natural Prescriptions.* New York: Carol Southern Books, 1994, p. 72.

60. Murray, Michael T., N.D. *Natural Alternatives to Over-the-Counter and Prescription Drugs.* New York: William Morrow and Co., 1994, p. 139.

61. Leung, Li-Hung, M.D. "A Stone That Kills Two Birds: Pantothenic Acid and the Treatment of Acne Vulgaris and Obesity," *Journal of Orthomolecular Medicine* 12(2): 99–114, 1997.

62. Ensminger, A., et al., *Foods and Nutrition Encyclopedia.* Clovis, Calif.: Pegus Press, 1983, pp. 413ff.

63. Zeisel, Steven H., M.D., Ph.D. "Choline: An Important Nutrient in Brain Development, Liver Function and Carcinogenesis," *Journal of the American College of Nutrition* 11(5): 473–481, 1992.

64. Davis, Adelle. *Let's Get Well.* New York: New American Library, 1965, pp. 173–174, 194.

65. Atkins, Robert C., M.D. *Dr. Atkins' Vita-Nutrient Solution,* New York: Simon and Schuster, 1998, pp. 78–79.

66. Kang, Soo-Sang, et al. "Hyperhomocysteinemias a Risk Factor for Occlusive Vascular Disease," *Annual Review of Nutrition* 12: 279–298, 1992.

67. Stampfer, Meir J., M.D., et al. "A Prospective Study of Plasma Homocysteine and Risk of Myocardial Infarction in U.S. Physicians," *Journal of the American Medical Association* 268(7): 877–881, Aug. 19, 1992.

68. Malinow, M. R., M.D. "Risk for Arterial Occlusive Disease: Is Hyperhomocysteinemia an Innocent Bystander?" *Canadian Journal of Cardiology* 7(9): VII–IX, Nov. 1991.

69. "Food and Mood," *Nutrition Action Health Letter,* Sept. 1992, pp. 5–7.

70. Ensminger, A., et al. *Foods and Nutrition Encyclopedia.* Clovis, Calif.: Pegus Press, 1983, pp. 1234ff.

71. Atkins, Robert C., M.D. *Dr. Atkins' Vita-Nutrient Solution,* New York: Simon and Schuster, 1998, pp. 80–82.

72. Matz, Robert, M.D. "Magnesium: Deficiencies and Therapeutic Uses," *Hospital Practice,* April 30, 1993, pp. 79–92.

73. Davis, Adelle. *Let's Get Well,* New York: New American Library, 1965, p. 53.

74. Giller, Robert M., and Kathy Matthews, *Natural Prescriptions.* New York: Carol Southern Books, 1994, pp. 72–73.

75. Grafton, Gilliam, et al. "Effect of MG2 and NA+ Dependent Inositol Transport/Role for MG2 in Etiology of Diabetic Complications," *Diabetes* 41: 35–39, 1992.

76. Holub, Bruce J., Ph.D. "The Nutritional Importance of Inositol in the Phospho-inositides," *New England Journal of Medicine* 326(19): 1285–1287, May 7, 1992.

77. Modlin, M. "Urinary Phosphorylated Inositols and Renal Stone," *Lancet,* Nov. 22, 1980, pp. 1113–1114.

78. Murray, Michael T., N.D. *Natural Alternatives to Over-the-Counter Prescription Drugs,* New York: William Morrow and Co., 1994, p. 136.

79. *Prevention's Healing with Vitamins,* Emmaus, Penn.: Rodale Press, 1996, p. 477.

80. Shamsuddin, AbulKalam, M., M.D., Ph.D. *IP-6: Nature's Revolutionary Cancer-Fighter.* New York: Kensington Books, 1998, pp. 85–86.

30 Vitamin C

Vitamin C is often prescribed by holistic physicians to prevent and/or treat diabetes. Since the vitamin is water-soluble, supplements should be spaced out during the day, since the vitamin is purged in urine and feces. In one study, vitamin C lowered blood sugar levels on average by 30% and daily insulin requirements by 27%; and sugar excretion in the urine could be almost eliminated. Vitamin C is also beneficial in preventing high blood pressure, cataracts, hardening of the arteries, and other complications that affect diabetics.

Type 2 diabetes is often caused or aggravated by a deficiency of certain vitamins and other essential nutrients in millions of cells in the pancreas, the liver, and the blood vessel walls, as well as other organs in those with a genetic predisposition to diabetic disorders, according to Matthias Rath, M.D. Optimum intake of vitamins and other nutrients can help prevent the onset of adult diabetes and correct, at least in part, existing diabetes and its complications, he added.[1]

Clinical studies indicate that in diabetic patients, vitamin C not only contributes to prevention of cardiovascular complications, it also helps to normalize the imbalance in the glucose metabolism, Rath said. A study by Professor R. Pfleger and colleagues at the University of Vienna showed that diabetic patients taking 300 to 500 mg/day of vitamin C could significantly improve glucose balance. Blood sugar levels could be lowered on average by 30% and daily insulin requirements by 27%; and sugar excretion in the urine could be almost eliminated.

"It is amazing that this study was published in 1937 in a leading European journal for internal medicine," Rath continued. "If the results of this important study had been followed up and documented in medical textbooks, millions of lives would have been saved and cardiovascular disease would no longer threaten diabetic patients."

The consumption of vitamin C above the Recommended Daily Allowance (60 mg/day; 100 mg/day for smokers) may provide important health benefits for those with Type 1 diabetes, reported the *Journal of the American College of Nutrition*. It has been known that vitamin C levels are lower in diabetics than in those without the disease. The vitamin normalizes red blood cell sorbitol concentrations in those with Type 1 diabetes. Sorbitol is a sugar alcohol that is produced in the body during the conversion to glucose.[2]

In a study at the University of Massachusetts at Amherst, 58 adults, ranging in age from 19 to 34, were given 100 mg/day or 600 mg/day of vitamin C. Nine of the volunteers were Type 1 diabetics, and 11 of the participants were nondiabetics. It was found that red blood cell sorbitol levels were significantly higher in the Type 1 patients. Either dose of the vitamin normalized the RBC-sorbitol levels in the Type 1 diabetics within 30 days.[3]

Vitamin C is effective in reducing sorbitol accumulation in the erythrocytes (red blood cells) of diabetics. Because of vitamin C's low toxicity, the researchers suggest that it is superior to pharmaceutical aldose reductase inhibitors, which block an enzyme that results in the accumulation of sugar by-products. The researchers added that there appears to be no advantage in the larger doses of the vitamin, since 100 mg/day effectively normalize RBC-sorbitol levels.

A research team at the University of Washington at Seattle reported that supplementing the diet of diabetics with vitamin C might protect them against oxidative damage of LDL-cholesterol (the bad kind), thus reducing their risk of developing hardening of the arteries.

In the study, susceptibility to low-density lipoprotein cholesterol oxidation relative to vitamin C and vitamin E was measured in 25 Type 2 diabetics and 22 healthy controls. The results found that vitamin C levels were low in the diabetics, while vitamin E levels were higher when compared to controls. Vitamin C can assist against vitamin E depletion, but when vitamin C levels are low, diabetics must depend on available stores of vitamin E, the researchers said.[4]

Supplementation with antioxidant vitamins significantly reduced the susceptibility of LDL-cholesterol to combine with copper, reported James W. Anderson, M.D., of the V.A. Medical Center in Lexington, Kentucky. In the study, 20 nondiabetics and 20 Type 2 diabetic men were given a placebo for 8 weeks, followed by 12 weeks of antioxidant supplements, including 24 mg/day of beta-carotene, 1,000 mg/day of vitamin C, and 800 IU/day of vitamin E, followed by 8 weeks of placebo.[5]

Anderson and colleagues reported that low-density lipoprotein cholesterol in diabetics was more susceptible to combining with oxygen (oxidation) and causing harm than LDL in nondiabetics.

At the Mahidol University in Bangkok, Thailand, researchers said that either elderly diabetics do not consume or absorb sufficient amounts of vitamin C, or the chronic manifestations of their disease alter the vitamin's status. The research team arrived at this conclusion by evaluating 26 elderly diabetics and 23 healthy controls. They found that healthy controls had significantly higher levels of vitamin C in their blood than did the diabetics. There was no difference between the groups in the amount of vitamin B_1, vitamin A, and vitamin E in their circulating blood.[6]

In studying 1,113 men and 1,451 women, with an average age of 70.4, it was found that men have lower average plasma vitamin C levels than women. The researchers added that smoking more than 10 cigarettes a day was associated with a lower plasma vitamin C concentration in men but not in women. While diabetics tended to have lower levels of vitamin C in their blood, the difference was significant only in women, the research team added.[7]

At the University of Sydney in Australia researchers evaluated 20 diabetics who were randomized to receive either 500 mg of vitamin C twice daily or a placebo for 12 months. The research team reported that the vitamin C therapy increased blood levels of vitamin C and reduced albumin excretion rate (AER) after 9 months. They added that vitamin C supplements given to diabetics may have long-term benefits in slowing the progression of diabetic complications.[8] Albumin is a protein and above normal levels may be a sign of kidney disease, especially for diabetics who have had the disease for a long time.

An increased intake of vitamin C lessens the risk of developing heart disease, according to researchers at the Harvard School of Medicine, Boston. The study evaluated 87,245 female nurses, between the ages of 34 and 59, who were symptom-free when the study began in 1980. The women reported on their vitamin C intake via questionnaires.

During 8 years, there were 437 heart attacks and 115 coronary deaths. In tabulating the results of the study, the researchers reported that those with the highest intake of vitamin C were better protected from heart disease than those with low intakes of the vitamin.[9]

A Danish study evaluated 4,224 men and women, aged 20 to 59, to determine antioxidant intake from diet and supplements in smokers, ex-smokers, and those who never smoked. Men who smoked more than 20 cigarettes a day had considerably lower beta-carotene and vitamin C intakes than men who never smoked, because of an almost 60% lower intake of fruit. Women who were moderate and heavy smokers also had lower intakes of vitamin C and fruit.[10]

In addition to getting exercise, following a healthful diet, avoiding cigarettes, and consuming only moderate amounts of alcohol, eating more fruits and vegetables high in vitamin C can help to lessen the risk of dying from heart disease and other chronic illnesses, according to Kay-Tee Khaw, M.D., and her colleagues at the University of Cambridge in England. Vitamin C helps to destroy the harmful free radicals that contribute to many chronic health problems.[11]

The researchers evaluated the vitamin C intakes of 20,000 men and women, ranging in age from 45 to 79, living in Norfolk and eastern England. A 4-year follow-up found that the levels of vitamin C in the blood were inversely related to deaths from all causes, including cardiovascular disease. The researchers, which reported their findings in *Lancet,* said that a daily increase equivalent to 50 g of fruits and vegetables was linked with a 20% decrease in the risk of death. "Those people with the highest levels of vitamin C in their blood have a 50% reduction in mortality," stated Alisa Welch, a nutritionist in the study.

Supplementing with vitamin C might be a useful therapy in the treatment of high blood pressure, according to researchers at the USDA Human Nutrition Research Center at Beltsville, Maryland. During the study, 20 volunteers, 12 of whom were borderline hypertensives, supplemented their regular diet with 1,000 mg/day of vitamin C or a placebo for two 6-week periods. The test group was not deficient in the vitamin. While the vitamin was associated with a significant reduction in systolic (beating) blood pressure and pulse pressure, it had no effect on diastolic (resting) blood pressure, total blood cholesterol, HDL-cholesterol, and total triglyceride levels.[12]

Researchers at the Medical College of Georgia at Augusta reported that there was a small, but significant, inverse relationship between diastolic and systolic blood pressure when healthy volunteers with normal blood pressure were given vitamin C. During the study, blood pressure and serum glucose were measured and food diaries and urine samples were tabulated for 13 men and 8 women, ranging in age from 41 to 45. They were given 500 mg of vitamin C twice daily along with their regular diet.

Following 4 weeks of treatment, blood pressure, dietary intake, urine samples, and glucose tolerance were again tested. The researchers said that average systolic blood pressure had dropped from 125 mmHg to 121 mmHg, and diastolic blood pressure went down from 80 mmHg to 77 mmHg due to the vitamin C supplementation. The researchers added that their study supports previous studies in suggesting a rationale for including vitamin C supplements in the prevention and possibly the treatment of mild high blood pressure.[13]

A panel of nutrition experts, which was sponsored by the Alliance for Aging Research, recommended that the Food and Drug Administration make recommendations on how much vitamin C, vitamin E, and beta-carotene people should take to prevent disease. Their recommendations are 250 to 1,000 mg/day of vitamin C, 100 to 400 IU/day of vitamin E, and 17,000 to 50,000 IU/day of beta-carotene. These nutrients are effective in preventing heart disease, cancer, cataracts, and other conditions associated with aging, the panel reported.[14]

Jeffrey Blumberg, Ph.D., of Tufts University, Boston, said that a study in Lixian, China, found that vitamin E and beta-carotene reduced the risk of cancer; two studies at Harvard University reported that beta-carotene and vitamin E reduced the risk of heart disease in both men and women; two Canadian studies found lower rates of infectious diseases and cataracts in people who took antioxidant vitamins.

References

1. Rath, Matthias, M.D. *Cellular Health Series: The Heart.* Santa Clara, Calif.: MR Publishing, 2001, pp. 97ff.

2. Cunningham, John J., Ph.D. "The Glucose/Insulin System and Vitamin C: Implications in Insulin-Dependent Diabetes Mellitus," *Journal of the American College of Nutrition* 17(2): 105–108, 1998.

3. Cunningham, John J., Ph.D., et al. "Vitamin C: An Aldose Reductase Inhibitor That Normalizes Erythrocyte Sorbitol in Insulin-Dependent Diabetes Mellitus," *Journal of the American College of Nutrition* 13(4): 344–350, 1994.

4. Brazg, R., et al. "Effects of Dietary Antioxidants on LDL Oxidation in Noninsulin-Dependent Diabetics," *Clinical Research* 40: 103A, 1992.

5. Anderson, J. W., et al. "Antioxidant Supplementation Effects on Low-Density Lipoprotein Oxidation for Individuals with Type 2 Diabetes Mellitus," *Journal of the American College of Nutrition* 18(5): 451–461, 1999.

6. Roongpisuthipong, C., et al. "Vitamin Status in Elderly Diabetic Subjects," *FASEB Journal* 5: 1299A, 1991.

7. Birolouez-Aragon, I., et al. "Association of Age, Smoking Habits and Diabetes with Plasma Vitamin C of Elderly of the POLA Study," *International Journal of Vitamin and Nutrition Research* 71(1): 53–59, 2001.

8. McAuliffe, A. V., et al. "Administration of Ascorbic Acid and an Aldose Inhibitor (Tolrestat) in Diabetes: Effect on Urinary Albumin Excretion," *Nephron* 80: 277–284, 1998.

9. Manson, J., et al. "A Prospective Study of Vitamin C and Incidence of Coronary Heart Disease in Women," *Circulation* 85: 865, 1992.

10. Zondervan, K. T., et al. "Do Dietary and Supplementary Intakes of Antioxidants Differ with Smoking Status?" *International Journal of Epidemiology* 25: 70–79, 1996.

11. Reaney, Patricia, "Study Links Vitamin C to Lower Death Rates," Reuters, March 2, 2001.

12. Osilesi, O., et al. "Blood Pressure and Plasma Lipids During Ascorbic Acid Supplementation in Borderline Hypertensive and Normotensive Adults," *Nutrition Research* 11: 405–412, 1991.

13. Feldman, E., et al. "Ascorbic Acid Supplements and Blood Pressure," *Annals of the New York Academy of Sciences* 669: 342–344, 1992.

14. Kritz, Fran. "FDA Urged to Back Antioxidants," *Medical Tribune,* March 23, 1994, p. 1.

31 Vitamin D

Vitamin D, a fat-soluble vitamin, is available from only a few common foods (fatty fish, egg yolks, liver, dairy products, fortified cereals, etc.) and it is formed in the body by exposure to the skin to ultraviolet rays of the sun. The most common forms of the vitamin are ergocalciferol (vitamin D_2) and cholecalciferol (vitamin D_3).

While it is necessary for regulating calcium and phosphorus in the body, the vitamin also plays a role in preventing rickets and osteomalacia.

The recommended daily amount of the vitamin is around 400 IU/day; however, older people may need up to 1,000 IU/day, depending on their diet and exposure to sunlight. The vitamin is available in a variety of over-the-counter supplements.

The vitamin is involved in both Type 1 and Type 2 diabetes. For example, children with a vitamin D deficiency are at risk for developing Type 1 diabetes. Vitamin D is related directly to the capacity to secrete insulin, and inversely to glucose tolerance; and glucose tolerance is more severe in those with low amounts of vitamin D in the blood. A deficiency in vitamin D is associated with cataract and heart disease, two complications of Type 2 diabetes.

The importance of vitamin D, a fat-soluble vitamin, lies in its role of regulating calcium and phosphorus. In the absence of vitamin D, mineralization of bone matrix is impaired, which results in rickets in children and osteomalacia in adults. Rickets, a bone disorder, has been known since 500

B.C., and it was first described in detail in London more than 300 years ago. The word "rickets" comes from the Old English word "wrikken," which means bent or twisted.[1]

Vitamins A, D, E, and K are fat-soluble, which means that they are dissolved in fats. Small amounts are stored in fats for later use. Vitamin B and C are water-soluble, meaning they are dissolved in water. They are released in urine and feces throughout the day, which is why they are best taken in divided doses during the day.

> ## Main Food Sources of Vitamin D
>
> Fatty fish, egg yolks, liver, cream, butter, cheese, fortified milk, fortified cereals, fortified bread, and fortified margarine.

Vitamin D is unique among the vitamins in that it occurs naturally in only a few common foods, and it can be formed in the body by exposure to the skin to ultraviolet (UV) rays of the sun. Hence, it is known as the "sunshine vitamin," the *Food & Nutrition Encyclopedia* states.

"Although about 10 sterol compounds with vitamin D activity have been identified, only two of these, known as provitamin D or precursors, are of practical importance from the standpoint of their occurrence in foods—ergocalciferol (vitamin D_2, calciferol or viosterol) and cholecalciferol (vitamin D_3)," the encyclopedia added.

Writing in the *New England Journal of Medicine,* Robert D. Utiger, M.D., said that vitamin D can be obtained from sunlight through the conversion of 7-dehydrocholesterol to provitamin D, which is then converted to vitamin D. Also, vitamin D from food sources or from the skin is converted to 25-hydroxyvitamin D in the liver and 1,25-dihydroxyvitamin D—the active hormone—in the kidneys.[2]

The serum half-life of 25-hydroxyvitamin D is longer than that of 1,25-dihydroxyvitamin D, in that it provides better assessment of vitamin D intake and storage, Utiger states. Blood levels of 25-hydroxyvitamin D decrease with age but go up slightly with sunlight exposure and vitamin D intake in foods and supplements.

In the Framingham Heart Study, 14% of women and 6% of men had low serum 25-hydroxyvitamin D stores, Utiger explains. For example, in 290 people with a mean age of 62, poor vitamin D intake and remaining indoors contributed to low 25-hydroxyvitamin D amounts in their blood. Utiger found that 66% of those with low 25-hydroxyvitamin D amounts had estimated vitamin D intakes that were less than adequate for their age group.

Utiger said that a vitamin D deficiency is related to increased parathyroid hormone secretion, increased bone loss, osteoporosis, and mild osteomalacia. The parathyroid glands release parathyroid hormone, which increases

How Safe Is Vitamin D?

Vitamin D intakes less than 2,000 IU (50 mcg) cause no known risk, and there is sufficient evidence to establish the safety of intakes up to 800 IU (20 mcg). In most adults, daily intake in excess of 50,000 IU (1.25 mg) is needed to produce toxicity, but much less may cause adverse effects in persons with certain diseases or idiopathic hypercalcemia (too much calcium in the blood).

In children, dietary vitamin D intakes as low as 2,000 to 4,000 IU (50 to 100 mcg) per day have led to adverse effects. The majority of dietary supplements that include vitamin D contain 400 IU (10 mcg), an amount known to be safe and recommended by many scientific authorities.

Source: John N. Hathcock, Ph.D. *Vitamin and Mineral Safety.* Washington, D.C.: Council for Responsible Nutrition, 1997, p. 7.

blood levels of calcium and magnesium, two minerals essential for bone health. He added that adults probably need 800 to 1,000 IU/day of the vitamin. This can be given as a single capsule of 5,000 IU or at a dose of 100,000 IU every four to six months. He said that the amount of the vitamin in supplemental multivitamins and calcium supplements should be increased substantially, and that all adults should be advised to take supplements of the vitamin.

Vitamin D has a dual role as vitamin and hormone, reports Robert Garrison, M.A., Ph.D., and Elizabeth Somer, M.A., R.D. Like other hormones, the vitamin's active metabolites are produced in the liver and kidneys, but have their effects on other tissues such as the intestinal mucosa and bone tissue. Vitamin D's activation in the skin is restricted by skin pigments and keratin, which screens UV light. Smog, fog, smoke, clothing, screens, and most glass screen the UV light, and, therefore, interfere with vitamin D formation. The vitamin is resistant to heat and oxidation; however, it is stable in mild acids and alkalis.[3]

An often-asked question is whether or not sunscreens inhibit the formation of vitamin D from the sun. In evaluating vitamin D levels and the use of sunscreen in more than 113 individuals 40 years of age or over, researchers at the University of Melbourne, Victoria, Australia, reported that over an Australian summer sufficient sunlight is received probably through both the sunscreen and the lack of total skin coverage. This assures adequate vitamin D production in those who are advised to use sunscreens regularly, they said.[4]

After reviewing 117 studies on vitamin D from 1971 to 1990, a research team at St. Michael's Hospital in Dublin, Ireland, reported that vitamin D fortification or supplementation is necessary to maintain optimal amounts of this vitamin in the elderly. The researchers said that while exposure to summer sun is critical in providing vitamin D, oral intake combined with either fortified foods or supplements is essential for maintaining proper tissue stores of the vitamin. Vitamin D intakes are, of course, lower during winter months, when the elderly wear clothes that prevent the formation of vitamin D through their skin.[5]

Low levels of vitamin D may be a significant risk factor for glucose intolerance, according to researchers at the Royal London School of

Medicine and Dentistry in London, England. The study evaluated 142 elderly Dutchmen, ranging in age from 70 to 88. It was found that the one-hour glucose tolerance test was inversely associated with blood concentrations of 25-hydroxyvitamin D. With the exclusion of newly diagnosed diabetics, total insulin concentration during the glucose test was inversely associated with the concentration of vitamin D.[6]

Researchers in Sweden reported that vitamin D supplementation was associated with a reduced risk of Type 1 diabetes. They added that most European studies indicate a positive effect of vitamin D supplementation for infants. They theorize that vitamin D may contribute to immune modulation and protect or arrest an ongoing immune process begun in susceptible children by early environmental exposures.[7]

In *Clinical Pearls,* health journalist Kirk Hamilton published his interview with B. J. Boucher, M.D., of the Royal London School of Medicine and Dentistry in England, concerning vitamin D and glucose intolerance. Boucher said that vitamin D is needed by the islet cells to secrete insulin normally. This may happen since it helps to ensure an adequate supply of calcium, upon which many enzymes related to insulin secretion and release are dependent.[8]

Boucher and his colleagues found that vitamin D is directly related to the capacity to secrete insulin and inversely to glucose tolerance. In their current study (reported above), they said that elderly Dutchmen had a vitamin D deficiency of 39%, and that glucose tolerance is more advanced in those with the lowest vitamin D. They also found that vitamin D status relates inversely to insulin sensitivity, and that in those depleted in insulin, or in whom it is not being produced in adequate amounts, it increases the risk of becoming diabetic.

In animal studies, at least, there is considerable evidence that vitamin D supplements can improve insulin secretion in the pancreas's islets, Boucher said. Further, vitamin D supplements given to humans over a considerable time can improve insulin secretion and glucose tolerance in those who have osteomalacia (softening of the bones), since these patients are severely deficient in vitamin D.

Low levels of vitamin D may be a significant risk factor for glucose intolerance, according to researchers at the Royal London School of Medicine and Dentistry in London, England. The study evaluated 142 elderly Dutchmen, ranging in age from 70 to 88. With the exclusion of newly diagnosed diabetics, total insulin concentration during the glucose test was inversely associated with the concentration of vitamin D.

Vitamin D can improve insulin resistance with a reduction in hyper-insulinemia (high levels of insulin in the blood), along with an improvement in glucose tolerance when given in the early stages of glucose intolerance in kidney disease. The latter develops when vitamin D is not properly formed, Boucher said.

Using data from the Keys Epidemiological Seven Countries Studies, David S. Grimes, M.D., and associates at the Royal Infirmary, Blackburn, England, recorded blood cholesterol levels and compared them to the recorded hours of sunshine at 136 locations in the United Kingdom. The body can produce vitamin D during exposure to sunlight. The vitamin is also synthesized in the skin from a cholesterol derivative when exposed to ultraviolet light (sunshine). A sunlight deficiency can increase blood cholesterol by allowing squalene (a precursor of sterols, such as cholesterol) metabolism to synthesize cholesterol instead of vitamin D, which would happen with greater sun exposure. The increased amounts of cholesterol in the blood during the winter is confirmed by this study, due to reduced sunlight exposure.[9]

Grimes said that sunlight influences our susceptibility to various disease, such as coronary artery disease. For example, there is a clear relationship between cholesterol and latitude, with cholesterol levels rising with increasing residential distance from the equator. He suggests that vitamin D slows the progression of heart disease. While free radicals can increase the rate of progression of heart disease, antioxidants such as vitamin C and selenium can also provide protection against the disease.

In studying 173 volunteers at high and moderate risk for coronary artery disease, vitamin D levels (specifically 1,25-dihydroxyvitamin D) were inversely related to the extent of vascular calcification. Vitamin D is also important in bone mineralization, which may explain the association between osteoporosis and vascular calcification (calcium deposits in blood vessels). Vascular calcification is found in more than 90% of patients with coronary heart disease.[10]

Writing in *Diabetes and Nutrition Metabolism,* O. Vaarala, et al., said that viruses are potential inducers of beta-cell damage, and that a number of viruses reportedly have been associated with Type 1 diabetes, such as the enteroviruses (polio, meningitis, etc.). Other viruses that may be involved with diabetes include mumps, measles, cytomegalo- (which causes cellular enlargement) and retroviruses (a group of tumor viruses); and cow's milk has been implicated in diabetes in several countries. In addition, they said, a vitamin D deficiency may contribute to Type 1 diabetes in childhood. Other factors in diabetes include excessive weight gain by the mother during pregnancy, older age of the mother, and amniocentesis (a surgical procedure to determine the sex of the child or chromosomal abnormalities).[11]

Arthur A. Knapp, M.D., a New York ophthalmologist, speaking at a meeting of the American Geriatrics Society, said that he treated some eye conditions of elderly people with massive doses of vitamin D. He believes that myopia, or shortsightedness, is not just an eye condition, but rather a manifestation of a vitamin D deficiency. He gave a group of patients vitamin D and calcium supplements for 5 to 28 months and found a decrease in the nearsightedness in over one-third of them, with a definite halt in the process in another 17%.[12]

Knapp said that a lack of vitamin D and calcium may be related to the formation of cataract. For example, laboratory animals kept on diets deficient in vitamin D and calcium invariably develop cataracts. Concerning human beings, there are some highly relevant facts linking vitamin D and calcium deficiencies and cataract. A drug used to decrease blood calcium in several diseases occasionally produces cataracts. Diabetics are known to suffer from a calcium imbalance, and they develop cataracts more often than nondiabetics. A condition called tetany, in which blood calcium levels are very low, often produces cataracts.

References

1. Ensminger, A., et al. *Foods and Nutrition Encyclopedia.* Clovis, Calif.: Pegus Press, 1983, pp. 2256ff.

2. Utiger, Robert D., M.D. "The Need for More Vitamin D," *New England Journal of Medicine* 338(12): 828–829, March 19, 1998.

3. Garrison, Robert, Jr., M.A., R.Ph., and Elizabeth Somer, M.A., R.D. *The Nutrition Desk Reference.* New Canaan, Conn.: Keats Publishing, 1995, pp. 78ff.

4. Marks, Robin, M.P.H., et al. "The Effect of Regular Sunscreen Use On Vitamin D Levels in an Australian Population," *Archives of Dermatology* 131: 415–421, April 1995.

5. McKenna, M. "Differences in Vitamin D Status Between Countries in Young Adults and the Elderly," *American Journal of Medicine* 93: 69–77, 1992.

6. Baynes, K. C. R., et al. "Vitamin D, Glucose Tolerance and Insulinemia in Elderly Men," *Diabetologia* 40: 344–347, 1997.

7. Dahlquist, G., et al. "Vitamin D Supplement in Early Childhood and Risk of Type 1 (Insulin-Dependent) Diabetes Mellitus," *Diabetologia* 42: 51–54, 1999.

8. Kirk, Hamilton. "Glucose Tolerance, Insulinemia and Vitamin D," *Clinical Pearls.* Sacramento, Calif.: I.T. Services, Inc., 1997, p. 305. Also, Boucher, B. J., M.D. "Vitamin D, Glucose Intolerance and Insulinemia in Elderly Men," *Diabetologia* 40: 344–347, 1997.

9. Grimes, David S., M.D. "Sunlight, Cholesterol and Coronary Heart Disease," *Quarterly Journal of Medicine* 89: 579–589, 1996.

10. Watson, Karol E., M.D., et al. "Active Serum Vitamin D Levels Are Inversely Correlated with Coronary Calcification," *Circulation* 96: 1755–1760, 1997.

11. Vaarala, O., et al. "Environmental Factors in the Aetiology of Childhood Diabetes," *Diabetes and Nutrition Metabolism* 12(2): 75–85, 1999.

12. Adams, Ruth. *The Complete Home Guide to All the Vitamins.* New York: Larchmont Books, 1975, pp. 196ff.

32 Vitamin E

Vitamin E has been thoroughly researched for more than 30 years as a necessary nutritional supplement for diabetes, heart disease, intermittent claudication (cramps in the legs), stroke, gangrene, hardening of the arteries, blood clots, nerve disorders, and other debilitating health conditions.

The vitamin is instrumental in lowering glycosylated hemoglobin, insulin levels, triglycerides, total cholesterol, LDL-cholesterol, VLDL-cholesterol, and apoprotein-b, another risk factor for ischemic heart disease. Since diabetics often have a vitamin E–poor diet, this supplement should be at the top of their to-take list. A variety of vitamin E supplements are available, and a health care professional should be consulted for the proper dosage.

In numerous studies published in medical journals, vitamin E is a potent antioxidant that protects diabetics and others from serious health problems. Antioxidants, such as vitamin E, are natural substances that inhibit the formation of free radicals, which can lead to serious illnesses. As the word implies, an antioxidant prevents substances from combining with oxygen (oxidation) to form free radicals. Although oxygen is an essential element, it can combine with various substances to become harmful.

When taking large amounts of vitamin E, diabetics should consult with their physician, since megadoses can raise blood pressure in susceptible individuals. It's best to begin with lower doses and gradually increase as needed. When taking vitamin E and selenium, take one in the morning and the other in the evening for better results.

Diabetics are especially susceptible to blood clots, according to Robert C. Atkins, M.D., who operates the Atkins Clinic in New York City. In addition to ridding the blood of harmful fats and improving circulation, vitamin E also thins the blood naturally, he said.[1]

"Thinning the blood is actually a misnomer," Atkins said. "Actually, blood tends to form clots through the process of platelet clumping. A clot that lodges in an artery can impede blood flow, causing a heart attack or, if the brain is affected, a stroke. When volunteers in a 1996 study took 400 IU of vitamin E daily, along with aspirin, they suffered fewer transient ischemic attacks (TIAs). These ministrokes interrupt blood flow to the brain only briefly but often portend a more serious stroke."

Blood platelets in diabetics contain less vitamin E than platelets of nondiabetics, says Atkins. When vitamin E levels are low, the risk of acquiring Type 2 diabetes rises by a ratio of nearly four to one. In one study, he said, Type 1 diabetics, when given 100 IU/day of vitamin E for 3 months, significantly reduced the tissue damage from high blood sugar, a process called glycation, as well as the accumulation of triglycerides, the diabetes-related heart disease risk factor. (Approximately 95% of fats in the body are triglycerides.)

In 1992, the cost of diabetic care in the United States exceeded $105 billion. Needless to say, it is considerably higher now. It has been suggested that accelerated non-enzymatic glycosylation and free radicals generated in oxidative reactions may be the reason hyperglycemia (high blood sugar) causes diabetic complications. Vitamin E supplementation may, therefore, benefit diabetics due to its antioxidant activity and its inhibiting of protein glycosylation by normalizing blood platelet activity.[2]

For example, protein glycosylation has been shown with the addition of 600 to 1,200 IU/day of vitamin E in diabetic patients. Vitamin E is involved in the production of prostacylin, a potent vasodilator and inhibitor of platelet aggregation. In one study, 900 IU/day of vitamin E for 4 months reduced oxidative stress and improved insulin action in 15 patients with Type 2 diabetes, compared with 10 controls.

In a related study, 900 IU/day of vitamin E for 3 months, given to 25 elderly diabetics, showed significant declines in plasma levels of hemoglobin A1C, triglycerides, total cholesterol, low-density lipoprotein cholesterol (LDL, the bad kind), and apolipoprotein-b, a risk factor for ischemic heart disease.

Glycosylated hemoglobin forms when sugar becomes attached to hemoglobin molecules, according to Robert H. Phillips, Ph.D. The more glucose (sugar) in the blood, the more hemoglobin becomes glycosylated. Hemoglobin is the iron-containing pigment in red blood cells. The hemoglobin molecules remain glycosylated until the blood cells die, which is normally about three months. Blood glucose levels are monitored with the glycosylated hemoglobin test, which measures the amounts of glycosylated hemoglobin, also called hemoglobin A1C, Phillips added.[3]

In an address at Washington State University at Spokane, Daniel Baker, Pharm.D., reported that glycosylated proteins and hemoglobin A1C decreased significantly in a group of diabetics given vitamin E. Those receiving 1,200 mg/day of the vitamin had the greatest reduction in glycosylated proteins and hemoglobin A1C. These findings suggest that the vitamin may be useful in preventing diabetic complications. Vitamin E may also keep platelets from sticking together, which can cause coronary disease. It may also help to prevent cataracts, Baker said. (Researchers often list vitamin E in milligrams or international units; the two have similar potencies.)[4]

Usually only a small amount of hemoglobin is glycosylated, but in poorly controlled diabetes, the level of glycosylated hemoglobin (hemoglobin A1C) is much higher, perhaps 9 to 12% more. A high reading suggests that blood glucose has been elevated over the previous month or six weeks. If the reading is in the normal range, it usually means that blood glucose has been normal during that same period. Constant self-monitoring, along with periodic measurements of hemoglobin A1C, are important in achieving overall control of diabetes.[5]

At the LSU Medical Center, Shreveport, Louisiana, Sushil K. Jain, Ph.D., supplemented 35 diabetic patients with either 100 IU/day of vitamin E or a placebo for 3 months. Results of this double-blind study showed that vitamin E lowered glycosylated hemoglobin, glucose, and triglycerides after vitamin E was given, when contrasted to before the vitamin was administered. Jain said that this amount of vitamin E significantly lowered glycosylated hemoglobin and triglyceride levels, but that it does not have any effect on red cell indices in Type 1 diabetics.[6]

Diabetics develop cardiovascular disease at an earlier age than do nondiabetics. In one study, researchers measured free radical and inflammatory activity in 75 volunteers, consisting of 25 Type 2 diabetics with cardiovascular disease, 25 Type 2 diabetics without this complication, and 25 healthy controls. The markers for inflammation included elevated levels of interleukin-lb and white blood cell stickiness, which contributes to inflammation.[7]

Following 3 months of supplementation with 1,200 IU/day of vitamin E, the diabetics were measured for free-radical and inflammatory activity. All diabetics had higher levels of free radicals and indicators of inflammation when compared to the controls.

However, the vitamin not only reduced levels of free-radical oxidation of cholesterol among all volunteers, but also reduced indicators of inflammation in all three groups. The researchers added that excess inflammation is regarded as a leading risk factor for cardiovascular disease, and vitamin E is a safe and inexpensive means of controlling inflammation in many people, especially diabetics.

Vitamin E supplements are useful therapy for reducing oxidative stress and improving insulin activity in Type 2 diabetics, according to researchers at the University of Naples and the University of Udine in Italy. The study involved giving 10 healthy controls and 15 Type 2 diabetics 900 mg/day of vitamin E for 4 months.[8]

Writing in the *European Journal of Endocrinology*, Paolo Pozzilli, M.D., said that he and his research team at St. Bartholomew's Hospital Medical College in London, England, have found that vitamin E and nicotinamide (vitamin B_3) are both likely to be effective in preserving beta-cell function in recent Type 1 diabetics up to one year after diagnosis. Beta cells in the pancreas make and release insulin. Both vitamins have few adverse side effects, and because they may act at different levels in the process leading to beta-cell destruction, a combination of the two nutrients may be considered for future trials concerning the disease.[9]

As soon as a Type 1 diabetic is diagnosed with the disease, the researchers recommend that nicotinamide therapy be given. Vitamin E may also be beneficial, but before both vitamins are given, a trial using the two together must be performed. The suggested vitamin E dosage is 15 mg per kg of body weight, while the B_3 therapy is 25 mg/kg body weight.

An article in *Circulation* pointed out that diabetics suffer oxidative stress related to glucose levels. Since vitamin E is an antioxidant and free-radical scavenger, it can reduce oxidative stress and curb the blood-clotting effect of thromboxane B_2. Thromboxanes are several substances formed from endoperoxides that cause the constriction of vascular and bronchial smooth muscle and promote blood coagulation.[10]

In the study, researchers evaluated 85 diabetics and 85 healthy controls, measuring their levels of isoprostane, thromboxane B_2, and glucose.

Isoprostane is a by-product of free radical chemical reactions, and increased levels suggest oxidative stress. As we have seen, thromboxane B_2 promotes blood clots, while glucose is the typical marker of diabetes and diabetic control.

Ten of the diabetics were given 600 IU/day of vitamin E for 2 weeks. It was found that diabetics had higher levels of both isoprostane and thromboxane B_2 when compared to healthy controls. In addition, high isoprostane levels correlated with high blood sugar and thromboxane B_2 levels. Results showed that the volunteers taking vitamin E found declines of 37% in isoprostane levels and 43% in thromboxane B_2 levels.

In a study of 29 diabetics (mean age of 12.4 years) and 21 nondiabetics (mean age of 10.9 years), the red blood cells of diabetic patients had 21% higher malondialdehyde, which suggests fatty acid oxidation, and 15% lower glutathione concentrations than in the healthy volunteers.[11]

The volunteers were given 100 IU/day of vitamin E or a look-alike pill for 3 months. It was found that vitamin E in the red blood cells was significantly correlated with the glutathione concentrations in those cells. In fact, vitamin B supplements increased glutathione concentrations by 9%, and lowered malondialdehyde amounts by 23% and hemoglobin A1C by 16% in the red blood cells of the diabetics. Glutathione, an antioxidant, aids in the structure of red blood cell membranes, and it assists the enzyme glutathione peroxidase in inactivating hydrogen peroxide and oxidized fats that can damage cells.

Antioxidants, such as vitamin E, can reduce the risk of developing ischemic stroke, according to an article in *Archives of Neurology*. In the study, male smokers, ranging in age from 50 to 69, took 50 IU/day of vitamin E, 20 mg/day of beta-carotene (provitamin A), both vitamins, or a placebo daily for 3 years. While vitamin E supplements reduced the risk of ischemic stroke, they increased the risk of subarachnoid hemorrhage in men with high blood pressure. It had no effect on stroke increase in men with normal blood pressure. Arachnoid is a membrane in the brain and spinal cord.[12]

Vitamin E decreased the likelihood of ischemic stroke among those with high blood pressure and diabetes, but without elevating the risk of subarachnoid hemorrhage. Beta-carotene supplements seemed to increase the risk of ischemic stroke among men with greater alcohol intake.

It has been known for some time that the body's production of prostaglandin E2 (PGE2) increases with age and apparently contributes to the age-associated increase in coronary artery disease. PGE2 is produced by COX-2, an enzyme that plays an important role in promoting inflammation. While various analgesic drugs inhibit COX-2 levels or activity, they have potentially dangerous side effects, such as allergic reactions and liver damage.[13]

As reported in the *Journal of Nutrition,* peroxynitrite, a type of free radical, increases the production of PGE2. But in a study using laboratory mice, vitamin E quenched peroxynitrite, which, in turn, reduced COX-2 activity. Therefore, the research team said, vitamin E appears to reduce the risk of heart disease by preventing the oxidation of cholesterol, by reducing the risk of blood clots, and by reducing the production of inflammatory PGE2.

Writing in the *American Journal of Clinical Nutrition,* a research team headed by D. Manzella reported that many diabetics experience cardiac autonomic neuropathy, which is thought to result in an unbalanced communication inside the body's complex nervous system, and it may be related to low levels of antioxidants in the body.[14]

The researchers asked 50 Type 2 diabetics to take 600 mg/day of vitamin E (equivalent to 600 IU) or a placebo for 4 weeks. It was found that those taking vitamin E noted improvements in heart rates as well as decreased blood levels of insulin and glycosylated hemoglobin. The lower levels of insulin suggested a more efficient use of glucose, while the lower glycosylated hemoglobin indicated better control of diabetes. While this study was limited to diabetics, it suggests the existence of another mechanism by which the vitamin may reduce autonomic nervous system in patients with Type 2 diabetes.

Oxidative stress seems to be elevated in insulin resistance syndrome and diabetes. This stress may inactivate nitric oxide (NO) and bring an increased risk of hardening of the arteries. NO, a colorless gas that interacts between cells, is involved in the dilation of blood vessels and penile erection, and it may affect immune reactions and memory. A shortage or inactivation of nitric oxide may cause a buildup of plaque in the arteries and result in hardening of the arteries. However, an excess of nitric oxide, which is a free radical, is toxic to brain cells, and it is responsible for the often fatal drop in blood pressure following septic shock; its medical importance is still being investigated.[15]

Inflammation of blood vessels is considered a major risk factor in heart disease, and C-reactive protein (a beta-globulin in the serum of people with various inflammatory, degenerative, and tumor diseases) is emerging as a measure of such inflammation. However, vitamin E supplements can reduce some of the signs of inflammation, a research team reported in *Free Radical Biology & Medicine.*[16]

Researchers took measurements of C-reactive protein and interleukin-6 (another indicator of inflammation) in 72 patients. The study involved three groups: diabetics with cardiovascular disease, diabetics without cardiovascular disease, and healthy volunteers. Initial measurements revealed that the diabetics with cardiovascular disease had elevated C-reactive protein levels. The volunteers were then given 1,200 IU/day of natural vitamin E (d-alpha tocopherol) for 3 months.

Following vitamin E therapy, people in all three groups benefited from a 30% reduction in C-reactive protein levels and a reduction in interleukin-6 levels. These changes might reduce the risk of cardiovascular disease, the researchers said.

As reported in the *American Journal of Clinical Nutrition,* free-radical damage (oxidation) to LDL-cholesterol and VLDL-cholesterol is thought to be a key factor in the development of coronary artery disease. Researchers divided 44 Type 1 diabetics into two groups: one group was given 750 IU/day of natural vitamin E for 1 year; the other group received a placebo for 6 months, followed by 750 IU/day of vitamin E for another 6 months.[17]

The research team found that all of the diabetics' blood showed that, after vitamin E supplementation, LDL and VLDL cholesterol were far more resistant to oxidative damage and there were fewer indicators of free-radical damage. There was no improvement when volunteers received a look-alike pill.

It was agreed that while various factors influence the early development of coronary artery disease, natural vitamin E reduces free-radical damage to LDL and VLDL cholesterol among diabetics, a change in turn that might reduce the risk of heart disease. Because the improvement in lipoprotein peroxidizability is reversible, lifelong supplementation with vitamin E should be considered in patients with Type 1 diabetes, the researchers said.

Reporting in *Current Opinion in Lipidology,* three prominent vitamin E researchers analyzed data from five clinical trials of vitamin E and heart disease. They reported that four of the five studies showed that vitamin E supplements, in dosages ranging from 50 to 800 IU/day, had significant benefits in reducing the risk of heart attacks in those with pre-existing heart disease.[18]

For example, one study found that the risk of nonfatal heart attack was lowered by 38%. In another study, nonfatal heart attacks were reduced by 77%. In one study, the vitamin reduced deaths from heart attacks by 20%, while in another study, vitamin E reduced the risk of a heart attack by 70%. The fifth study found no benefit from vitamin E, but that study had a number of design defects. The researchers said that high doses of the vitamin did not appear to increase the risk of hemorrhagic (bleeding) strokes.

Age-related macular degeneration is probably due to increased levels of oxidative stress, according to Jeffrey Blumberg, Ph.D., of Tufts University, USDA Human Nutrition Research Center on Aging, Boston. An increase in vitamin E supplementation, carotenoids, vitamin C, and selenium can significantly lower the risk of this complicated eye problem.[19]

An 8-month, double-blind study involved 36 Type 1 diabetics who had had diabetes for less than 10 years, and 9 nondiabetics, ranging in age from 18 to 45. The test group was given 1,800 IU/day of vitamin E or a placebo for 4 months, and then the volunteers' protocols were reversed for an additional 4 months. The researchers found that the vitamin normalized retinal function and improved kidney function in Type 1 diabetics who had had the disease for a short time. The research team added that vitamin E may be beneficial in reducing the risk of diabetic retinopathy and nephropathy; in other words, eye and kidney disease.[20]

At a small-town hospital in Pennsylvania, a nurse reported on the case of a 59-year-old woman with diabetes who was admitted with ulceration of her right foot. She had not received any medication prior to admittance. The doctors immediately gave her insulin and 800 IU/day of natural vitamin E. Then they packed the ulcerated area with cotton saturated with vitamin E. Two months later all wounds had healed.[21]

In various issues of *The Summary*, the Shute Brothers (Evan and Wilfrid, both doctors) described the value of vitamin E in treating gangrene, in which diabetics often have to have a foot or leg amputated. They reported that A. J. DeLiz, M.D., of New York, was faced with treating 20 schizophrenic patients, all of whom were suffering from circulatory problems in their feet and legs. All were diabetic, and 3 had gangrene. He began by giving the patients 20 capsules daily of vitamin E (100 IU), and later increased the dosage to 40 capsules. Four months later all of the patients were without leg pains.[22]

A Hungarian physician, F. Gerloczy, reported "spectacular" results using vitamin E to treat 10 cases of thrombosis of the arteries, 16 cases of thrombophlebitis, and 12 out of 15 cases of Buerger's disease (inflammation of blood vessels). He gave the vitamin in enormous doses, up to 24,000 IU daily. Not all cases were successful, but a patient who had had a leg ulcer for 20 years was completely healed after 6 weeks with vitamin E supplements plus vitamin E rubbed on the skin.[23]

Another case involved a 53-year-old diabetic who had a perforating ulcer on his foot. It was dark purple, the color of a gangrenous foot. On 375 IU/day of vitamin E, he healed completely in 71 days, and within several months his insulin requirement had decreased to about one-third of what it had been, and he returned to work.[24]

References

l. Atkins, Robert C., M.D. *Dr. Atkins' Vita-Nutrient Solution.* New York: Simon & Schuster, 1999, pp. 108–109.

2. "Diabetes and Vitamin E," *Diabetes* 44(2), February 1995.

3. Phillips, Robert H., Ph.D. *Coping With Diabetes.* New York: Avery/Penguin-Putnam, 2000, p. 24.

4. Baker, Daniel, Pharm.D., and R. Keith Campbell. "Vitamin and Mineral Supplementation in Patients with Diabetes Mellitus," *Diabetes Educator* 18(5):420–427, Sept./Oct. 1992.

5. Tapley, Donald F., M.D. et al. *The Columbia University College of Physicians and Surgeons Complete Home Medical Guide.* New York: Crown, 1985, pp. 1493–1494.

6. Jain, Sushil K., Ph.D., et al. "Effect of Modest Vitamin E Supplementation on Blood Glycolated Hemoglobin and Triglyceride Levels and Red Cell Indices in Type 1 Diabetic Patients," *Journal of the American College of Nutrition* 15(5):1458–1461, 1996.

7. Devaraj, S., et al. "Low-Density Lipoprotein Postsecretory Modification, Monocyte Function and Circulating Adhesion Molecules in Type 2 Diabetic Patients with and without Macrovascular Complications: The Effect of Alpha-Tocopherol Supplementation," *Circulation* 102:191–196, 2000.

8. Paolisso, G., et al. "Pharmacologic Doses of Vitamin E Improve Insulin Action in Healthy Subjects and in Non-Insulin-Dependent Diabetic Patients," *American Journal of Clinical Nutrition* 57:650–656, 1993.

9. Hamilton, Kirk. "Insulin Dependent Diabetes Mellitus, Vitamin E and Nicotinamide." *Clinical Pearls with the Experts Speak.* Sacramento, Calif.: I. T. Services, 1997, p. 315. Also, Pozzillini, Paolo, M.D. "Vitamin E and Nicotinamide Have Similar Effects in Maintaining Residual Beta Cell Function in Recent Onset Insulin-Dependent Diabetes," *European Journal of Endocrinology* 137:234–239, 1997.

10. Davi, G., et al. "In Vivo Formation of 8-iso-prostaglandin E2 Alpha and Platelet Activation in Diabetes Mellitus," *Circulation* 99:224–229, 1999.

11. Jain, S. K., et al. "Vitamin E Supplementation Restores Glutathione and Malondialdehyde to Normal Concentrations in Erythrocytes of Type 1 Diabetic Children," *Diabetes Care* 23(9):1389–1394, Sept. 2000.

12. Leppala, J. M., et al. "Vitamin E and Beta-Carotene Supplementation in High Risk of Stroke," *Archives of Neurology* 57:1503–l509, 2000.

13. Wu, D., et al, "Vitamin E and Macrophage Cyclooxygenase Regulation in the Aged," *Journal of Nutrition* 131:3825–3885, 2001.

14. Manzella, D., et al. "Chronic Administration of Pharmacologic Doses of Vitamin E Improves the Cardiac Autonomic Nerve System in Patients with Type 2 Diabetes," *American Journal of Clinical Nutrition* 73:1052–1057, 2001.

l5. *Stedman's Medical Dictionary,* 26th edition. Baltimore, Md.: Williams & Wilkins, 1995, p. 1211.

16. Devaraj, S., et al. "Alpha Tocopherol Supplementation Decreases Serum C-Reactive Protein and Monocyte Interleukin-6 in Normal Volunteers and Type 2 Diabetic Patients," *Free Radical Biology and Medicine* 29:790–792, 2000.

17. Engelen, W., et al. "Effects of Long-Term Supplementation with Moderate Pharmacologic Doses of Vitamin E Are Saturable and Reversible in Patients with Type 1 Diabetes," *American Journal of Clinical Nutrition* 72:1142–1149, 2000.

18. Jialal, I., et al. "Is There a Vitamin E Paradox?" *Current Opinion in Lipidology* 12:49–53, 2001.

19. Blumberg, Jeffrey, Ph.D. "The Requirement for Vitamins and Aging and Age-Associated Degenerative Conditions," *Vitamin Intake in Human Nutrition* 52:108–115, 1995.

20. Bursell, S. E., et al, "High Dose Vitamin Supplementation Normalizes Retinal Blood Flow and Creatine Clearance in Patients with Type 1 Diabetes," *Diabetes Care* 22:1215–1251, 1999.

21. Adams, Ruth, and Frank Murray. *Improving Your Health with Vitamin E.* New York: Larchmont Books, 1978, p. 122.

22. Ibid., p. 19.

23. Ibid., pp. 19–20.

24. Ibid., p. 120.

33 Chromium

In numerous studies, the mineral chromium has improved insulin sensitivity without significant changes in body fat. Symptoms of chromium deficiency include impaired glucose tolerance, low blood sugar, high levels of sugar in the blood, glucose in the urine, neuropathy, and other conditions. Low levels of the mineral in the blood are associated with diabetes, cataracts, and cardiovascular disease. Doses of up to 1,000 mcg/day have been used in laboratory and research studies with few, if any, side effects. Chromium has been shown to lower insulin requirements by at least 30%.

Chromium is a critical component of glucose tolerance factor (GTF), which contains niacin, glycine, glutamic acid, cysteine, and chromium. Animal studies have found that a deficiency in chromium brings glucose intolerance, and it may also facilitate the binding of insulin to the cell membrane. GTF is a compound that helps insulin to transport glucose from the blood to the cells.[1]

Writing in *Diabetes and Metabolism*, Richard A. Anderson, Ph.D., said that in a double-blind study involving 29 Type 2 diabetics 1,000 mcg/day of chromium improved insulin sensitivity without significant changes in body fat. Also, in 48 Type 1 diabetics and 114 Type 2 diabetics, Type 1 diabetics *reduced their insulin dosage* by 30%, and their blood sugar variations were considerably smaller after 10 days of supplemental chromium picolinate at 200 mcg/day.

He added that 200 mcg of chromium picolinate three times daily reduced glycosylated hemoglobin from 11.3% to 7.9% after 3 months of supplementation in a 28-year-old woman who had had Type 1 diabetes for 18 years. In another study, which involved supplementation with 250 mcg/day of chromium chloride, 25 diabetics with hardening of the arteries saw improvements in high-density lipoprotein cholesterol (HDL, the good kind) and triglycerides following 6 months of supplementation.[2]

Anderson said that in studies that have shown no beneficial effects using chromium, the dosages were usually 200 mcg or less, which is not adequate for those with diabetes, especially if it is in a form with low absorption. In another study, Anderson said that 30 women with gestational diabetes, between 20 and 24 weeks of gestation, were divided into three groups. Each was given 0.4 or 8 mcg of chromium per kilogram of body weight for 8 weeks or a placebo. Chromium supplements enhanced glucose tolerance and lowered hyperglycemia (high levels of glucose in the blood); the higher dosage was the most beneficial. Steroid-induced diabetes was held in check in 47 of 50 volunteers who were given 200 mcg of chromium picolinate three times a day. Secondary diabetes, which is relatively rare, occurs when steroids and other medications damage the pancreas.

At a meeting of the Federation of American Societies for Experimental Biology in New Orleans in 1989, Gary W. Evans, Ph.D., and his colleagues, Raymond I. Press, M.D., and Jack Geller, M.D., of the Mercy Hospital Medical Center, San Diego, California, discussed a double-blind study involving chromium picolinate. The study involved 11 diabetics who were not taking insulin, who were given 200 mcg/day of chromium or a placebo for 42 days. While on the mineral, the volunteers' fasting blood glucose, glycosylated hemoglobin, total cholesterol, and low-density lipoprotein cholesterol (LDL, the bad kind) dropped considerably.

Eight of the 11 patients reported a positive response to the mineral. Their blood glucose range went down by 24%; glycosylated hemoglobin dropped by 19%; total cholesterol went down 13%; and LDL-cholesterol dropped 11%.[3]

Chromium is a critical component of glucose tolerance factor (GTF), which contains niacin, glycine, glutamic acid, cysteine, and chromium. Animal studies have found that a deficiency in chromium brings glucose intolerance, and it may also facilitate the binding of insulin to the cell membrane.

"Most chromium is removed from grains when they are refined," states the *Nutrition Desk Reference.* "Low chromium levels in a highly refined diet, combined with an increased intake of sugars and other processed carbo-hydrates that require chromium for metabolism, might predispose some individuals to a chromium deficiency and aggravate adult-onset diabetes."

Writing in the *Journal of Nutrition*, Walter Mertz, Ph.D., said that thirty-five years of research has shown that chromium plays a significant role in the progression of glucose intolerance and the increased risk of developing diabetes and car-diovascular disease. In thirteen of fifteen stud-ies, evaluating chromium supplementation's effect on glucose tolerance shows benefits by maintaining glucose levels that produced less insulin. He added that monitoring the effects of glucose tolerance is the only way to discover if there is a chromium deficiency.[4]

A chromium deficiency results in insulin resistance, which can therefore improve with chromium supplementation. Marginal deficien-cies of chromium are common in the United States and other countries, and this is a major cause of insulin resistance in many populations. Mertz insists that insulin resistance is a signifi-cant risk factor for cardiovascular disease and may be more important in the cause of cardio-vascular disease than the role of LDL-cholesterol. Since chromium deficiency is difficult to detect, many physicians ignore the potential benefits of chromium supplementation.

"Most chromium is removed from grains when they are refined," states the Nutrition Desk Reference. *"Low chromium levels in a highly refined diet, combined with an increased intake of sugars and other processed carbohydrates that require chromium for metabolism, might predispose some individuals to a chromium deficiency and aggravate adult-onset diabetes."*

In a study in Beijing, China, 188 volunteers with Type 2 diabetes, between the ages of 35 and 55, with hemoglobin A1C values of 8 to 12%, were given either a placebo, low-dose chromium (200 mcg/day), or high-dose chromium (1,000 mcg/day) for 4 months. The researchers reported that hemoglobin A1C values went down significantly in the high-dose group at 2 months, and in both supplemented groups at 4 months when compared to controls. Fasting blood glucose was lower at 2 and 4 months in the high-dose group, but not significantly in the low-dose group and placebo group.

The researchers also found that fasting insulin amounts fell signifi-cantly in the chromium-supplemented volunteers, as did the 2-hour oral glucose tolerance insulin values. Fasting and 2-hour insulin values also went down in the placebo group, but not significantly.[5]

In another study, Chinese volunteers with Type 2 diabetes were divided into three groups of 60 each and given a placebo, 100 mcg, or 500 mcg of chromium picolinate twice daily for 4 months. Researchers at the U.S. Department of Agriculture in Beltsville, Maryland, reported that improvements in the glucose/insulin ratio were very significant in those given 500 mcg of the mineral twice daily, with less or no improvement in those given 100 mcg twice daily after 2 and 4 months. The mineral improves insulin binding, insulin receptor number, insulin internalization, beta-cell sensitivity, and insulin receptor enzymes, with an overall increase in insulin sensitivity, researchers concluded.[6]

Based on another study involving the U.S. Department of Agriculture, Richard A. Anderson, Ph.D., and colleagues, recommend that those with Type 2 diabetes, impaired glucose tolerance, or hyperlipidemia (high levels of fats in the blood) take 400 to 600 mcg/day of chromium.

In one study, Anderson and colleagues gave 200 mcg/day, 1,000 mcg/day of chromium or a placebo to 180 Type 2 diabetics. They found that, after 2 months, glycosylated hemoglobin improved significantly in the high-dose chromium group. After 4 months of therapy, there was a significant improvement in both chromium groups concerning glycosylated hemoglobin, with an average of 6.6% in the high-dose group, 7.5% in the low-dose group and 8.5% in the placebo group. In addition, high-doses of the mineral improved fasting and 20-hour after-eating glucose values after 2 to 4 months. Total cholesterol went down after 4 months. Both groups taking the mineral had reductions in fasting and 2-hour after-eating insulin levels after 2 and 4 months. No side effects were reported.[7]

Chromium supplements enhance glucose tolerance and the usual symptoms of low blood sugar, reported Jorgen Clausen, M.D., of the Institute for Life Sciences and Chemistry, Roskilde University in Denmark. In the study, 20 hypoglycemic volunteers were given 125 mcg/day of chromium in the form of yeast. During the treatment period, glucose tolerance improved in 40% of the patients. Following 1 month of treatment, glucose tolerance was improved in 72% of the patients. The volunteers also reported improvement in symptoms of chilliness (47%) and disappearance of chilliness entirely (15%). Clausen reported that in all patients, 50 to 90% of the typical symptoms of low blood sugar improved, such as trembling, emotional instability, and disorientation.[8]

At Academia Sinica in Beijing, China, researchers determined that elderly diabetics probably lack chromium and that it is lost and excreted in an increasing amount with aging. The study involved 57 diabetics, compared with 55 healthy fasting controls. Chromium amounts in the blood and urine for the diabetics were 0.22 to 0.36 mcg/dl and 4.54 to 5.90 mcg/dl in the two groups studied; there was significantly lower than 0.66 to 0.84 mcg/dl and 7.80 to 9.68 mcg/dl in the two groups of healthy controls. Chromium levels in female diabetics were significantly higher than in the males.[9]

The estimated safe dietary level of chromium is between 50 and 200 mcg/day; however, most diets contain less than 60% of the suggested minimum intake of 50 mcg/day, according to Richard A. Anderson, Ph.D. Doses of up to 1,000 mcg/day have been used in supplements in laboratory work without toxicity, he said. Chromium losses in the urine include daily stresses such as chronic exercise, high sugar diets, lactation, and physical trauma.[10]

Joeffrey Gordon, M.D., a San Diego, California researcher, reported that taking chromium picolinate lowers total cholesterol, LDL-cholesterol, and triglycerides, as well as improving the LDL-HDL ratio. He determined this by treating 10 patients with high cholesterol levels, using 200 mcg/day of chromium picolinate, 1 to 2 g/day of niacin, along with dietary suggestions.

After 4 weeks of therapy, total cholesterol levels had gone down from 301 mg/dl to 229 mg/dl (a drop of 29%), LDL-cholesterol decreased from 219 mg/dl to 160 mg/dl (a decrease of 27%), and triglyceride levels dropped from 158 mg/dl to 90 mg/dl (a decrease of 43%). HDL-cholesterol in the blood remained unchanged, but there was a substantial improvement in the LDL-HDL ratio. He did not evaluate the effect of niacin.[11]

Chromium may be a secondary factor in the further progression of cataract changes in the lens of diabetics, according to researchers in Nantes, France. These observations came after evaluating the chromium concentrations in 61 human lenses and 38 blood samples. An analysis of chromium in a human lens shows a significant difference between elderly and diabetic populations, the researchers said. The mean chromium concentrations in diabetic cataracts was 0.137 compared to 0.345 in the normal population.[12]

In an Israeli study involving Type 2 diabetics, it was reported that almost half of the volunteers were able to reduce dosages of their antidiabetic medication after chromium supplements were given. Diabetics whose glucose levels are not well controlled with traditional medications may benefit from 300 to 1,000 mcg/day of chromium picolinate added to their dietary regimen, according to an article in *Hospital Practice*. Note that it takes about four hours for the mineral to become effective. The research team said that the best food sources of the mineral include meat, cheese, whole grains, brewer's yeast, liver, wheat germ, spinach, apples, potatoes, and carrots.[13]

In a double-blind study, 29 male and female volunteers, who were at a high risk for developing Type 2 diabetes, were given either 1,000 mcg/day of chromium picolinate or a placebo for 8 months, reported a research team from the University of Vermont College of Medicine at Burlington. The results showed that the mineral significantly improved the action of insulin in those who had a family history of Type 2 diabetes. This suggested a direct effect on chromium picolinate on muscle insulin action.[14]

Reporting in *Diabetes*, David F. Horrobin, Ph.D., said that those with diabetes should take a full range of nutritional supplements, especially chromium, vitamin C, vitamin B$_6$, zinc, and alpha-lipoic acid.[15]

It is known that there are alterations of tissue concentrations of specific minerals in diabetic patients, according to S. Bhanot, M.D., of the University of British Columbia, Vancouver, Canada. As a general rule, all diabetics tend to have low magnesium stores and high amounts of zinc in the blood, among other things. Type 2 diabetics tend to be deficient in chromium, either as a cause or result of their condition. Since chromium potentiates insulin's action, diabetics can benefit from chromium supplementation, Bhanot said.[16]

The beneficial effects of barley on blood glucose and water consumption in diabetics, mentioned earlier in the book, might be attributed to its high chromium content, according to a study at King's College in London, England. Barley is often used in Iraq to treat diabetes because of its ability to modulate glycemic response to the ingestion of carbohydrates, as well as to inhibit weight loss and excessive water consumption. Barley contains about 5.69 mcg of chromium per gram. In the study, diabetic rats were fed a diet containing barley, starch, or sucrose. Only the barley-supplemented diet resulted in improved diabetic parameters.[17]

References

1. Garrison, Robert, Jr., M.A., R.Ph., and Elizabeth Somer, M.A., R.D. *The Nutrition Desk Reference*. New Canaan, Conn.: Keats Publishing, 1995, pp. 183–184.

2. Anderson, Richard A., Ph.D. "Chromium in the Prevention and Control of Diabetes," *Diabetes and Metabolism* (Paris) 26(1): 22–27, 2000.

3. Press, Raymond I., M.D., et al. "The Effect of Chromium Picolinate on Serum Glucose, Glycosylated Hemoglobin and Cholesterol of Adult Onset Diabetics." Paper read

at a meeting of the Federation of American Societies for Experimental Biology, New Orleans, Louisiana, March 21, 1989.

4. Mertz, Walter, Ph.D. "Chromium in Human Nutrition: A Review," *Journal of Nutrition* 123: 626–633, 1993.

5. Hellerstein, M. K. "Is Chromium Supplementation Effective in Managing Type 2 Diabetes?" *Nutrition Reviews* 56(10): 302–306, 1998.

6. Anderson, Richard A., Ph.D. "Nutritional Factors Influencing the Glucose/Insulin System: Chromium," *Journal of the American College of Nutrition* 16(5): 404–410, 1997.

7. Baker, Barbara. "Chromium Supplements Tied to Glucose Control," *Family Practice News,* July 15, 1996, p. 5.

8. Clausen, Jorgen, M.D. "Chromium Induced Clinical Improvement in Symptomatic Hypoglycemia," *Biological Trace Element Research* 17: 229–236, 1988.

9. Ding, W., et al. "Serum and Urine Chromium Concentrations in Elderly Diabetics," *Biological Trace Element Research* 63: 231–237, 1998.

10. Anderson, Richard A., Ph.D. "Chromium As An Essential Nutrient for Humans," *Regulatory Toxicology and Pharmacology* 26: S35–S41, 1997.

11. Gordon, J. "An Easy and Inexpensive Way to Lower Cholesterol," *Western Journal of Medicine* 154: 3, 1991.

12. Pineau, A., et al. "A Study of Chromium and Human Cataractous Lenses and Whole Blood of Diabetic, Senile and Normal Populations," *Biological Trace Element Research* 32: 133–138, 1992.

13. Kuritzky, L., et al. "Improving Management of Type 2 Diabetes Mellitus: Chromium," *Hospital Practice,* Feb. 15, 2000, pp. 113–116.

14. Cefalu, W. T., et al. "Effect of Chromium Picolinate on Insulin Sensitivity In Vivo," *Journal of Trace Elements and Experimental Medicine* 12: 71–83, 1999.

15. Horrobin, David F., Ph.D. "Essential Fatty Acids in the Management of Impaired Nerve Function in Diabetes," *Diabetes* 46(Suppl. 2): S90–S93, 1997.

16. Bhanot, S., M.D. "Essential Trace Elements of Potential Importance in Nutritional Management of Diabetes Mellitus," *Nutrition Research* 14(4): 593–604, 1994.

17. Mahdi, G., et al. "Role of Chromium in Barley in Modulating the Symptoms of Diabetes," *Annals of Nutrition and Metabolism* 35: 65–70, 1991.

34 Magnesium

Approximately three-fourths of the U.S. population has a magnesium deficiency. Such a deficiency is related to diabetes, irregular heartbeat, heart attack, hardening of the arteries, high blood pressure, migraine headaches, toxemia of pregnancy, kidney stones, and other life-threatening situations.

Low magnesium levels, along with elevated calcium in the blood, increase the possibility of blood clots, which have been implicated in the development of diabetes, heart attack, and eclampsia, or the convulsions during pregnancy.

At a meeting of the American Diabetes Association, it was reported that low blood levels of magnesium may be a strong predictor of Type 2 diabetes in Caucasians. A magnesium deficiency is prominent in patients with diabetes, according to Robert K. Rude, M.D. This association has been known since 1946. For diabetics with a magnesium deficiency, oral doses of 300 mg/day are often recommended, although that dosage may need to be increased to 600 mg/day.

As reported in Diabetologia, *magnesium supplements can improve beta-cell response and insulin action in Type 1 diabetics. Suggested daily intakes range from 240 to 480 mg.*

Magnesium is a co-factor in more than 300 enzymatic reactions, yet three-fourths of the U.S. population may have a dietary magnesium deficiency, according to Burton M. Altura, Ph.D., State University of New York Health Sciences Center, Brooklyn College of Medicine, New York. Even more problematic is the fact that it is possible to have a normal blood level of the mineral and still have a total body deficit, he said.

A magnesium deficiency is difficult to assess; however, two relatively new techniques may improve our understanding of a magnesium deficiency. These are the ion-selective electrode and nuclear magnetic resonance spectroscopy. This is important because a magnesium deficiency is related to arrhythmias, heart attacks, hardening of the arteries, high blood pressure, diabetes mellitus, migraine headaches, toxemia of pregnancy, and kidney stones, among others.[1]

A magnesium deficiency is often related to lack of the mineral in the diet, malabsorption of the mineral, or expelling of magnesium by the kidneys due to drugs or genetic factors, states Altura. Fifty-five percent of magnesium in the blood is ionized (converted to other ions), compared to 33% that is bound to protein. It is important for magnesium stores to be evaluated in alcoholics, diabetics, patients with cardiovascular disease, those on long-term diuretics (substances that increase urination) or digitalis, and women who are pregnant or breast-feeding.

Low magnesium levels with elevated calcium increase the stick-togetherness of platelets and blood clots, which have been implicated in the development of diabetes, heart attack, and eclampsia (convulsions during pregnancy), according to Mildred S. Seelig, M.D. Low magnesium levels can increase the release of thromboxane, one of a number of substances which can cause blood clots.[2]

Researchers at the University of Texas Southwestern Medical Center at Dallas evaluated 1,089 pregnant women who were given phenytoin (Dilantin) for eclamptic convulsions, compared to 1,049 women who received magnesium sulfate. Preeclampsia is a potentially serious complication of pregnancy, which often develops after the twenty-eighth week of pregnancy. Its most serious form (eclampsia) may bring on seizures and coma, which endanger both mother and fetus. Early symptoms include excessive fluid retention, an abnormal rise in blood pressure, and protein in the urine. It is theorized that magnesium sulfate may not act as an anticonvulsant but serve as a vasodilator and subsequent reaction of cerebral ischemia.

The research team found that 10 of the women given the drug had convulsions compared to none getting the mineral. The magnesium therapy consisted of an initial 10 g dose of 50% magnesium sulfate given intramuscularly, then a maintenance dose of 5 g every 4 hours. For the pregnant women with severe preeclampsia, an additional 4 g initial dose was administered intravenously. The Dilantin regimen consisted of an initial 1,000 mg dose infused over 1 hour, and then a 500 mg oral dose 10 hours later.[3] With each regimen, the anticonvulsive procedures were continued for 24 hours postpartum. The researchers concluded that magnesium sulfate is superior to Dilantin in preventing eclampsia in pregnant women with high blood pressure.

At a meeting of the American Diabetes Association in 1997, it was reported that low blood levels of magnesium may be a strong *predictor* of Type 2 diabetes in white individuals. While studying blood levels of the mineral in 12,398 nondiabetic, middle-aged African-American and white volunteers over a 6-year period, there was no association between magnesium levels and the development of diabetes in African-Americans, but there was one in the whites.[4]

At the conclusion of the study, there were 807 new cases of Type 2 diabetes in the whites, with the largest increase in risk for Type 2 diabetes (94%) associated with those who had the lowest levels of magnesium in the blood. Magnesium deficiency can adversely affect insulin metabolism, according to researchers from Johns Hopkins University in Baltimore, Maryland.

In evaluating 26 fasting, nonpregnant females, 20 normal pregnant females, and 13 diet-controlled gestational diabetic women, Mordechai Berdicef, M.D., said that, compared with nonpregnant controls, total and ionized magnesium were considerably lower in both normal pregnant and gestational diabetic women. Also, gestational diabetic women had significantly lower intracellular magnesium values when compared with nonpregnant and normal pregnant volunteers. Ionized calcium rates were similar in all groups, which resulted in significant elevation of ionized calcium/magnesium ratios in both pregnant groups.

These results confirm magnesium depletion as a factor in pregnancy and in gestational diabetes. The research team concluded that magnesium depletion, or calcium excess, may predispose one to vascular complications in pregnancy.[5] (Researchers usually recommend a 2:1 ratio of calcium to magnesium—if 800 mg of calcium, then 400 mg of magnesium. However, in some instances, other researchers have recommended a 1:1 ratio.)

A magnesium deficiency is prominent in patients with diabetes mellitus, according to Robert K. Rude, M.D. This can result in an increased risk for cardiac arrhythmia, hypertension, heart attack, and altered glucose metabolism. Actually, this association between low magnesium levels and diabetes has been known since 1946. For those patients with a magnesium deficiency, oral doses of 300 mg/day can be given, but the doses may have to be increased to 600 mg/day to achieve the desired therapeutic effect. To avoid diarrhea, a complication in susceptible individuals, Rude recommends the mineral be taken in divided doses. For those with impaired kidney function, magnesium therapy should be reviewed by their doctor.[6]

In evaluating 6,781 deaths in Taiwan from diabetes mellitus from 1990 to 1994, compared with 6,781 deaths from other causes, Chun-Y Yang, Ph.D., and colleagues said that there was a significant protective effect of magnesium in drinking water and the risk of dying from diabetes.[7] (It has long been known that people who live in areas with hard water—which is rich in minerals—are often protected from heart disease.)

Researchers at Uppsala University Children's Hospital in Sweden reported that diabetic children have a chronic magnesium deficiency and insufficient liver synthesis of certain proteins in the blood. Their conclusions came after evaluating 34 children who were followed for 5 years from the onset of their diabetes. During that time, magnesium levels in their blood decreased to significantly lower levels than those in matched controls after 2 and 5 years. However, zinc levels in the blood were higher in the diabetic children than in the controls. The diabetics had slightly reduced amounts of serum albumin.[8]

Low blood levels of magnesium are found in about 25% of diabetic patients, according to Lorraine Tosiello, M.D., of Overlook Hospital in Summit, New Jersey. Also, low levels of the mineral have been chronicled in childhood insulin-dependent diabetics and in adults with Type 1 and Type 2 diabetes. Low levels of magnesium are associated with insulin resistance in nondiabetic elderly patients. Tosiello noted that a magnesium deficiency is related to gastrointestinal loss of the mineral, excess excretion by the kidneys, nutritional deficiencies, endocrine disorders (internal secretions), redistribution problems and chronic alcoholism, alcoholism withdrawal, major burns, and liquid protein diets.[9]

At Thomas Jefferson University, Philadelphia, J. Caddell said that infants with respiratory distress syndrome and SIDS (sudden infant death syndrome) are at high risk for magnesium deficiency because of premature birth, and because many times they are infants of adolescent diabetic mothers, who are at risk of magnesium deficiency. That is because adolescent and fetal growth increase magnesium requirements. A magnesium deficiency brings increased clumping together of platelets and increased production of thromboxane A2, which can also cause platelets to stick together.[10]

Health problems associated with low levels of intracellular magnesium include high blood pressure and aging, which are also associated with insulin resistance, according to a team of researchers from the University of Naples in Italy. Low levels of magnesium are especially noted in patients with diabetes mellitus, which shows up as impaired insulin response in Type 2 diabetics.[11]

Magnesium supplements can improve beta-cell response and insulin action in insulin-dependent diabetics. Suggested daily intakes of the mineral are between 240 and 480 mg. Further, a magnesium deficiency may account for the atherosclerotic tendency in diabetics; that is, the development of hardening of the arteries. In patients given 3 g/day of magnesium supplements for 3 weeks, it was reported that these noninsulin-dependent diabetics showed improved glucose and arginine-induced insulin secretion along with insulin sensitivity.

In a study involving 7 Type 2 diabetics with high blood pressure and low blood levels of magnesium, the participants were given 260 mg twice daily for 6 weeks. The 7 volunteers without diabetes or high blood pressure received a placebo. The magnesium supplement increased blood levels of the mineral in the diabetic patients and led to a subsequent fall in blood pressure from an average of 157/96 mmHg to 128/77 mmHg. High blood pressure was controlled in the diabetics without medication, except for the magnesium. Platelets became less sticky and thromboxane was decreased. (In a healthy young adult, the systolic [beating] or highest pressure is recorded as 120 mm of mercury, and the diastolic [resting] or lowest reading is 80 mm of mercury. This is given as a blood pressure reading of 120/80.)

Jerry Nadler, M.D., notes that magnesium can be used by Type 2 hypertensive diabetics with normal kidney function, but those with abnormal kidney function should confer with their physician about using the mineral. He added that the effect of magnesium on Type 1 diabetics is not known.[12]

S. E. Browne, M.D., initially used magnesium sulfate intramuscularly and intravenously in his practice to treat patients with gangrene, leg ulcers, Raynaud's disease, chilblains, intermittent claudication, peripheral vascular disease, congestive heart failure, angina, myocardial infarction, and cerebrovascular disease. He reported that magnesium has a significant vasodilating effect (widening of blood vessels) and can result in considerable flushing after intravenous injections of 4 to 12 mmol (millimole, one-thousandths of a gram-molecule) of magnesium. It has excellent therapeutic results in all forms of arterial disease, he reported. This rapid infusion maintains a very high initial blood level of the mineral, and it produces significant results that cannot be obtained by oral or other means. Of 8 patients with leg ulcers, 5 healed quickly after failing to respond to other therapies, he said.[13]

Magnesium is essential for glucose balance, and it helps in glucose transport and regulates energy production in the liver. The mineral also is needed for the release of insulin and the maintenance of the pancreatic beta cells associated with insulin production and release. Magnesium deficiency not only contributes to the atrophy of beta cells, but also it increases the affinity and number of insulin receptors, according to *Diabetes Research and Clinical Practice*.[14] Insulin receptors are sites on cell walls that react to insulin, which allows the cell to open and let glucose in.

As mentioned, blood and tissue levels of magnesium are lower in diabetics, while the most frequent cause of low magnesium levels, other than acute ketoacidosis (sometimes called diabetic coma), is diabetes itself. The cause of a magnesium deficiency is complicated, but it includes increased urination with glucose in the urine, an opposite association between plasma magnesium and blood glucose, an under-secretion of insulin and adrenalin, modification of vitamin D metabolism, and a lack of vitamin B_6.

Magnesium supplements restore low blood and tissue levels, produces a protective effect against cardiovascular disease, and might aid in the prevention of vascular complications associated with diabetes, as well as in the development of the disease, the researchers said.

Magnesium deficiency occurs in about 11% of hospitalized patients and in 52% of patients in coronary care units, according to researchers at Northeastern Ohio Universities College of Medicine at Rootstown. Among diabetics, deficiency in the mineral ranges from 25% to 39%. Alcoholism, various drugs, and endocrine abnormalities can further contribute to the magnesium deficiency, they added.[15]

At the National Public Health Institute in Helsinki, Finland, Johan Eriksson, M.D., Ph.D., gave 56 diabetics 600 mg/day of magnesium for 90 days. In another 90-day study, 2,000 mg/day of vitamin C was given. He reported that there was a decrease in systolic and diastolic blood pressure in Type 1 diabetics given the mineral. And vitamin C improved glycemic control among Type 2 diabetics in both fasting blood glucose and hemoglobin A1C levels. Vitamin C also reduced cholesterol and triglyceride levels in Type 2 patients.[16] (Fasting blood glucose refers to the amount of blood sugar present after fasting for eight or more hours. Those with uncontrolled diabetes have fasting glucose readings of 126 mg/dl or

Top Food Sources of Magnesium

Nuts, whole grains, green leafy vegetables, meat, fish and seafood, poultry, dried fruit, chocolate and cottonseed, peanut and soybean flours.

higher. In those without diabetes, the reading is 70 to 115 mg/dl. Hemoglobin A1C is formed when glucose is attached to hemoglobin molecules. The amount registered is an indicator of blood sugar levels for the 8 to 12 weeks prior to taking this test.)

In a study involving 89 Type 2 diabetics and 31 volunteers without the disease, researchers in Japan found that low oxygen uptake in Type 2 diabetics was significantly correlated with plasma and red blood cell magnesium levels, but not with urinary excretion of the mineral. Uptake in this instance refers to the amount of oxygen absorbed by the tissues. A deficiency of the mineral in Type 2 diabetics may be related to environmental or genetic factors and may result in low oxygen uptake and decreased work capacity, they added.[17] Although not discussed in this study, oxygen delivered by the bloodstream is necessary for the muscles to oxidize blood sugar into carbon dioxide. This might explain the decreased work capacity due to fatigue.

In studying 12 Type 1 diabetics, compared with 12 healthy controls, researchers in Turkey found that red blood cell magnesium levels were much lower in the diabetics and that magnesium losses in the urine were elevated. The researchers found no correlation between urine magnesium concentrations and glycosylated hemoglobin or fasting plasma glucose levels.[18]

Magnesium supplements are available in a variety of formulations in health food stores and other outlets. The mineral is often combined with calcium and other minerals in supplements. The so-called Recommended Daily Allowance for the mineral is around 350 mg/day for men and 280 mg/day for women, but as we have seen, larger amounts may be prescribed by health care professionals for diabetes and other disorders.

References

1. Altura, Burton M., Ph.D., et al. "Magnesium Growing in Clinical Importance," *Patient Care,* Jan. 15, 1994, pp. 130–136.

2. Seelig, Mildred S., M.D., et al. "Low Magnesium: A Common Denominator in Pathologic Process in Diabetes Mellitus, Cardiovascular Disease and Eclampsia," *Journal of the American College of Nutrition* 11(5): 608/Abstract 39, Oct. 1992.

3. Lucas, Michael J., M.D., et al. "A Comparison of Magnesium Sulfate with Phenytoin for the Prevention of Eclampsia," *New England Journal of Medicine* 333(4): 201–205, July 27, 1995. Also, Duley, Lelia, and Richard Johanson. "Magnesium Sulfate for Preeclampsia and Eclampsia: The Evidence So Far," *British Journal of Obstetrics and Gynecology* 101: 565–567, July 1994.

4. Kahn, Jason. "Magnesium Levels May Predict Risk of Type 2 Disease in Whites," *Medical Tribune,* July 1997, p. 16.

5. Bardicef, Mordechai, M.D., et al. "Extracellular and Intracellular Magnesium Depletion in Pregnancy and Gestational Diabetes," *American Journal of Obstetrics and Gynecology* 172(3): 1009–1014, 1995.

6. Rude, Robert K., M.D. "Magnesium Deficiency and Diabetes Mellitus: Causes and Effects," *Postgraduate Medicine* 92(5): 217–223, 1992.

7. Yang, Chun-Y, Ph.D., et al. "Magnesium in Drinking Water and the Risk of Death from Diabetes Mellitus," *Magnes Res.* 12(2): 131–137, 1999.

8. Tuvemo, T., et al. "Serum Magnesium and Protein Concentrations During the First Five Years of Insulin-Dependent Diabetes in Children," *Acta Pediatrica*: Suppl. 418: 7–10, 1997.

9. Tosiello, Lorraine, M.D. "Hypomagnesemia and Diabetes Mellitus," *Archives of Internal Medicine* 156: 1143–1148, June 10, 1996.

10. Caddell, J. "Hypothesis: The Role of Magnesium Deficiency in Idiopathic Respiratory Syndrome of Prematurity (RDS); Links Between RDS and Sudden Infant Death Syndrome (SIDS)," *Journal of the American College of Nutrition* 11(5): 627/Abstract 102, Oct. 1992.

11. Paolisso, G., et al. "Magnesium and Glucose Homeostasis," *Diabetologia* 33: 501–514, 1990.

12. Nadler, Jerry, M.D. "Magnesium Lowers Blood Pressure in Type 2 Diabetes," *Practical Cardiology* 16(10): 4, October 1990.

13. Browne, S. E., MB. "The Case for Intravenous Magnesium Treatment of Arterial Disease in General Practice: Review of 34 Years of Experience," *Journal of Nutritional Medicine* 4: 169–177, 1994.

14. Elamin, A., and T. Tuveno. "Magnesium and Insulin-Dependent Diabetes Mellitus," *Diabetes Research and Clinical Practice* 10: 203–209, 1990.

15. Trehan, Shruti, M.D., et al. "Magnesium Disorders: What to Do When Homeostasis Goes Awry," *The Consultant,* November 1996, pp. 2485–2497.

16. Eriksson, Johan, M.D., Ph.D. "Magnesium and Ascorbic Acid Supplementation in Diabetes Mellitus," *Annals of Nutrition and Metabolism* 39: 217–223, 1995.

17. Kobayashi, T., et al. "Plasma and Erythrocyte Magnesium Levels Are Correlated with Oxygen Uptake in Patients with Non-Insulin-Dependent Diabetes Mellitus," *Endocrine Journal* 45(2): 277–283, 1998.

18. Guriek, A., et al. "Intracellular Magnesium Depletion Relates to Increased Urinary Magnesium Loss in Type 1 Diabetes," *Hormone and Metabolic Research* 30: 99–102, 1998.

35 Selenium

Selenium deficiencies are often difficult to detect because vitamin E and the sulfur-containing amino acids (cysteine and methionine) may act as partial substitutes for the mineral in some of its functions. The metabolic roles of selenium and vitamin E overlap, so that each nutrient may replace the other in helping to prevent cancer, cataract, heart disease, diseases of the liver, cardiovascular or muscular diseases, and aging.

The mineral stimulates the enzyme glutathione peroxidase, a powerful scavenger of free radicals, which can damage cells. Selenium deficiencies are often found in people who live in areas where there are low amounts of the mineral in the soils. In the U.S., the average daily intake of selenium is around 60 mcg/day. The suggested daily amount for adults is 50 to 200 mcg/day. Larger amounts need to be monitored by a physician.

When you take selenium, it is absorbed in the intestines, mostly in the duodenum, where it is bound to a protein and transported in the blood to the tissues. There it is incorporated into tissue protein as selenocysteine and selenomethionine. In the latter process, selenium replaces the sulfur in the amino acids cysteine and methionine. Most of the mineral is excreted in the kidneys, although smaller amounts exit via feces and sweat.[1]

"It is not surprising that deficiencies of selenium are sometimes hard to detect, because vitamin E and the sulfur-containing amino acids—

cysteine and methionine—may act as partial substitutes for the mineral in some of its functions," states the *Foods & Nutrition Encyclopedia*. "Other nutrients, such as fat and protein, may also affect the body's need for selenium."

The metabolic roles of selenium and vitamin E overlap, so that each nutrient may replace the other to a limited extent in preventing certain types of disorders, the encyclopedia continued. But there are also unique functions for each nutrient, so each must be supplied in the diet to ensure good nutrition. As reported by the National Research Council in Washington, D.C., selenium is involved in such human medical problems as cancer, cataract, diseases of the liver, and cardiovascular or muscular diseases, along with the aging process.

Some researchers have suggested that deficiencies of selenium and vitamin E might contribute to heart disease, since these nutrients help to maintain adequate levels of coenzyme Q in the heart muscle. If CoQ (specifically CoQ10) is lacking, the production of energy in the heart and other muscles may diminish so that these tissues can no longer carry their workloads. Death rates in the United States from heart disease have consistently been highest in the states with low selenium in the soils (Washington, Oregon, Michigan, Florida, Ohio, Indiana, New England states, and others).

The selenium content of the lens of the eye increases from birth to death, but it has been found that lenses with cataracts may contain less than one-sixth of the normal amounts of the mineral. Lack of selenium to activate the enzyme glutathione peroxidase may block the destruction of peroxides in the lens of the eye, such that these toxic substances may accumulate in sufficient amounts to damage the lens. As reported in the *Journal of Nutritional Medicine*, Joseph Bittner, M.D., said that, in 1977, he had reversed macular degeneration in two patients using intravenous injections of selenium and zinc. Improvements also were noted when the two minerals were taken orally. Vitamin E and taurine, the amino acid, also were included in the therapy.[2]

The liver is susceptible to damage by toxic substances released during fat metabolism unless it is supplied with selenium, vitamin E, and/or methionine and cysteine to prevent the buildup of peroxides.

Recommended daily amounts of selenium are 50 to 200 mcg/day, but the average intake in the American diet is estimated at 60 mcg/day. Researchers often use larger amounts in supplements for specific health conditions.

Selenium, which is available in breads, cereals, fish, poultry, and meat, stimulates glutathione peroxidase and thus is a powerful scavenger against damaging free radicals, according to the *British Medical Journal*. Selenium is a constituent of an important antioxidant enzyme—glutathione peroxidase—which destroys free radicals. Taking selenium supplements below 800 mcg/day, or eating Brazil nuts, the richest food source of the mineral, is a reasonable option for those facing a selenium deficiency, the journal reported.[3]

Selenium and the enzyme glutathione peroxidase protect cell membranes from damage by oxidation and thus are an important antioxidant source, according to researchers at Karolinska Hospital in Stockholm, Sweden. Dietary recommendations between 50 and 200 mcg/day are recommended, but deficiency symptoms are noted in less than 10 mcg/day. A deficiency in the mineral has been reported for cardiomyopathy (disorder of the heart muscle). Low levels of selenium in Finnish soils have been associated with an increased risk of ischemic heart disease, and low levels of the mineral have been noted in smokers.[4]

> *In studying 150 Type 1 diabetics, between the ages of 11 and 60, it was found that the selenium content in diabetic patients was significantly lower than in the controls. In general, selenium, but not zinc and copper, concentrations in the blood are off normal in diabetic patients, the researchers said.*

In studying 150 Type 1 diabetics, between the ages of 11 and 60, it was found that the selenium content in diabetic patients was significantly lower than in the controls. In general, selenium, but not zinc and copper, concentrations in the blood are off normal in diabetic patients, the researchers said.[5]

In evaluating 364 patients with various complaints, compared with 50 healthy volunteers, researchers reported that there was a strong association between blood levels of selenium for healthy people, alcoholics, and cancer patients. However, blood levels of the mineral were much lower in diabetics, those with infections, and the senile. Age, kidney function, and albumin (protein in blood plasma) levels are also associated with low levels of the mineral, the researchers said.[6]

Selenium is known to help several insulin-like actions in humans, such as stimulating glucose uptake and metabolic processes such as glycosis (enzymatic breakdown of a carbohydrate such as glucose); gluconeogenesis (formation of glucose from fats and proteins); and fatty acid synthesis.[7]

A research team in Vienna, Austria, evaluated 20 Type 1 diabetics and 20 healthy controls, and found that selenium levels were low in the red blood cells of the diabetics and that glutathione peroxide activity in red blood cells was also low. Diabetics with normal kidney function had significantly reduced amounts of vitamin A. The researchers said that reduced selenium levels in the red blood cells of diabetics could contribute to unnecessary bleeding.[8]

During 1986 and 1987, researchers at Erasmus University Medical School, the Interuniversity Reactor Institute, and Zuiderziekenhuis Hospital in the Netherlands found that patients with heart attack had long-term low selenium levels, as indicated by the amount of the mineral found in their clipped toenails, which probably accounted for an increased risk for a coronary episode. The toenails often indicate how much selenium is stored in the body.

The researchers said that heart patients had lower levels of selenium when compared to the controls. As toenail selenium concentrations decreased, risk of myocardial infarction increased. The researchers concluded that low selenium levels were present before the heart attack, and this might have played a role in its development.[9]

At the Clinic for Internale Medicine in Rostock, Germany, Bode Kuklinski, M.D., said that in a 1-year, double-blind, controlled trial following a heart attack, no patient died following antioxidative treatment, but 20% of the controls expired. The treatment involved selenite (selenium), coenzyme Q10, selenocysteine, beta-carotene, vitamin C, vitamin E, zinc, and vitamin B_6.

Researchers found that kidney excretion of albumin was lowered during administration of vitamin E, thioctic acid (alpha-lipoic acid), and selenite in diabetic late syndrome patients. The term "late syndrome" refers to late complications in long-term diabetic patients with retinopathy (diseases of the retina), nephropathy (kidney disease), and neuropathy (disorder of the nerves). Peripheral diabetic neuropathy improved in 60% of the patients. In those with intensive alcoholic liver damage, the possibility of dying from the disorder was reduced to 6% using antioxidant therapy, while in the control group, lethality (death) was 40%.[10]

"It is our own experience in experimental work that convinced us to use antioxidant therapy," Kuklinski said. "In the meantime, a lot of severely ill patients living in a country where they are confronted with enormous environmental pollution every day could be stabilized with therapeutics that basically are free of side effects. As long as enrichment of food is not common here (Germany) and people eat with a low concentration of essential nutrients, we have to support at least basic essentials to assist the body in the healing process."

In an article in *ACTA Ophthalmology*, researchers at Hospital of Anbelholm in Sweden discussed the case of a 35-year-old male who had subcapsular cataract, atopic eczema, asthma, and other complications. He was treated with 600 mcg/day of selenium, 1,200 mg/day of vitamin E, 80 mg/day of vitamin B_6, 15 mg/day of vitamin B_2, and 2 g/day of vitamin C. At the beginning of the therapy, the right eye measured 2/10 and the left eye was 3/10. Five months later, vision in the right eye was 4/10 and 8/10 in the left eye. After 2 months of treatment, signs of atopic dermatitis had vanished and there were no signs of asthma.

The authors suggest it is reasonable to try selenium and vitamin E treatment in other kinds of cataracts, such as senile and diabetic cataracts. The use of selenium is safe, assuming the patient has normal kidney function, the researchers said.[11]

References

1. Ensminger, A., et al. *Foods and Nutrition Encyclopedia*. Clovis, Calif.: Pegus Press, 1983, pp. 1976ff.

2. Wright, Jonathan V., M.D., et al. "Improvement of Vision in Macular Degeneration Associated with Intravenous Zinc and Selenium Therapy," *Journal of Nutritional Medicine* 1: 133–138, 1990.

3. Rayman, Margaret P. "Dietary Selenium: Time to Act," *British Medical Journal* 314: 387–388, Feb. 8, 1997.

4. Bluhm, G. "Selenium and Cardiovascular Disease," *Trace Elements in Medicine* 7(3): 139–145, 1990.

5. Ruiz, C., et al. "Selenium, Zinc and Copper in Plasma of Patients with Type 1 Diabetes Mellitus in Different Metabolic Control States," *Journal of Trace Elements in Medicine and Biology* 12: 91–95, 1998.

6. Simonoff, M., et al. "Serum and Erythrocyte Selenium in Normal and Pathological States in France," *Trace Elements in Medicine* 5(2): 64–69, 1998.

7. Stapleton, S. R. "Selenium: An Insulin-Minetic," *Cell. Mol. Life Sci.* 57: 1874–1879, 2000.

8. Osterode, W., et al. "Nutritional Antioxidants, Red Cell Membrane Fluidity and Blood Viscosity in Type 1 (Insulin Dependent) Diabetes Mellitus," *Diabetes Medicine* 13: 1044–1050, 1996.

9. Kok, F., et al. "Decreased Selenium Levels in Acute Myocardial Infarction," *Journal of the American Medical Association* 261: 1161–1164, 1989.

10. Hamilton, Kirk. "Pancreatitis (Acute) and Sodium Selenite," *The Experts Speak*. Sacramento, Calif.: I.T. Services, 1996, p. 174. Also, Kuklinski, Bodo, M.D. "Reducing the Lethality in Acute Pancreatitis with Sodium Selenite," *Med. Klin.* 90 (Suppl.): I-36–41, 1995.

11. Ahlrot-Westerlund, Britt, M.D., et al. "Cataracts, Vitamin E, and Selenomethionine," *ACTA Ophthalmology,* April 1988, pp. 237–238.

36 Vanadium

Vanadium in its various forms has been used to treat diabetes since the early 1900s. Daily requirements for the mineral are about 10 mcg/day, and the average Western diet contains about 15 to 30 mcg/day, depending on who is counting. An intake of up to 100 mcg/day is said to be safe; however, researchers are using megadoses of vanadium to treat Type 1 and Type 2 diabetics. The mineral can improve glycemic control and lower fasting plasma glucose levels, cholesterol, and triglyceride levels, as well as hemoglobin A1C.

This mineral is a natural element that has worked for many diabetics, according to Robert M. Giller, M.D. It is available in buffered form and it has insulin-like properties, which increase the uptake of glucose and protein by the muscles and liver.[1]

Vanadium has been studied for more than 40 years, yet it is not classified as an essential nutrient for human beings, according to Barbara F. Harland, Ph.D., R.D., and B. A. Harden-Williams, M.S., of Howard University in Washington, D.C. Pharmacologic doses of the mineral 10 to 100 times the normal intake can alter cholesterol and triglyceride metabolism, as well as the shape of red blood cells, and stimulate glucose oxidation and glycogen synthesis in the liver.[2]

The estimated intake of the mineral in the American diet is 10 to 60 mcg/day, the authors said. Vanadium levels in the diet range from 30.9 in the Southeast to 50.5 mg/kg dry weight in the West. Vanadium seems to assist in the metabolism of glucose by mimicking the action of insulin or altering the activity of the multifunctional enzyme glucose-6-phosphatase.

Vanadium enhances the stimulatory effect of insulin on DNA synthesis in cultured cells, the authors state. Pharmacological doses of vanadium also have been shown to block the formation of cholesterol in both animals and humans.

Daily requirements for vanadium have not been established, but the suggested intake is about 10 mcg/day, according to researchers at the University of British Columbia in Canada. Food sources include mushrooms, parsley, dill, and black pepper. The elevated levels of the mineral in processed foods is apparently due to the stainless steel processing equipment, they added.[3]

Vanadium toxicity can be prevented by giving EDTA (ethylenediaminetetraacetic acid), vitamin C, chromium, protein, ferrous iron, chloride, and aluminum hydroxide, which apparently inhibits the mineral's absorption.[4]

In the early 1900s, French physicians used vanadium as a cure-all for diabetes, anemia, chronic rheumatism, and tuberculosis. Vanadium treatment has been shown to reduce blood glucose levels and maintain normal glycemic states at least three months after withdrawal of treatment.[5]

Writing in *Anti-Fat Nutrients,* Dallas Clouatre, Ph.D., reported that problems with carbohydrate metabolism play a role in the tendency to put on excess weight. One of the main substances involved in fat storage is the hormone insulin, so it is reasonable to assume that foods and nutrients that make insulin more effective and can mimic insulin's actions in the body might aid in controlling appetite and weight gain. A great deal of scientific evidence is being directed at various nutrients that appear to perform these functions. They include vanadium, chromium, *Gymnema sylvestre,* bay leaves, allspice, cinnamon, cloves, and turmeric, Clouatre said.[6]

An article in *Science* in 1985 suggested that vanadium controlled diabetes in laboratory animals. Other studies have confirmed these results, and it is now known that the mineral plays a significant role in controlling blood sugar levels.

"In the 1932 edition of *Dorland's Medical Dictionary,* it listed vanadium as a treatment for diabetes and neurasthenia (nervous exhaustion); with the addition of selenium, it was also suggested as a treatment of cancer," Clouatre added. "In the 1956 edition of *Dorland's,* hardening of the arteries was added to the illnesses for which vanadium was recommended."

At Temple University Hospital, Philadelphia, a research team gave 50 mg of vanadyl sulfate (vanadium), taken orally twice daily for 4 weeks, which resulted in a 20% reduction in fasting glucose concentrations and a decrease in glucose output in the liver in 8 Type 2 diabetics. However, patients given the mineral for longer than 1 month should be evaluated for its metabolic effects, the researchers said.[7]

A research team at the University of Texas Health Science Center at San Antonio, studied 11 Type 2 diabetics (4 women and 7 men, all 59 years old), who had had diabetes for four years. Their hemoglobin A1C registered 8.4%.[8] Readings between 6 and 7% are considered satisfactory.

Each volunteer was given 150 mg/day of vanadyl sulfate for 6 weeks, with each 25 mg tablet of the mineral equaling 8 mg of elemental vanadium. This amount was increased over a 2-week period to 50 mg three times daily, at breakfast, lunch, and dinner.

Vanadium significantly improved their glycemic control, and their fasting blood glucose level was reduced from 194 to 155 mg/dl; hemoglobin A1C went down from 8.1 to 7.8%. In addition, vanadyl sulfate reduced glucose production by about 20%, which correlated with a reduction in fasting plasma glucose. The mineral also lowered blood levels of cholesterol from 223 to 202 mg/dl, and LDL-cholesterol (the bad kind) was lowered from 141 to 129 mg/dl (milligrams per deciliter).

Long-term treatment with vanadium brings a marked and sustained decrease in glucose in the blood, triglycerides, and cholesterol, according to researchers at the University of British Columbia, Vancouver, Canada. Vanadium supplements have blood-pressure-lowering effects because of their ability to counter insulin resistance and weaken hyperinsulinemia (excess insulin in the blood), they added.[9]

Sodium vanadate at 125 mg/day can lower insulin requirements in Type 1 diabetics, and lower their cholesterol, according to J. J. Cunningham of the University of Massachusetts at Amherst. Chromium, vitamin B_3 (niacin), vitamin C, vitamin E, and zinc can also benefit Type 1 diabetics, he said.[10]

Researchers at the Albert Einstein College of Medicine, Bronx, New York, reported that vanadyl sulfate given at 100 mg/day to 7 Type 2 diabetics and 6 nondiabetics, lowered fasting glucose and hemoglobin A1C in diabetics. There was no change in blood levels of glucose in either group. As we know, hemoglobin A1C is a substance in red blood cells that carries oxygen to the cells and sometimes binds with glucose.[11]

References

1. Giller, Robert M., M.D., and Kathy Matthews. *Natural Prescriptions.* New York: Carol Southern Books, 1994, p. 116.

2. Harland, Barbara F., Ph.D., R.D., and B. A. Harden-Williams., M.S. "Is Vanadium of Human Nutritional Importance Yet?" *Journal of the American Dietetic Association* 94(8):891–895, Aug. 1994.

3. French, Rodney J., BSc., and Peter J. H. Jones, Ph.D. "Nutritional Aspects of Vanadium," *The Nutrition Report* 11(7): 49, 56, July 1993.

4. Harland, Barbara F., Ph.D., R.D., and B. A. Harden-Williams, M.S. "Is Vanadium of Human Nutritional Importance Yet?" *Journal of the American Dietetic Association* 94(8):891–895, Aug. 1994.

5. French, Rodney J., BSc., and Peter J. H. Jones, Ph.D. "Role of Vanadium in Nutrition: Metabolism, Essentiality and Dietary Considerations," *Life Sciences* 52(4): 339–346, 1993.

6. Clouatre, Dallas, Ph.D. *Anti-Fat Nutrients.* San Francisco, Calif.: Pax Publishing, 1993, pp. 20ff.

7. Boden, Guenther, et al. "Effect of Vanadyl Sulfate on Carbohydrate and Lipid Metabolism in Patients with Non-Insulin-Dependent Diabetes Mellitus," *Metabolism* 45(9): 1130–1135, Sept. 1996.

8. Cusi, K., et al. "Vanadyl Sulfate Improves Hepatic and Muscle Insulin Sensitivity in Type 2 Diabetes," *Clinical Endocrinology and Metabolism* 86(3): 1410–1417, 2001.

9. Verma, Subodh, Ph.D., et al. "Nutritional Factors That Can Favorably Influence the Glucose/Insulin System: Vanadium," *Journal of the American College of Nutrition* 17(1): 11–18, 1998.

10. Cunningham, J. J. "Micronutrients As Nutraceutical Interventions in Diabetes Mellitus," *Journal of the American College of Nutrition* 17(1): 7–10, 1998.

11. Halberstam, Meyer. "Oral Vanadyl Sulfate Improves Insulin Sensitivity in NIDDM But Not in Obese Nondiabetic Subjects," *Diabetes* 45: 659–666, May 1996.

37 Zinc

It has been estimated that 50% of Americans have zinc intakes that are less than 75% of the Recommended Daily Allowance, which is around 15 mg/day. A zinc deficiency is often found in Type 1 and Type 2 diabetics. The mineral is important in the synthesis of insulin, and those with high concentrations of glucose in their blood have low levels of zinc that may result in oxidative stress that damages cells irreversibly. A zinc deficiency is related to poor eyesight, macular degeneration, senile dementia, dermatitis, abnormal pregnancy, and abnormal sense of taste and smell, among other things.

The most likely cause of zinc deficiency, such as in diabetics, is a diet low in bioavailable zinc. A deficiency in the mineral causes dermatitis, abnormal pregnancy, immature sexual glands, poor eyesight, abnormal sense of taste and smell, macular degeneration, senile dementia, and other health problems.

According to the U.S. Department of Agriculture, 50% of those who follow the Dietary Guidelines for Americans have zinc intakes that are less than 75% of the Recommended Daily Allowance (15 mg/day). Meat, poultry, and fish provide about 50% of the zinc in the omnivore diet, and red meat has twice as much zinc as white meat. Cereals and legumes provide about 30% of dietary zinc, but phytate and fiber in those foods may impede zinc absorption. Foods prepared from cow's milk provide only about 20% of dietary zinc.[1]

Obese patients, who are at high risk in developing diabetes, often have abnormal zinc and copper levels, according to a study at Surgical Research Laboratories in Tennessee. The research team measured copper and zinc levels in the blood, urine, liver, and skeletal tissues of 37 obese patients. Blood, liver, and urinary copper levels were significantly above normal, but blood levels of zinc were low and urinary zinc was elevated, which meant it was not being retained by the body.[2]

Moderate zinc deficiency occurs frequently in Type 2 diabetics, according to researchers at Ohio State University at Columbus. Their study involved giving 40 menopausal women with diabetes 30 mg/day of zinc and other nutrients.[3]

At Umea University in Sweden, researchers studied 2,957 cases of diabetes compared to 7,165 controls, ranging in age from 3 to 14, to study the relationship between zinc in the drinking water and risk of diabetes. They reported that a high concentration of the mineral in ground water (hard water) was associated with a significantly decreased risk of diabetes. In other words, people got reasonable amounts of zinc in the diet, presumably from the water. There was an even stronger association between zinc and diabetes in rural areas where drinking water came from local wells.[4] The so-called hard water contains a variety of minerals compared with "soft" water.

In a French study, 20 mg of zinc gluconate increased the assimilation of glucose due to its insulin-like effect.[5]

In 10 volunteers with advanced cirrhosis of the liver and impaired glucose tolerance, or diabetes, long-term supplementation with 20 mg of zinc, three times daily, for 60 days, improved the dispersion of glucose by more than 30%, according to researchers at the Universita di Bologna in Italy. Insulin sensitivity, which was reduced before the treatment began, did not change. The involvement of glucose was almost halved in cirrhosis patients before treatment and increased after zinc therapy. The normalization of zinc levels after long-term zinc supplementation in advanced cirrhosis patients improved their ability to handle glucose. The researchers added that poor zinc status may contribute to the impaired glucose tolerance and diabetes found in cirrhosis patients.[6]

Zinc is an important mineral in the synthesis and action of insulin. Hyperglycemia (an abnormally high concentration of glucose in the blood) in Type 1 and Type 2 diabetics causes loss of zinc from the body. Researchers have found that low levels of zinc may result in oxidative stress that damages the cells irreversibly, thereby making some of the complications of diabetes even worse.[7]

In a study of 110 diabetics who had had fasting glycosylated hemo-globin of less than 7.5% for at least 5 years, the volunteers were randomly assigned to four groups that were given either 30 mg of zinc gluconate, 400 mcg of chromium picolinate, 30 mg of zinc and 400 mcg of chromium, or a placebo. The ages of the diabetics ranged from 51 to 55 years.[8]

At the beginning of the study, it was thought that more than 30% of the volunteers may have been zinc deficient. Following supplementation, there was a significant reduction of plasma thiobarbituric acid reactive substances (TBARS) in the chromium group by 13.6%, in the zinc group by 13.6%, and in the zinc-chromium group by 18.2%. There were no changes in the placebo group. TBARS are a marker for lipid peroxidation. High levels of lipid peroxides often indicate free-radical damage in both Type 1 and Type 2 diabetics. Lipid peroxidation indicates an interaction of fats with oxygen, which can lead to the destruction of cells. There were no adverse side effects with zinc supplementation or copper status, HDL-cholesterol, or interactions between zinc and chromium.

At the University of Vienna in Austria, researchers evaluated 158 patients: 77 were Type 1 diabetics; 39 of 81 patients with Type 2 diabetes had peripheral vascular disease or coronary artery disease. Compared to controls, TBARS levels were elevated in the diabetics and Type 2 patients had higher levels than Type 1. Type 2 patients with angiopathy (disease of the blood vessels) had higher TBARS levels than those without the disor-der. Raised levels of lipoperoxides, which are thought to be carcinogenic, contribute to the formation of free radicals in diabetes, which can destroy cell membranes.[9]

As reported in the *Journal of the American College of Nutrition*, researchers evaluated 3,575 volunteers, between the ages of 25 and 64, including 1,769 men and women in rural India and 1,806 urban people. The research team found that the prevalence of coronary artery disease, diabetes, and glucose intolerance was significantly higher among those consuming lower amounts of zinc. Low amounts of zinc in the blood were associated with a higher prevalence of high blood pressure, high amounts of triglycerides, and low high-density lipoprotein cholesterol levels.[10]

After eating, insulin and blood glucose levels declined as zinc intake increased in rural men and urban men and women, the researchers said. Serum zinc levels rose with increased zinc intakes in the diet in all vol-unteers.

References

1. Sandstead, Harold H., and Norman G. Egger. "Is Zinc Nutriture a Problem in Persons with Diabetes Mellitus?" *American Journal of Clinical Nutrition* 66: 681–682, 1997.

2. Bhattacharyas, R. D., et al. "Significantly Altered Copper and Zinc Levels in Serum, Liver, Urine and Skeletal Muscle of Morbidly Obese Patients," *Journal of the American College of Nutrition* 7: 401, 1988.

3. Blostein-Fujii, Ashley, et al. "Short-Term Zinc Supplementation in Women with Non-Insulin-Dependent Diabetes Mellitus: Effects on Plasma 5′-Nucleotidase Activities, Insulin-Like Growth Factor I Concentrations and Lipoprotein Oxidation Rates in Vitro," *American Journal of Clinical Nutrition* 66: 639–642, 1997.

4. Haglund, Bengt, Ph.D., et al. "Evidence of a Relationship Between Childhood-Onset Type 1 Diabetes and Low Groundwater Concentrations of Zinc," *Diabetes Care* 19(8): 873–875, Aug. 1996.

5. Brun, Jean-Frederic, et al. "Effects of Oral Zinc Gluconate on Glucose Effectiveness and Insulin Sensitivity in Humans," *Biological Trace Element Research* 47: 385–391, 1995.

6. Marchesini, G., et al. "Zinc Supplementation Improves Glucose Disposal in Patients with Cirrhosis," *Metabolism* 47(7): 792–798, July 1998.

7. Chausmer, Arthur R., M.D., Ph.D. "Zinc, Insulin and Diabetes," *Journal of the American College of Nutrition* 17(2): 109–115, 1998.

8. Anderson, R. A., et al. "Potential Antioxidant Effects of Zinc and Chromium Supplementation in People with Type 2 Diabetes Mellitus," *Journal of the American College of Nutrition* 20(3): 212–218, 2001.

9. Griesmacher, Andrea, M.D., et al. "Enhance Serum Levels of Thiobarbituric-Acid-Reactive Substances in Diabetes Mellitus," *American Journal of Medicine* 98: 469-475, May 1995.

10. Singh, R. B, et al. "Current Zinc Intake and Risk of Diabetes and Coronary Artery Disease and Factors Associated with Insulin Resistance in Rural and Urban Populations of North India," *Journal of the American College of Nutrition* 17(6): 564–570, 1998.

38 Other Minerals of Importance to Diabetics

A number of minerals, including calcium and lithium, are being used to treat diabetes and the various complications associated with the disease. For example, calcium is associated with a drop in high blood pressure. Lithium is said to have a hypoglycemic effect when it is combined with treatments for reducing blood glucose levels; however, its use should be monitored by a physician, since it has been used in the past as a salt substitute.

Up to 60% of diabetics have hemochromatosis, which is an iron overload disorder, but this condition can be alleviated by periodically donating blood.

Calcium: A high-calcium, low-fat diet lowers blood pressure in both hypertensive and normotensive (normal) people, according to researchers at Tufts University in Boston. In the study, the volunteers were given daily diets containing less than 20% fat, along with 1,600 and 2,000 mg of calcium. Nonfat milk was the main source of calcium. Blood pressures were recorded before breakfast during the 34-day study.

The researchers found that systolic (beating) and diastolic (resting) blood pressures decreased 11 and 12%, respectively, in men, but only 1% in women. Improvements were noted in both young and elderly men.[1]

At Wayne State University in Michigan, 6 Type 2 diabetics with high blood pressure (hypertension) were taken off hypertensive drugs and supplemented with 600 mg/day of calcium for 3 months. The researchers found that forearm blood flow increased, left ventricular mass was reduced, and blood pressure decreased following supplementation.[2]

For nonvegetarians who do not incorporate milk products in their diet, Ralph Golan, M.D., recommends 500 to 1,000 mg/day of calcium. The so-called RDA for the mineral is 800 to 1,200 mg/day, with up to 1,500 mg/day recommended for pregnancy/lactation and menopause. Since magnesium assists in calcium uptake, he recommends a 1:1 ratio of the two minerals.

However, he does advise twice as much magnesium as calcium for treating hardening of the arteries, coronary heart disease, heart rhythm disturbances, high blood pressure, nervous irritability, and other conditions.[3] For vegetarians, he recommends 300 to 500 mg/day of calcium, with more for those with acute insomnia and muscle and menstrual cramps.

Iron: Hemochromatosis (too much iron in the blood) is a disorder that affects about 1.5 million Americans, with an estimated prevalence of 1 in 200 to 250. Ten percent of those with the problem are carriers for the gene. It is more common in Caucasians and Hispanics than in other races, and it is usually controlled by periodic blood donations, which reduces the amount of iron in the blood.[4]

The preferred screening test is transferrin saturation. If the reading is a level of 50, this necessitates a test for levels of serum ferritin or stored iron. Patients should consult their doctor about taking iron supplements unless they are deficient in the mineral.

Diabetes is present in up to 60% of patients with hemochromatosis, according to researchers at the University of Minnesota at Minneapolis. Insulin resistance with hyperinsulinemia is apparently the earliest detectable abnormality in hemochromatosis, followed by the impaired secretion of insulin as iron is selectively deposited in the beta cells in the pancreas. Type 2 diabetes has a strong genetic component, while idiopathic hemochromatosis is a genetic disease, they added.[5]

Recent studies suggest that mild iron overload is unlikely to be a major factor contributing to Type 2 diabetes, the research team said. There is some beneficial effect in Type 2 diabetic patients with increased serum ferritin (iron) in the absence of hemochromatosis, which show benefit with deferoxamine and iron chelating therapy. However, deferoximaine is expensive.

The authors admitted that Type 2 diabetes is a disease with multiple causes. It is possible the accumulation of iron during adulthood leads to glucose intolerance, and Type 2 diabetes is an attractive hypothesis for this based on the potential reversibility of the disease. However, it is improbable that such a simple explanation could explain a complex disease such as Type 2 diabetes, they said.

Restless leg syndrome has been linked to iron deficiency, uremia, pregnancy, diabetes mellitus, rheumatoid arthritis, and polyneuropathy (nerve disorder), reported an article in *Archives of Internal Medicine*.[6]

At the opposite end of the iron spectrum is low iron, or anemia. Of the many types of anemia, iron-deficiency anemia is best known and it is a major nutritional problem worldwide, according to Robert Garrison, Jr., M.A., R.Ph., and Elizabeth Somer, M.A., R.D. With this condition, red blood cells contain less hemoglobin, have a reduced capacity to carry oxygen, and are small and pale in color. The limited iron supply to tissues causes diminished energy production and characteristic symptoms such as lethargy, tiredness, apathy, reduced brain function, pallor, headache, heart enlargement, spoon-shaped nails, and depleted iron stores.[7]

Reduced iron in the blood is one of the final stages of iron deficiency, the authors state. Symptoms of a mild to moderate deficiency include hyperglycemia (high levels of glucose in the blood), increased oxygen use, impaired growth, and a compromised immune function. Women are especially vulnerable to an iron deficiency due to monthly blood losses during menstruation, estimated to be on average 28 mg of iron monthly.

The recommended intake of iron for men and women ranges from 10 to 15 mg/day, with 30 mg/day for pregnant women and 15 mg/day for breast-feeding women. Among the best food sources of iron are liver, organ meats, dried fruits, lima beans, legumes, dark green leafy vegetables, sardines, prune juice, and oysters.

Lithium: At the Second Affiliated Hospital-Human Medical University in China, a research team said that lithium carbonate is an effective supplementary medication for oral hypoglycemia agents and/or insulin in treating diabetics. The dosage of 100 mg/day produced no significant side effects. In Chinese literature, lithium was used clinically before insulin was commercially available.[8]

In the study, 33 Type 2 diabetics and 5 Type 1 diabetics, ranging in age from 20 to 70, were evaluated for the effect of lithium on low blood sugar. Depending on the severity of the disease, the volunteers were treated by diet only, with oral hypoglycemic drugs, or with insulin. After their blood glucose levels were stabilized, the people were given 100 mg/day of lithium carbonate.

Fasting blood glucose and blood glucose levels after meals decreased significantly in the diabetics following lithium therapy. An exception was the fasting blood glucose in the Type 2 diabetics who were treated with diet and no medications. The researchers concluded that lithium could improve glucose metabolism in most diabetics. Lithium is said to have a hypoglycemic effect when it is combined with treatments for reducing blood glucose levels. However, when given at a dose of 300 mg four times daily, lithium can cause restless leg syndrome, so lithium intake should be monitored by a physician.[9]

Sodium/Potassium: Researchers at the University of Palermo and the University of Naples in Italy have found that a moderate reduction in dietary sodium, combined with an increased intake of potassium can lower blood pressure in patients with high blood pressure.

Hypertensive volunteers were given a standard diet for 2 weeks and then randomly assigned to the same standard diet plus 7 g of sodium chloride or 7 g of inorganic mineral low-sodium, high-potassium salt daily. The body weight, urinary excretion, heart rate, and arterial blood pressures were monitored for all participants. The results indicated that modest reductions in sodium and increases in potassium intake *reduced* blood pressure by 17 mmHg in systolic (beating) and 6 mmHg in diastolic (resting) pressures.[10]

References

1. Ferland, G., et al. "Effects of a High Calcium, Low-Fat Diet on Systolic and Diastolic Blood Pressure of Healthy Humans," *FASEB Journal* 6: A1174, 1992.

2. Zemel, M., et al. "Dietary Calcium Supplementation Increases Forearm Blood Flow and Reduces Left Ventricular Mass in Hypertensive Non-Insulin-Dependent Diabetics," *Hypertension* 12: 344, 1988.

3. Golan, Ralph, M.D. *Optimal Wellness.* New York: Ballantine Books, 1995, pp. 133–134.

4. Waldron, Theresa. "CDC Recommends Routine Screening for 'Iron Overload,'" *Medical Tribune,* April 17, 1997, pp. 1, 5.

5. Redmon, J. Bruce, M.D., and R. Paul Robertson, M.D. "Iron and Diabetes: An Attractive Hypothesis But," *Mayo Clinic Proceedings* 69: 90–92, 1994.

6. O'Keeffe, S. T. "Restless Leg Syndrome: A Review," *Archives of Internal Medicine* 156(3): 243–248, Feb. 12, 1996.

7. Garrison, Robert, Jr., M.A., R.Ph., and Elizabeth Somer, M.A., R.D. *The Nutrition Desk Reference.* New Canaan, Conn.: Keats Publishing, 1995, pp. 197ff.

8. Hu, Min, et al. "Assisting Effects of Lithium on Hypoglycemic Treatment in Patients with Diabetes," *Biological Trace Element Research* 60: 131–137, 1997.

9. Heiman, E. M. "Lithium-Aggravated Nocturnal Myoclonus and Restless Leg Syndrome," *American Journal of Psychiatry* 143(9): 1191–1192, Sept. 1986.

10. Bompiani, G., et al. "Effects of Moderate Low Sodium/Low Potassium Diet on Essential Hypertension: Results of a Comparative Study," *International Journal of Clinical Pharmacology* 26: 129–132, 1988.

39 Alpha-Lipoic Acid

Alpha-lipoic acid is a vitamin-like substance that is found in beef and spinach, but diabetics need an over-the-counter supplement to provide sufficient dosage for benefit. Over fifteen trials in Germany, using at least 600 mg/day of alpha-lipoic acid, have shown beneficial results. A short-term, 3-week study, using 600 mg/day of the nutrient intravenously can reduce the chief symptoms of diabetic polyneuropathy, which affects peripheral nerves, causing leg pain, numbness, and muscle weakness. The supplement prevents beta-cell destruction leading to Type 1 diabetes, and it enhances glucose uptake in Type 2 diabetes.

Alpha-lipoic acid has been shown to have a number of beneficial effects, both in prevention and treatment of diabetes, reported Lester Packer, Ph.D., and colleagues at the University of California at Berkeley and ASTA Medica in Frankfurt Am Main, Germany. The supplement may act in a number of ways that are especially protective in diabetes.

For example, it prevents beta-cell destruction leading to Type 1 diabetes, and it enhances glucose uptake in Type 2 diabetes. In addition, it prevents glycation reactions in some proteins. Its antioxidant effects may be especially useful in slowing the development of diabetic neuropathy and cataracts, and this may be especially significant in alleviating diabetes-induced reduction in intracellular vitamin C levels, they said.[1]

Few of these improvements will surface over the course of weeks or months, they added. This has been demonstrated in trials for treatment of neuropathy, which lasted up to 12 weeks, in which objective improvement was not observed but clear subjective improvement was present, even in double-blind studies. It is unrealistic to expect dramatic effects in weeks, since diabetic complications develop over years and decades, they said.

Alpha-lipoic acid has been shown to have a number of beneficial effects, both in prevention and treatment of diabetes, reported Lester Packer, Ph.D., and colleagues at the University of California at Berkeley and ASTA Medica in Frankfurt Am Main, Germany. The supplement may act in a number of ways that are especially protective in diabetes. It prevents beta-cell destruction leading to Type 1 diabetes, and it enhances glucose uptake in Type 2 diabetes. There is no doubt that all diabetics should supplement their diets with alpha-lipoic acid, according to Richard A. Passwater, Ph.D. It can mean all the difference in the world, he said.

There is no doubt that all diabetics should supplement their diets with alpha-lipoic acid, according to Richard A. Passwater, Ph.D. It can mean all the difference in the world, he said. They should also consider supplementing with chromium picolinate. It is imperative that diabetics monitor their blood sugar levels closely and have appropriate adjustments made to their medication doses to prevent lowering their blood sugar levels too far, he added.[2]

Burt Berkson, M.D., of Las Cruces, New Mexico, has said that alpha-lipoic acid is an effective treatment for the prevention, treatment, and reversal of Type 2 diabetes. First, the supplement is a powerful antioxidant that neutralizes hazardous free radicals, which causes many diabetic complications. Second, the substance improves the efficiency of insulin and lowers blood sugar or glucose levels. Third, alpha-lipoic acid slows the aging process, which is accelerated by diabetes.[3]

At its most fundamental biological level, alpha-lipoic acid serves as a coenzyme in the Krebs Cycle. The Krebs Cycle breaks down glucose in every cell and converts it to energy; however, without alpha-lipoic acid, this breakdown cannot occur. For the process to occur, insulin must shuttle glucose from the blood into the cells.

In Type 2 diabetes, the body overproduces insulin in response to diets that are high in refined carbohydrates (breads, pastas, pizzas, cookies, etc.). After years of such a diet, glucose-burning cells stop responding to the insulin, which leads to a condition called insulin resistance, and glucose is increasingly stored as triglycerides in fat cells.

At a July 1994 symposium at the Diabetic Research Institute in Munich, Germany, researchers discussed the role of alpha-lipoic acid in treating polyneuropathy. This condition affects between 25 and 50% of diabetics. The researchers reported that hyperglycemia (elevated levels of sugar in the blood) is the most important factor in the development of polyneuropathy, and that increased levels of oxygen free radicals contribute to the loss of neurologic function in diabetes.[4]

Polyneuropathy affects peripheral nerves, such as cranial nerves in the brain and spinal nerves. Hands and feet are also affected. The condition is caused by toxic exposure, nutritional deficiency, especially for vitamin B_1 (thiamine), vitamin B_6 (pyridoxine), and pantothenic acid, another B vitamin sometimes referred to as B_5, and malabsorption. Symptoms include leg pain, numbness, and muscle weakness.

The researchers reported that alpha-lipoic acid (thioic acid) stimulates the glucose carriers to increase sugar uptake in the cells, but in the case of diabetes, cellular sugar intake is impaired. In one study, alpha-lipoic acid therapy at 100 mg/IV or chronic treatment at 500 mg/IV for 14 days increased the glucose utilization of diabetics by 20 to 50%.

Another study, using 600 mg/day of the vitamin-like supplement by mouth for 30 days in 10 polyneuropathy patients found that ATP production in the muscle of diabetics was improved because the supplement improved the energy supply. Adenosine triphosphate (ATP) contains phosphate bonds that function as the energy source of cells.

In a rat model, it was found that alpha-lipoic acid prevented the development of polyneuropathy entirely. However, when the treatment was stopped, polyneuropathy returned in a short time.

As a potent antioxidant, alpha-lipoic acid is able to regenerate the body's own antioxidants, such as vitamins C and E and glutathione. In a study in which 23 volunteers received 600 mg/IV and then 600 mg/day by mouth, compared to a treatment with vitamin B_1, alpha-lipoic acid brought lasting improvement in the clinical symptoms of peripheral diabetic neuropathy. However, there was no improvement in nerve function in one study during 15 weeks of treatment.

Using a specific fat cell, a research team evaluated the effect of alpha-lipoic acid, dihydrolipoic acid (to which the body converts alpha-lipoic acid), and N-acetylcysteine (NAC), another antioxidant, on the cellular transport of glucose. The effective transport of glucose to the cells is needed to burn during normal metabolic processes. The effect of these antioxidants on insulin concentrations was also measured.

In the first experiment, the research team found that glucose transport was increased when the fat cells were exposed to alpha-lipoic acid and dihydrolipoic acid, but not with NAC. This suggests that the two forms of lipoic acid prevent insulin resistance, or poor insulin function, the main symptom of Type 2 diabetes. In the second experiment, all of the antioxidants reduced levels of insulin.

In another study, researchers gave 600 mg/day of alpha-lipoic acid for 3 weeks to 10 diabetics with polyneuropathy. Symptoms of the disorder were evaluated with measurements of blood flow and clinical assessments of the symptoms.[5]

The researchers reported that clinical symptoms of the diabetic complication polyneuropathy improved significantly following alpha-lipoic acid therapy. In addition, the supplement improved the movement of blood cells in capillaries, which is thought to influence nerve function.

Writing in the New Mexico Supplement to the *Western Journal of Medicine*, Burton M. Berkson, M.D., Ph.D., said that he believes that alpha-lipoic acid reverses several types of acute and chronic liver disease. Other studies show that the supplement can be used as an antioxidant, as a chronic disease protectant, as a radio-protectant, for organ regeneration, and as an hypoglycemic agent for adult onset diabetes (Type 2), and that it may be able to reverse certain types of neoplastic disease (cancer).[6]

He added that Russian researchers have studied alpha-lipoic acid in the treatment of heart disease. They found it is an excellent antioxidant, preventing damage to molecules that rid the body of excess cholesterol; and it stimulates enzymes that break down fats. The research also found that the supplement increased oxygen transport to the heart by 70%.

"In 1995, at a European Conference," Berkson said, "several speakers described the reversal of diabetic neuropathies using alpha-lipoic acid. They concluded that this was probably due to the chemical's hypoglycemic and antioxidant effects. In German studies, researchers revealed that thioctic [alpha-lipoic] acid can actually regenerate nervous tissue and protect healthy neurons from the direct effect of high blood sugar."

In an alpha-lipoic acid in diabetic neuropathy study at Heinrich-Heine University in Dusseldorf, Germany, 328 Type 2 diabetics with symptoms of peripheral neuropathy (nerve damage) were given an injection of either a placebo or alpha-lipoic acid, using 3 doses of 1,200 mg, 600 mg, and 100 mg for 3 weeks. Dosages of 1,200 mg and 600 mg, versus the placebo, brought relief in the feet from the start of the trial to day 19. With regard to pain, burning, paresthesia (tingling), and numbness, all these symptoms were lower in the 600 mg group versus placebo after 19 days.[7] Pain was greatly reduced in the alpha-lipoic acid group that got 1,200 and 600 mg, compared to placebo, after 19 days of treatment.

In another study, patients with Type 2 diabetes and cardiac autonomic neuropathy were randomly given a daily oral dose of 800 mg of alpha-lipoic acid (39 patients), while 34 volunteers were given a placebo for 4 months. Two of the four parameters of heart rate variability at rest were greatly improved in the alpha-lipoic acid group versus the placebo group. No side effects of significance were reported.

The research team concluded that intravenous treatment with alpha-lipoic acid at 600 mg/day for 3 weeks is safe and effective in reducing the symptoms of diabetic peripheral neuropathy; oral treatment with 800 mg/day for 4 months may improve cardiac autonomic dysfunction in Type 2 diabetes.

In the Dusseldorf study just discussed, improvements were recorded in 71% of the 1,200 mg group, 82% in the 600 mg group, and 65% in the 100 mg group, as well as 58% in the placebo group.[8]

In another related study, 65 volunteers were given 2 oral doses of alpha-lipoic acid at 600 and 1,200 mg/day or a placebo for 2 years. While the trial was said to be "not sufficiently rigorous" to determine the efficacy of alpha-lipoic acid, the research team said that there was clinically meaningful improvement in neuropathic function in the Type 1 and Type 2 diabetics.[9]

In a third related trial, in which 509 volunteers were given alpha-lipoic injections for 3 weeks (600 mg/day), followed by 600 mg of oral supplement three times daily, the researchers concluded there was no difference between the placebo and treatment groups. However, during the intravenous period, Neuropathy Impairment Scale scores were significantly reduced.[10]

In a study involving lab rats with diabetes, the researchers gave them alpha-lipoic acid and then measured changes in different types of nerves. Alpha-lipoic acid improved nerve function in the animals' toes but not in the sciatic nerves, which extend down the leg. The polyneuropathy in their toes was similar to polyneuropathy found in human toes.[11]

In a study involving laboratory rats that had been made diabetic, researchers tested alpha-lipoic acid, vitamin E, and vitamin C to see if they could reduce kidney damage. The research team measured the animals' urinary albumin excretion, glomerular volume, glomerular content of immunoreactive transforming growth factor-beta, and other signs of kidney damage. The glomerulus is a tuft of capillaries in the kidney.[12]

It was reported that alpha-lipoic acid was far more effective than the two vitamins in preventing kidney disease. In fact, diabetic rats given alpha-lipoic acid supplements did not experience the increases in markers of kidney disease, when compared with untreated animals.

In another human study, 31 volunteers were asked to take 600 mg/day of alpha-lipoic acid or 400 IU/day of vitamin E for 2 months, followed by the same amounts of both supplements for an additional 2 months. The research team reported that alpha-lipoic acid significantly slowed free-radical oxidative damage to cholesterol, which might promote the development of coronary artery disease. Alpha-lipoic acid is both water- and fat-soluble and works well with fat-soluble vitamin E in halting free-radical buildup.[13]

In Germany, alpha-lipoic acid is an approved "drug" for the treatment of nerve disorders in diabetics, but recent research has also studied the benefit of the nutrient to lower blood sugar (glucose) levels in diabetics. A research team from Israel and Germany studied the effect of alpha-lipoic acid on diabetic rats, which have elevated glucose levels, and compared them with animals given a placebo.[14]

The researchers reported that alpha-lipoic acid substantially lowered blood glucose levels after fasting and meals, thus reducing the principal symptom of diabetes and probably lowering the risk of diabetic complications. It was also found that blood glucose levels were about 23% lower after feeding and some 45% lower after fasting, when compared to the rats on placebo. It seems that alpha-lipoic acid improved the transport of glucose in muscle cells, where most of the glucose is burned for energy.

In another study involving diabetic rats, a research team suggested that alpha-lipoic acid, as a potent antioxidant, protects nerve cells by protecting against free-radical damage. Diabetics often suffer from oxidative stress because of large amounts of damaging free radicals and small amounts of protecting antioxidants. While blood flow to the nerves of the animals was 50% of normal, alpha-lipoic acid protected the nerves from damage by reducing oxidative stress. High doses of the supplement restored normal blood flow in diabetic rats after 1 month, but it did not affect blood flow in rats without diabetes.[15]

In another animal model, researchers studied how alpha-lipoic acid alone and in combination with insulin increased glucose uptake by muscle cells from normal, lean rats and from obese rats. As we know, insulin is the hormone that promotes glucose uptake by cells.[16]

The research team reported that alpha-lipoic acid stimulated glucose uptake in muscles from lean rats by 76% and by 48% in muscles from obese animals. Insulin further enhanced glucose uptake by 30 to 55%.

References

1. Packer, Lester, Ph.D., et al. "Alpha-Lipoic Acid As a Biological Antioxidant," *Free Radical Biology and Medicine* 19(2): 227–250, 1995.

2. Passwater, Richard A., Ph.D. *Lipoic Acid: The Metabolic Antioxidant.* New Canaan, Conn.: Keats Publishing, 1995, pp. 41–42.

3. Challem, Jack. "Beat Diabetes with Alpha-Lipoic Acid," *GreatLife,* Nov. 2001, pp. 34ff.

4. Hamdorf, G., M.D. "Thioctic Acid—A Rational Remedy for the Treatment of Diabetic Polyneuropathy," *Experimental Clinical Endocrinology and Diabetes* 104: 126–127, 1995.

5. Haak, E. S., et al. "The Effect of Alpha-Lipoic Acid on the Neurovascular Reflex Arc in Patients with Diabetic Neuropathy Assessed by Capillary Microscopy," *Microvascular Research* 58: 28–34, 1999.

6. Hamilton, Kirk. "Hepatic Necrosis and Thioctic Acid." *The Experts Speak*. Sacramento, Calif.: I.T. Services, 1996, pp. 124–125. Also, Berkson, Burton, M.D., Ph.D. "Fungal Toxicology, Mushroom Poisoning and Thioctic Acid," New Mexico Supplement to the *Western Journal of Medicine* 162(5): 2, May 1995.

7. Ziegler, Dan, M.D., and F. Arnold Gries. "Alpha-Lipoic Acid in the Treatment of Diabetic Peripheral and Cardiac Autonomic Neuropathy," *Diabetes* 46 (Suppl. 2): S62–S66, Sept. 1997.

8. Ziegler, Dan, M.D., et al. "Treatment of Symptomatic Diabetic Peripheral Neuropathy with the Anti-Oxidant Alpha Lipoic Acid," *Diabetologia* 38(12): 1425–1433, 1995.

9. *Free Radical Research* 31(3): 171–179, 1999.

10. *Annals of Neurology* 38(3): 478–482, 1995.

11. Stevens, M. J., et al. "Effects of D1-Alpha-Lipoic Acid on Peripheral Nerve Conduction, Blood Flow, Energy Metabolism and Oxidative Stress in Experimental Diabetic Neuropathy," *Diabetes* 49: 1006–1015, 2000.

12. Melhem, M. F., et al. "Effects of Dietary Supplementation of Alpha-Lipoic Acid on Early Glomerular Injury in Diabetes Mellitus," *Journal of the American Society of Nephrology* 12: 124–133, 2001.

13. Marangon, K., et al. "Comparison of the Effect of Alpha-Lipoic Acid and Alpha-Tocopherol Supplementation on Measures of Oxidative Stress," *Free Radical Biology and Medicine* 27: 1114–1121, 1999.

14. Khamaisi, M., et al. "Lipoic Acid Reduces Glycemia and Increases Muscle GLUT4 in Streptozotocin-Diabetic Rats," *Metabolism* 46: 763–768, 1997.

15. Low, P. A., et al. "The Roles of Oxidative Stress and Antioxidant Treatment in Experimental Diabetic Neuropathy," *Diabetes* 46(Suppl. 2): S38–S42, 1997.

16. Henriksen, E. J., et al. "Stimulation by Alpha-Lipoic Acid of Glucose Transport Activity in Skeletal Muscle of Lean and Obese Zucker Rats," *Life Sciences* 61: 805–812, 1997.

40 Amino Acids

Amino acids are links of protein that are needed for human nutrition. Complete protein is available only from animal sources and a few legumes. Amino acids that can be synthesized in the body are called non-essential amino acids. Those that have to be supplied by the diet are referred to as essential amino acids.

Of the twenty-two amino acids, both essential and non-essential ones are being used to treat a variety of disorders, such as diabetes. For example, taurine, an amino acid cousin, keeps blood sugar lower in Type 1 diabetics. Arginine improves insulin sensitivity in Type 2 diabetics. Glutamine and arginine may improve immune function. Many more beneficial uses for amino acids supplements will be forthcoming when pharmaceutical companies decide that this research is profitable.

In order for a protein to be synthesized in the body, all of its constituent amino acids must be available. Amino acids synthesized in the body are called non-essential, or dispensable, amino acids. If the body cannot synthesize an amino acid from materials normally available, it must be supplied by diet or supplements. It is an essential amino acid.[1]

Cysteine and methionine are the principal sources of sulfur in the diet, and sulfur is needed for the formation of coenzyme A and taurine in the body. Methionine can convert to cysteine, but not the other way around. Lysine is involved in the synthesis of carnitine, which stimulates fatty acid synthesis within cells. Histidine is a powerful blood vessel dilator.

The body can convert phenylalanine to tyrosine, but not vice versa. Most of the phenylalanine not used in protein synthesis is converted to tyrosine. The latter is involved in the manufacture of the hormones norepinephrine and epinephrine by the adrenal glands, and the hormones thyroxine and triiodothyronine by the thyroid gland.

Tryptophan is necessary for the production of serotonin, an important neurotransmitter of the brain. Serotonin counteracts the effects of epinephrine and norepinephrine and improves the duration of sleep. Serotonin is also a powerful constrictor of blood vessels in tissues, including blood platelets, and cells of the intestinal mucosa. Some vitamin B_3 can be manufactured from tryptophan, but this is not enough to meet the body's need for niacin.

There are twenty-two amino acids, including nine essential and thirteen non-essential ones, although arginine is not considered essential for human beings. The remaining essential amino acids not discussed here are isoleucine, leucine, threonine, and valine. Cysteine and tyrosine are non-essential amino acids. Taurine and carnitine are not considered essential or non-essential amino acids, but may be needed for some health problems.

The proportions in which the essential amino acids are required are as important as the amounts, according to Ruth M. Leverton. The body prefers that these amino acids be available from food in about the same proportions each time for use in maintenance, repair, and growth. Meat, fish, poultry, eggs, milk, cheese, and some legumes contain complete protein.[2]

"Often the proteins in grains, nuts, fruit and vegetables are classed as partially complete or incomplete because the proportionate amount of one or more of the essential amino acids is low or because the concentrations of all of the amino acids are too low to be helpful in meeting the body's needs," Leverton said.

When animal sources are not readily available, as in some developing countries, foods can sometimes be combined to make a complete protein. For example, corn can be combined with wheat to increase the proportion of tryptophan.

"Just as hands and feet are mirror images of each other, amino acids occur as mirror image forms (optical isomers)," said Robert A. Ronzio, Ph.D. "The left-hand forms are designated as 'L,' and the right-handed opposites are designated as 'D.' Only L-amino acids are supplied by food and synthesized in the body, and only the 'L' forms occur in proteins. Therefore, unless indicated otherwise, an amino acid can be assumed to be the 'L' form when mentioned in nutrition literature. The only common amino acid that does not exist as optical isomers is glycine, the simplest of amino acids."[3]

Evidence has been accumulating concerning the beneficial effects of amino acids, reported *Lancet*. For example, glutamine and arginine may improve immune function. Glutamine, a non-essential amino acid, when included in a study of intensive-care patients, lowered six-month mortality. The beneficial effect occurred during the convalescing of the patients. The researchers added that there is a lack of defined dose-response relation with regard to glutamine or arginine.[4]

"The absence of large, multicenter trials in nutritional support of these amino acids is astonishing in view of the beneficial effects so far reported," the authors said. "The most likely explanation is the reluctance of pharmaceutical companies to put huge investments into international multicenter trials when the financial profits are going to be limited."

Although Type 1 and Type 2 diabetes are two distinct diseases, taurine is useful in stabilizing blood sugar in both, according to Robert C. Atkins, M.D. For those with Type 2, taurine improves cellular sensitivity to insulin. For patients with Type 1, 1.5 g/day of the substance keeps blood sugar lower over the long term and reduces abnormal platelet activity. Diabetics often have below normal levels of taurine, which might compound their susceptibility to retinopathy and heart damage, he said.[5]

Although the mechanism by which it works is unknown, researchers at the University of Graz in Austria found that L-arginine improves insulin sensitivity in overweight patients, in Type 2 diabetics, and in healthy people. The study involved 7 healthy volunteers, 9 obese patients, and 9 Type 2 diabetics. The research team said that L-arginine (a non-essential amino acid), given at 0.52 mg/kg/minute restored the impaired insulin-mediated vasodilation that is seen in overweight people and those with Type 2 diabetes.

The Austrians said that their study shows that defective insulin-mediated vasodilation (the dilation of blood vessels) in obesity and Type 2 diabetes can be normalized by intravenous infusions of L-arginine given over 3 hours. A holistic physician should be asked if an equivalent amount of the amino acid can be given orally.[6]

An increase in dietary protein associated with a decrease in carbohydrate could be useful in Type 2 diabetes, according to an article in the *Journal of the American College of Nutrition*. When protein is eaten, it is broken down into amino acids. In the liver, most of the absorbed amino acids are deaminated (separated). The nitrogen is converted to urea and excreted in urine, while the remaining carbon elements can be converted to glucose. For example, 3.5 g of glucose can be produced from every gram of nitrogen produced from ingested protein. In other words, 28 g of glucose can be formed from the ingestion of 50 g of protein.[7]

Researchers have determined that protein results in a modest increase in circulating insulin in normal people but a large increase in Type 2 diabetics, as well as increasing circulating glucagon concentrations. Glucagon is a hormone that raises glucose (sugar) in the blood. It has a significant anti-insulin effect and increases blood sugar levels by releasing glucose that is stored as glycogen in the liver and muscles.

At the University of Sassari in Italy, a research team evaluated 39 Type 1 diabetics and 34 controls for levels of taurine before and after 1.5 g/day were given for 90 days. It was reported that platelet taurine concentrations were lower in diabetic patients than in the controls. Oral administration of taurine decreased platelet aggregation, which may reduce diabetic complications such as micro- and macro-angiopathies, which are associated with increases in platelet aggregation.

The study suggests that normal concentrations of taurine could be important in restoring normal clotting and subsequently preventing blood vessel damage in Type 1 diabetics. The amino acid has antioxidant capability, which may protect cell membranes and other cellular components.[8]

References

1. Ensminger, A., et al. *Foods and Nutrition Encyclopedia.* Clovis, Calif.: Pegus Press, 1983, pp. 60ff.

2. Leverton, Ruth M. "Amino Acids." Washington, D.C.: *USDA—The Yearbook of Agriculture,* 1959, pp. 64ff.

3. Ronzio, Robert A., Ph.D. *The Encyclopedia of Nutrition and Good Health.* New York: Facts on File, Inc., 1997, p. 19.

4. Wernerman, J. "Documentation of Clinical Benefit of Specific Amino Nutrients," *Lancet,* Sept. 5, 1998, pp. 756–757.

5. Atkins, Robert C., M.D. *Dr. Atkins' Vita-Nutrient Solution.* New York: Simon & Schuster, 1998, p. 186.

6. Wascher, T. C., et al. "Effects of Low-Dose L-arginine on Insulin-Mediated Vasodilation and Insulin Sensitivity," *European Journal of Clinical Investigation* 27: 690–695, 1997.

7. Cannon, M. D., and F. Q. Nuttal. "The Metabolic Response to Dietary Protein in Subjects with Type 2 Diabetes," *Journal of the American College of Nutrition* 16(5): 478/ Abstract 33, 1997.

8. Franconi, Flavia. "Plasma and Platelet Taurine Are Reduced in Subjects with Insulin Dependent Diabetes Mellitus: Effects of Taurine Supplementation," *American Journal of Clinical Nutrition* 61: 1115–1119, 1995.

41 Coenzyme Q10

Coenzyme Q10 (ubiquinone) is an antioxidant that is being used to treat a variety of disorders affecting diabetics, including cardiomyopathy, myocardial infarction, angina pectoris, arrhythmias, blood clots, and other complications. Heart disease is a major problem for diabetics. CoQ10 is also recommended to reduce high blood sugar levels and to decrease large amounts of insulin in the blood. Using CoQ10 therapy, one diabetic was able to control her disease with only diet restrictions. The supplement may be more effective that some vitamins in controlling various heart disorders.

Coenzyme Q10 (CoQ10) is present in the mitochondria, or "energy factories," of human cells, and it is a co-factor in several enzyme systems related to energy production, according to Per H. Langsjoen of Scott and White Clinic in Temple, Texas. Since myocardial cells have a high percentage of mitochondria, and energy needs are great, it is believed that a deficiency of CoQ10 would have a significant effect on myocardial function.[1]

In a study of 19 patients with cardiomyopathy (a disorder of the heart muscle) who were treated with CoQ10, Langsjoen reports, there was a subsequent improvement in heart function and clinical status.

A longer study was undertaken involving patients with chronic dilated cardiomyopathy, in which 126 men and women were given 33.3 mg of CoQ10 t.i.d. (three times daily) or a placebo. All of the patients, of whom 75% were 60 to 80 years of age, had symptoms of heart disease before the study began, and all had been prescribed various medications. In 99% of the patients, heart failure was deemed the main complaint, and 86% were experiencing pulmonary edema. Other complaints were chest pain, arrhythmias, thromboembolism (blood clots), and heart blocks.

As the study began, CoQ10 levels in the heart patients were significantly below that of the 54 control patients. It was found that 71% of the patients improved on the CoQ10 therapy within 3 months. After 6 months, 16% more had improved. There was no improvement in 13%. There were no major complaints, although 2 patients did experience minor itching.

CoQ10 is similar to vitamin B_3 (niacin) in its chemical concept. However, it should be pointed out that CoQ10's therapy may need a period of time to kick in. CoQ10 therapy is effective and safe for treatment of dilated cardiomyopathy for at least six years, said Langsjoen.

The biomedical and clinical applications of CoQ10 continue to generate tremendous interest throughout the world, says heart specialist Stephen T. Sinatra, M.D. There have been 10 international symposia on the biomedical and clinical aspects of CoQ10 from 1976 through 1998. These symposia have comprised more than 450 papers presented by more than 250 physicians and scientists from 18 countries, who have investigated CoQ10 supplementation in a wide range of medical disorders, he said. The majority of these clinical studies have demonstrated CoQ10's positive impact on heart disease, and they have been remarkably consistent in their conclusions: treatment with CoQ10 significantly improved a wide variety of cardiovascular diseases while producing no adverse effects or drug interactions.[2]

Sinatra, a cardiologist, has been using CoQ10 for over a decade. He points to a study of 115 patients with hypertensive heart disease, in which CoQ10 resulted in clinical improvement, lowering of elevated blood pressure, improved diastolic function, and a decrease in myocardial thickness in 53% of the patients. In a study involving 7 patients with heart problems, all of them reported improvement in symptoms of fatigue and shortness of breath on an average of 200 mg/day of CoQ10.

"I recommend that when patients fail to respond to standard levels of CoQ10—90 to 150 mg/day—it is best to obtain a blood level," Sinatra said. "If a serum CoQ10 level is not feasible, treat the patient clinically by doubling or even tripling the dose according to their clinical symptoms, as cardiologists frequently do with diuretics and/or ACE inhibitors when treating congestive heart failure. We must also keep in mind that the higher doses of CoQ10 are required for patients with 'right-sided' cardiac symptoms, particularly since rather serious myocardial CoQ10 deficiencies have been found in cases with high right atrial pressures."

CoQ10 (or ubiquinone) could represent one of the major medical advances in the treatment of heart disease, Sinatra said. CoQ10 is a naturally occurring substance in foods and is synthesized in all cells of the body. While the average dietary intake approximates 5 to 10 mg/day, the dominant source in man is biosynthesis. This is a complex process involving tyrosine, an amino acid, and at least seven vitamins and several minerals.

"As an antioxidant," Sinatra continued, "CoQ10 inhibits lipid peroxidation in both cell membranes and serum low-density lipoproteins, and it also protects proteins and DNA from oxidative damage."

Writing in *Dr. Atkins' Vita-Nutrient Solution*, Robert C. Atkins, M.D., reported that CoQ10, at a dose of 60 mg/day, can help to reduce high blood sugar within six months. Since hardening of the arteries is a frequently encountered complication of diabetes, CoQ10 is doubly important, he added.[3]

Doses of between 30 and 600 mg/day of CoQ10 have been shown to benefit some patients with angina pectoris (chest pain), according to the *European Journal of Clinical Nutrition*. In addition, doses of between 60 and 200 mg/day provide some benefit in treating angina pectoris, reducing blood pressure, and other complications. The nutrient may also be useful when given one week before cardiovascular surgery.[4]

At the University of Firenze Medical School in Florence, Italy, 18 patients with essential hypertension (high blood pressure) were taken off all high blood pressure medications for 2 weeks and given either 100 mg/day of CoQ10 or a placebo for 10 weeks. For 2 weeks no supplements were given, and then the two groups switched to the protocol they had not been taking for an additional 10 weeks.[5]

It was reported that, after 10 weeks of CoQ10 therapy, systolic blood pressure (when the heart is beating) dropped about 10 points, while the diastolic pressure (when the heart rests between beats) dropped 7 points on average. The researchers concluded that CoQ10 is beneficial as a hypertensive agent.

In another study at the University of Firenze Medical School, researchers report that CoQ10 has shown potential in treating congestive heart failure, angina pectoris, high blood pressure, and arrhythmias. Their study involved 5 men and 5 women with a mean age of 61.[6]

The patients with essential arterial hypertension were given 50 mg of CoQ10 twice daily for 10 weeks. At the end of the study, systolic blood pressure went down from 161.5 mmHg on average to 142.2 mmHg. Diastolic pressure decreased from 98.5 mmHg to 83.1 mmHg. Total blood cholesterol dropped from 227 to 203, while HDL-cholesterol (the good kind) increased from 42 mg/dl to 45.9 mg/dl.

At Hamamatsu University in Japan, 12 patients, with an average age of 56, with stable angina pectoris, were given 50 mg of CoQ10 three times daily for 4 weeks. The researchers found there was a reduction in anginal frequency and nitroglycerine use and an increase in exercise time. One patient had a loss of appetite, but continued the therapy.[7]

In an article in *American Journal of Cardiology*, Ram B. Singh, M.D., discussed a study in which two capsules of CoQ10 were given twice daily to patients with myocardial infarction (heart attack). He found the supplement more effective than vitamins in controlling arrhythmias, angina and left ventricular failure, as well as other cardiac events. He also found that the supplement can decrease hyperinsulinemia (too much insulin in the blood) and possibly lipoprotein-A, which is thought to be a risk factor for coronary disease.[8]

A 35-year-old woman with diabetes, aspiration pneumonia, respiratory failure, and other complications was treated with antibiotic therapy, but after 1 week, her consciousness remained unclear. Later, she was given 160 mg/day of CoQ10 for 6 months. In a 1-year follow-up, the patient only needed diet restriction to control her diabetes, reported an article in *European Neurology*.[9]

In *Cortlandt Forum*, Gerard K. Nash, D.O., said research showed that heart failure patients with CoQ10 deficiency had a favorable 8-year survival rate when CoQ10 supplements are given.[10]

Italian researchers evaluated 48 chronic hemodialysis patients and found that 62% had abnormally low levels of CoQ10. They added that low CoQ10 levels may contribute to the defective serum antioxidant activity and increase the risk of peroxidative damage in uremic patients with chronic hemodialysis.[11]

Coenzyme Q10 treatment is indicated in high-risk cardiac surgery patients who have CoQ10 deficiency, according to Karl Folkers, Ph.D., of the University of Texas at Austin, a pioneer in CoQ10 research. He said that CoQ10 is a natural co-factor of the heart, a potent free-radical scavenger, and a superoxide inhibitor.[12]

The study involved 10 high-risk patients during heart surgery compared to 10 placebos (people who did not have a high risk), who were given 100 mg/day of the supplement 14 days prior to and 30 days after surgery.

The recovery course, 3 to 5 days, was uncomplicated in the CoQ10 group, Folkers said.

In 34 patients with various thyroid disorders, including Graves' disease and multiple malignancies, there were raised levels of vitamin E but reduced levels of CoQ10 in the thyroid tissue of patients with Graves' disease and follicular and papillary thyroid cancers.[13]

Researchers in Denmark pointed out that a defective myocardial energy supply due to a poor utilization of oxygen may be a common final pathway in the progression of myocardial disease. However, CoQ10 is a natural antioxidant to combat the problem. After taking myocardial tissue samples from 45 patients with a variety of cardiomyopathies, it was found that CoQ10 was significantly lower in those with more advanced heart failure when compared to those with milder cases of the disease.[14]

The researchers said that myocardial tissue CoQ10 deficiency might be restored significantly with oral supplementation in selected cases. In an open trial conducted by S. A. Mortensen, M.D., CoQ10 therapy at 100 mg/day resulted in almost two-thirds of the patients having clinical improvement. Double-blind studies have confirmed the efficacy of CoQ10 as an adjunctive treatment in heart failure, Mortensen said.

References

1. Langsjoen, Per H., et al. "Long-Term Efficacy and Safety of Coenzyme Q10 Therapy for Idiopathic Dilated Cardiomyopathy," *American Journal of Cardiology* 65: 521–523, Feb. 15; 1990.

2. Sinatra, Stephen T., M.D. "Coenzyme Q10—A Cardiologist's Commentary," *Natural Medicine Journal* 2(2); 9–15, Feb. 1999.

3. Atkins, Robert C., M.D. *Dr. Atkins' Vita-Nutrient Solution.* New York: Simon and Schuster, 1998, p. 248.

4. Overvad, K., et al. "Coenzyme Q10 in Health and Disease," *European Journal of Clinical Nutrition* 53: 764–770, 1999.

5. Digiesi, V., et al. "Effect of Coenzyme Q10 on Essential Arterial Hypertension," *Current Therapeutic Research* 47(5): 841–845, May 1990.

6. Digiesi, V., et al. "Mechanism of Action of Coenzyme Q10 in Essential Hypertension," *Current Therapeutic Research* 51(5): 668–672, May 1992.

7. Kamikawa, T., et al. "Effects of Coenzyme Q10 on Exercise Tolerance in Chronic Stable Angina Pectoris," *American Journal of Cardiology* 56: 247–251, Aug. 1, 1985.

8. Hamilton, Kirk. "Acute Myocardial Infarction and Antioxidants," *Clinical Pearls 1998. The Experts Speak.* Sacramento, Calif.: I.T. Services, Inc., 1998, pp. 17–18. Also, Singh, Ram B. "Interventional Therapy with Mega Dose of Antioxidant Vitamins in Patients with Acute Myocardial Infarction: Could We Throw Caution to the Wind?" *American Journal of Cardiology* 80: 823–824, Sept. 15, 1997.

9. Liou, C. W., et al. "Correct of Pancreatic B-Cell Dysfunction with Coenzyme Q10

in a Patient with Mitochondrial Encephalomyopathy, Lactic Acidosis and Stroke-Like Episodes Syndrome and Diabetes Mellitus," *European Neurology* 43: 54–55, 2000.

10. Nash, Gerard K., D.O. "Whatever Happened to Coenzyme Q10," *Cortlandt Forum*, Feb. 1992, p. 48.

11. Triolo, Luigi, et al. "Serum Coenzyme Q10 and Uremic Patients and Chronic Hemodialysis," *Nephron* 66: 153–156, 1994.

12. Judy, W. V., et al. "Myocardial Preservation in Therapy with Coenzyme Q10 During Heart Surgery," *Clinical Investigator* 71: S155–S161, 1993.

13. Mano, Toshiki, et al. "Vitamin E and Coenzyme Q Concentrations in the Thyroid Tissues of Patients with Various Thyroid Diseases," *American Journal of Medical Science* 315(4): 230–232, 1998.

14. Mortensen, S. A., M.D. "Prospectives on Therapy of Cardiovascular Disease with Coenzyme Q10 (Ubiquinone)," *Clinical Investigator* 71: S116–S123, 1993.

42 The Benefits of Herbs for Diabetes

Many physicians treating diabetics apparently are not aware that there are dozens of herbs that can lower blood pressure, improve glucose metabolism, lower blood sugar levels, and reduce sugar in the urine and other complications of the disease. Herbs can help to prevent heart disease and hardening of the arteries, reduce pain in diabetic neuropathy, and treat diabetics with cirrhosis of the liver, among other things. These natural plants have few, if any, side effects, and are user-friendly for most diabetics.

Writing in the *Journal of the American Osteopathic Association*, R. P. Mozersky said that a number of herbs and supplements have proved useful in dealing with diabetes. For example:[1]

- One capsule containing 400 mg of a standardized onion extract improves glucose utilization.

- Bitter gourd improves glucose utilization when used as a 5 ml tincture two to three times a day to a total as high as 50 ml/day.

- *Gymnema sylvestre* lowers blood pressure when given as three-fourths of a teaspoon in a glass of hot water as a tea.

- Fenugreek improves glucose utilization when taken as 625 mg capsules, two to three times daily.

- Stevia, a sweetener, improves glucose utilization when taken at 200 mg twice daily.

- St. John's wort helps to control depression, and possibly diabetic neuropathy, when taken as one 425 mg standard extract capsule containing 0.35 hypericin twice daily.

- Ivy gourd enhances glucose metabolism when taken as six tablets a day in divided doses.

Mozersky added that these supplements may also benefit diabetics:

- Vitamin E, at 200 to 400 IU/day.

- Vitamin C, at 500 to 1,000 mg/day.

- Vitamin B_6, which improves glucose metabolism and enhances nerve function, although the dosage depends on whether or not the patient is taking other medications.

- Biotin, another B vitamin, which improves glucose metabolism at 200 to 400 mcg/day.

- Inositol, related to the B-complex, which improves glucose metabolism at 500 mg b.i.d. (twice a day).

In studying 370 women and 256 men in Morocco, 61% had diabetes, 23% were hypertensives, and 16% were hypertensive diabetics; yet almost 67.5% of the patients regularly used medicinal plants to control their disease. For diabetics, 41 plants were used, the most popular being *Trigonella foenum-graecum L.* (fenugreek), *Globularia alpum L.*, *Artemisia* (herba-alba), *Citrulis colocynthis L.*, and *Tetraclinis articulata Benth.*[2]

For high blood pressure, the patients were using 18 different herbs, including garlic, *Olea europea L.*, *Arbutus unedo L.*, *Urtica doica L.*, and *Petroselinum crispum.* Among the 18 herbs used for high blood pressure, 14 were also selected by the diabetics.

Bitter Melon *(Momordica charanta)*: Indian researchers have reported on the ability of bitter melon, also known as balsam pear, to reduce blood sugar, reported James A. Duke, Ph.D. In animal studies, the herb delayed the development of diabetic complications. In a later human trial, those with diabetes who consumed 2 oz. of bitter melon juice a day saw their blood sugar levels decline by 54%. Dried fruits and seeds from the plant also help to reduce blood sugar.[3]

Capsaicin: While capsaicin cream (from chili peppers) has been recommended for treating arthritis, it is also useful in dealing with diabetic neuropathy, according to researchers at Case Western Reserve University School of Medicine in Cleveland, Ohio. Purified capsaicin depletes Substance P, which contributes to pain in inflammation.[4]

Fenugreek: At the National Institute of Nutrition in Jamai-Osmania, Hyderbad, India, 10 Type 1 diabetics were given 100 mg of fenugreek seed powder, divided into 2 equal dosages and placed in the diets. The patients, ranging in age from 12 to 37, were given this therapy for two 10-day periods. The fenugreek diet considerably reduced fasting blood sugar levels, improved glucose tolerance, and led to a 54% reduction in daily urinary glucose excretion. Cholesterol, LDL-cholesterol, VLDL-cholesterol, and triglyceride levels also went down, while HDL-cholesterol remained unchanged.[5]

Fig Leaves *(Ficus carica)*: Drinking a decoction of fig leaves lowered the required insulin dose by 12% in a group of 6 men and 4 women, 22 to 38 years of age, who had had Type 1 diabetes for nine years. The fig leaf decoction was taken for 1 month, followed by consuming a nonsweet commercial tea for the second month in a crossover design. Following a meal, the amount of glucose in the blood was significantly lower during the fig leaf supplement when compared with the tea.[6]

Garlic Oil: A research team at John Bastyr College of Naturopathic Medicine in Seattle, Washington, reported that garlic oil could be effective as part of a program to control and prevent hardening of the arteries and coronary artery disease, since it lowers cholesterol, blood pressure, and platelet aggregation.[7]

In the study, 20 healthy volunteers were randomly divided into two groups, and rotated for 4-week periods through two different sequences of oral garlic oil or placebo (18 mg/day). The amount of platelet aggregation dropped a lot, and serum cholesterol levels and blood pressure also declined with the garlic oil therapy.

Ginseng: At various clinical trials, ginseng has been used regarding diabetes, cancer risk, high blood pressure, and colds and flu. For example, in one Korean study involving 26 volunteers with high blood pressure, those receiving 4.5 g/day of red ginseng for 8 weeks experienced a decrease in 24-hour mean systolic (beating) blood pressure, and a slight decline in diastolic (resting) blood pressure.[8]

While the World Health Organization has recorded two incidents in which ginseng interacted with phenelzine, a monoamine oxidase (MAO) inhibitor, there have been relatively few adverse effects using the herb. MAO inhibitors are drugs designed to treat depression, high blood pressure, and other conditions. Standardized extracts should contain 4% ginsenosides. Those who use this form should take 100 mg twice daily. For those who use nonstandardized raw ginseng in powder form, the recommended dose is 1 to 2 g/day for as long as three months.

Researchers at the University of Oulu in Finland treated 36 Type 2 diabetics for 8 weeks, giving them 100 mg/day or 200 mg/day of ginseng or a placebo. They reported that the ginseng elevated mood, improved mental and bodily processes, and reduced fasting blood sugar and body weight. The larger dosage improved glycosylated hemoglobin and other parameters.[9]

A study reported in *Archives of Internal Medicine* involved 10 nondiabetics (6 males and 4 females, mean age of 34), and 9 Type 2 diabetics (5 males and 4 females, mean age of 62). The participants were randomly selected to receive 3 g of ginseng or look-alike pills, either 40 minutes before or together with a 25-g glucose challenge. The placebo capsules contained only corn oil. The results showed no difference in the nondiabetic volunteers in after-eating sugar levels between placebo and ginseng, when given the glucose challenge, but when ginseng was taken 40 minutes before the glucose challenges, significant reductions were recorded.

In Type 2 diabetics, the same was true, whether the ginseng was taken before or together with the glucose challenge. It was found that American ginseng reduced after-meal glucose levels in both treatment groups. The researchers recommended that American ginseng might be suggested for nondiabetics with meals to avoid low blood sugar.[10]

Researchers at the University of Oulu in Finland treated 36 Type 2 diabetics for 8 weeks, giving them 100 mg/day or 200 mg/day of ginseng or a placebo. They reported that the ginseng elevated mood, improved mental and bodily processes, and reduced fasting blood sugar and body weight. The larger dosage improved glycosylated hemoglobin and other parameters.

Gurmar *(Gymnema sylvestre)*: In a study involving 22 Type 2 diabetics, who were given 400 mg/day of gurmar in addition to conventional oral hypoglycemia agents for 18 to 20 months, there was a reduction in glycosylated hemoglobin levels from 12 to 8.5%.[11]

In another study, involving 27 Type 1 diabetics, whose condition was followed for up to 30 months, volunteers were given 400 mg/day of gurmar for 6 to 8 months. Their average insulin requirement dropped from 60 to 45 units/day, or almost 30%, and their serum lipids returned to near normal levels. It is thought that the herb may regenerate or revitalize pancreatic beta cells. There may be an increase in insulin levels or a decrease in insulin resistance, but these mechanisms are still hypotheses, according to *Family Practice News.*

Jackass Bitters *(Neurolaena lobata)*: When this plant's ability to control Type 2 diabetes becomes better known, jackass bitters will become easier to find, said James A. Duke, Ph.D. Its use in treating diabetes surfaced in 1989, when a Florida physician sent a sample to Walter Mertz, M.D., then director of the USDA Health Nutrition Research Center in Beltsville, Maryland, wondering what the plant was.[12]

"One of the physician's patients, a woman with Type 2 diabetes, had picked up the herb on a trip to Trinidad," Duke reported. "She put it in vermouth and took small sips of the concoction twice a day. Within six months, her blood sugar normalized. . . . Animal studies have found that a tincture a little stronger than what the woman was taking–the equivalent of about a shot glass a day–significantly lowers blood sugar levels."

Marshmallow *(Althaea officinalis)*: This root is very high in soluble plant fiber known as pectin (35% on a dry-weight basis). Taking pectin is an effective way of keeping blood sugar levels down, according to James A. Duke, Ph.D., a leading expert on herbs.[13]

Milk Thistle *(Silybum marianum)*: At Hospital Monfalcone in Italy, Mari Velussi, M.D., and colleagues studied 60 cirrhotic diabetic patients, ranging in age from 45 to 70, who were getting insulin and who had high insulin levels. The patients received either 600 mg/day of silymarin or no silymarin for 6 months; silymarin is a component in this herb.

After 6 months of therapy, the silymarin-treated diabetics had the mean levels of fasting glucose, daily blood glucose, daily glycosuria (sugar in the urine), glycosylated hemoglobin, daily insulin need, fasting insulinemia, blood malondialdehyde, and basal and glucagon-stimulated C peptide counted. All of these parameters were lower than in the untreated patients and lower than when the study began.[14]

Velussi said that these results suggest that milk thistle can reduce lipoperoxidation of liver cells in diabetics with cirrhosis of the liver, and increase production of insulin inside the body and thus decrease the need for insulin injections. Lipid peroxides are toxic molecules that can harm the body. Silymarin apparently restores the plasma membrane of liver cells and increases the sensitivity of insulin receptors. The herbal therapy should probably be continued beyond a 6-month period.

Red Wine: A moderate amount of red wine during meals may help to prevent cardiovascular disease in diabetics, according to *European Journal of Clinical Investigation.* The study involved 20 Type 2 diabetics (12 males and 8 females). Their average age was 55.1 years, and they had had diabetes for 9.2 years. The patients were evaluated during fasting consumption of 300 ml of red wine, or during a meal in which they were given red wine or abstained.

The researchers reported that red wine consumption during a meal significantly preserved antioxidant defenses in the blood and reduced low-density lipoprotein cholesterol oxidation and development of blood clots. The beneficial nutrient in red wine is thought to be resveratrol.[15]

Tulasi *(Ocimum sanctum)*: Twenty-seven Type 2 diabetics received 1 g of tulasi powder, which was consumed in a fasting state each morning for 30 days. Following 1 month of tulasi therapy, there was a 20.8% lowering of blood glucose, 11.2% lowering of glycated proteins, 13.5% lowering of total amino acids, and 13.7% lowering of uronic acid, which is an oxidation product of sugars. The latter is combined in many polysaccharides and in urine. In addition, total cholesterol was reduced 11.3%, LDL-cholesterol went down 14%, VLDL-cholesterol was reduced 16.3%, and triglycerides were reduced 16.4%. There was no change in HDL-cholesterol.[16]

Eugenol, a major component of the essential oil in tulasi leaves, has been found to inhibit lipid peroxidation. It is suspected that eugenol protects the beta cells from free radical damage, thus allowing increased insulin secretion.

References

1. Mozersky, R. P. "Herbal Products and Supplemental Nutrients Used in the Management of Diabetes," *Journal of the American Osteopathic Association* Suppl. 12:S4–S9, Dec. 1999.

2. Ziyyat, A., et al. "Phytotherapy of Hypertension and Diabetes in Oriental Morocco," *Journal of Ethno-pharmacology* 58: 45–54, 1997.

3. Duke, James A., Ph.D. *Anti-Aging Prescriptions.* Emmaus, Penn.: Rodale, Inc., 2001, p. 349.

4. Deal, Chad L., M.D. "The Use of Topical Capsaicin in Managing Arthritis Pain: A Clinician's Prospective," *Seminars in Arthritis and Rheumatism* 23(6): 48–52, June 1994.

5. Sharma, R. D., et al. "Effect of Fenugreek Seed on Blood Glucose and Serum Lipids in Type 1 Diabetes," *European Journal of Clinical Nutrition* 44: 301–306, 1990.

6. Serraclara, Alicia, et al. "Hypoglycemic Action of an Oral Fig Leaf Decoction in Type 1 Diabetic Patients," *Diabetes Research and Clinical Practice* 39: 19–22, 1998.

7. Barrie, Stephen A., N.D., et al. "Effects of Garlic Oil on Platelet Aggregation, Serum Lipids and Blood Pressure in Humans," *Journal of Orthomolecular Medicine* 2(1): 187–192, 1987.

8. Pettit, J. L. "Ginseng," *Clinician Reviews* 10(8): 86–92, Aug. 2000.

9. Sotaniemi, Eero, M.D., Ph.D., et al. "Ginseng Therapy in Non-Insulin Dependent Diabetic Patients," *Diabetes Care* 18(10): 1373–1375, Oct. 1995.

10. Vuksan, V., et al. "American Ginseng (Panax Quinquefolius L.) Reduces Postprandial Glycemia in Nondiabetic Subjects and Subjects with Type 2 Diabetes Mellitus," *Archives of Internal Medicine* 160: 1009–1013, April 10, 2000.

11. Walsh, N. "Asian Herb for Diabetes To Be Tested in Clinical Trial," *Family Practice News* 22: 37–38A, April 1, 2001.

12. Duke, James A., Ph.D. *Anti-Aging Prescriptions.* Emmaus, Penn.: Rodale, Inc., 2001, pp. 350–351.

13. Duke, James A., Ph.D. *The Green Pharmacy.* Emmaus, Penn.: Rodale Press, 1997, p. 165.

14. Velussi, Mari, M.D. "Silymarin Reduces Hyperinsulinemia, Malondialdehyde Levels and Daily Insulin Need in Cirrhotic Diabetic Patients," *Current Therapeutic Research* 53(5): 533–545, May 1993.

15. Coriello, A., et al. "Red Wine Protects Diabetic Patients from Meal-Induced Oxidative Stress and Thrombosis Activation: A Pleasant Approach to the Prevention of Cardiovascular Disease in Diabetes," *European Journal of Clinical Investigation* 31(4): 322–328, 2001.

16. Rai, V., et al. "Effect of Ocimum Sanctum Leaf Powder on Blood Lipoproteins, Glycated Proteins and Total Amino Acids in Patients with Non-Insulin-Dependent Diabetes Mellitus," *Journal of Nutritional and Environmental Medicine* 7: 113–118, 1997.

43 Other Supplements and Techniques to Help Diabetics

Researchers are using a variety of relatively unknown over-the-counter substances in dealing with diabetes. Ask your doctor for recommendations. For example, brewer's yeast, which is rich in the B-complex vitamins and glucose tolerance factor, improves glucose tolerance in Type 2 diabetics. 5-HTP, a cousin of the amino acid tryptophan, helps diabetics to decrease their fat and energy intakes, along with their body weight. Phosphatidylcholine helps to reduce blood cholesterol levels, a significant problem in cardiovascular diseases. Acupuncture can also greatly help reduce the symptoms and complications of diabetes.

Brewer's Yeast: Supplementation with brewer's yeast, an excellent source of glucose tolerance factor (GTF), has been shown to improve glucose tolerance of Type 2 diabetics, increase their sensitivity to insulin, and lower their level of blood fats, according to Melvyn Werbach, M.D.

GTF occurs pre-formed in certain foods, especially brewer's yeast, and human beings have a varying ability to synthesize it from inorganic chromium, vitamin B_3, and amino acids. Werbach added that there are many commercial GTF products on the market and their actual GTF activity is variable and largely unproven. Unless you can find out how potent a GTF supplement is, he recommends that you obtain your GTF from brewer's yeast. As a supplement, he suggests 9 g/day of brewer's yeast during a trial period of eight weeks.[1]

5-HTP: At the University of Rome in Italy, a research team headed by Filippo Rossi-Fanelli, M.D., evaluated 25 overweight Type 2 diabetics. The volunteers were given either 750 mg/day of 5-hydroxy-tryptophan (5-HTP) or a look-alike pill for 2 weeks. The amount of the amino acid tryptophan in the brain was significantly reduced in the diabetics when compared to the healthy controls. Those getting 5-HTP significantly decreased their daily energy intake by reducing carbohydrate and fat intake and also lowered their body weight.[2]

Phosphatidylcholine (PC): This supplement should be considered an important supportive therapy for the treatment of lipid disorders in diabetics, according to an article in *La Clinica Therapeutica*. In the study, 29 diabetics were divided into 2 groups. PC was given at a dose of 1,200 mg/day in the form of three 200-mg capsules at two main meals.

The PC therapy led to a rapid fall in blood cholesterol, which was evident after 30 days of treatment and was statistically significant at 90 days, resulting in a 15.1% reduction in cholesterol. There was an increase in HDL-cholesterol (the beneficial kind) of 13% after 90 days, and a significant decrease in LDL-cholesterol (the bad kind) from 60 days onward.[3]

Acupuncture: Researchers at the University of Manchester in England evaluated 46 patients with the mean age of 57.2 years. Thirty-four of the volunteers were Type 1 diabetics, while 10 were Type 2 diabetics who had had the disease for 13.2 years. Two patients did not complete the study. Twenty-one of the patients were on a diet and oral hypoglycemic drugs, while 23 were taking insulin.[4]

The volunteers, complaining of chronic painful peripheral neuropathy, were treated with acupuncture analgesia. Sixty-three percent were already receiving standard medical treatment for neuropathy. The patients were given 6 courses of classical acupuncture for 10 weeks, using traditional Chinese medicine acupuncture points.

Of the 44 patients who completed the study, 77% showed significant improvement in their primary and/or secondary symptoms. During an 18 to 52 week follow-up, 67% were able to stop or reduce their medications significantly. During the follow-up period, only 24% of the patients required further acupuncture treatment. The researchers said that 77% of the patients reported significant improvement, and 21% said their symptoms had cleared completely. Only 1 volunteer reported side effects.

References

1. Werbach, Melvyn, M.D. *Healing with Food.* New York: HarperCollins, 1993, pp. 111, 121.

2. Cangianno, C., et al. "Effects of Oral 5-Hydroxy-Tryptophan on Energy Intake and Macronutrient Selection in Non-Insulin Dependent Diabetic Patients," *International Journal of Obesity* 22: 648–654, 1998.

3. Arsenio, L., et al. "An Investigation Into the Therapeutic Effects of Phosphatidylcholine in Diabetes with Dyslipidemia," *La Clinica Therapeutica* 114(2): 117–127, July 31, 1985.

4. Abuaisha, B. B., et al. "Acupuncture for the Treatment of Chronic Painful Peripheral Diabetic Neuropathy: A Long-Term Study," *Diabetes Research and Clinical Practice* 39: 115–121, 1998.

Glossary

A

ACE inhibitors: Drugs that can lower blood pressure and slow the progression of kidney disease.

Acetone: A chemical found in the blood when the body uses fat instead of glucose for energy. When acetone forms, it usually means that the cells do not have enough insulin, or cannot use the insulin that is in the blood, to use glucose (sugar) for energy. Acetone exits in the urine, and someone with lots of acetone in the body can have breath that smells fruity.

Acidosis: Too much acid in the body. For diabetics, this can lead to diabetic ketoacidosis.

Acute diabetic ketoacidosis (DKA): A serious condition found in Type 1 diabetics due to insufficient insulin. Symptoms include high blood glucose levels (over 240 mg/dl), ketones in the urine, shortness of breath, nausea, and in extreme cases, coma.

Adrenal glands: Two organs sitting on top of the kidneys that release hormones such as adrenalin (epinephrine). This and other hormones, such as insulin, control the body's use of glucose (sugar).

Adult-onset diabetes mellitus: Former term for Type 2 diabetes.

After-eating blood glucose: Blood taken one to two hours after eating to see the amount of glucose (sugar) in the blood.

Albumin: A water-soluble protein that is found in tissues and fluids.

Albuminuria: The presence of protein in the urine.

Alpha cell: A type of cell in the pancreas, in the area called islets of Langerhans, which make and release a hormone called glucagon, which raises the level of glucose in the blood.

Amino acids: A group of twenty-two essential and non-essential nitrogen-containing compounds that form the basic structure of proteins.

Aminos: Compounds that contain nitrogen.

Amylase: A pancreatic or salivary enzyme necessary for breaking down starch so that it can be absorbed.

Amyotrophy: A type of diabetic neuropathy that brings muscle weakness and wasting.

Angina pectoris: Chest pain that may also involve the arm, jaw, and shoulder.

Angiopathy: A disease of the blood vessels (arteries, veins, and capillaries) that occurs when someone has diabetes for a long time. In macroangiopathy, fat and blood clots build up in large blood vessels, stick to the vessel walls, and block the flow of blood. In microangiopathy, the walls of the smaller blood vessels become so thick and weak that they bleed, leak protein, and slow the flow of blood through the body. Cells, such as those in the eye, do not get enough blood and may be damaged.

Antibodies: Proteins that the body makes to protect itself from foreign substances. For diabetics, the body sometimes makes antibodies to work against pork or beef insulins because they are not exactly the same as human insulin or because they have impurities. The antibodies can keep the insulin from working well and may cause a diabetic to have an allergic reaction to the beef or pork insulins.

Anticoagulants: Blood thinners that inhibit the formation of clots.

Antioxidant: A substance, such as vitamin E, that prevents free-radical or oxidative damage.

Apolipoprotein-A: A fairly newly defined risk factor for hardening of the arteries, including coronary and cerebrovascular vessels. It is similar to LDL-cholesterol.

Apolipoprotein-B: A single protein found in LDL-cholesterol, which allows LDL to attach itself to cells. LDL-cholesterol, the so-called bad kind, is associated with cardiovascular disease by way of oxidation and free radical damage. When LDL mixes with oxygen and becomes oxidized, it can clog arteries and lead to cardiovascular disease.

Arrhythmia: Irregular heartbeat.

Arteriole: The smallest blood vessel.

Artery: A blood vessel that carries oxygen-rich blood away from the heart.

Ascorbic acid: Vitamin C.

Atherosclerosis: Commonly called hardening of the arteries, this is a process in which cholesterol, triglycerides, and other fatty substances are deposited in artery walls, causing a blockage of an artery.

Autonomic neuropathy: Damage that is caused by elevated blood sugar levels.

B

Basal metabolic rate: The energy necessary for internal or cellular work when the body is resting.

Benign: Harmless.

Beta-carotene: Provitamin A. One of the carotenoids in plants that can be converted into vitamin A in the body.

Beta cell: A cell in the pancreas in the islets of Langerhans, which make and release insulin, a hormone that controls the level of glucose (sugar) in the blood.

Bilirubin: Breakdown product of the hemoglobin molecule in red blood cells.

Biotin: A B-complex vitamin.

Blood brain barrier: A barrier that prohibits the passage of substances from the blood to the brain.

Blood glucose: The main sugar that the body makes from proteins, fats, and carbohydrates, mostly from carbohydrates. Glucose is the major source of energy for living cells and is carried to the cells via the bloodstream. Cells cannot use glucose without the help of insulin.

Blood glucose monitoring: A way of testing how much glucose is in the blood. A drop of blood, usually taken from the fingertip, is placed on the end of a specially coated strip, called a testing strip, which has a chemical on it that makes it change color according to how much glucose (sugar) is in the blood.

Telling whether the level of glucose is low, high, or normal can be determined by comparing the color on the end of the strip to a color chart that is printed on the side of the test strip container, or by inserting the strip into a small machine, called a meter, which reads the strip and shows the level of blood glucose in a digital window display.

Blood testing is more accurate than urine testing in monitoring blood glucose levels, since it shows what the current level of glucose is, rather than what the level was an hour or so previously.

Blood pressure: The force of the blood on the walls of the arteries. The higher, or systolic, pressure occurs each time the heart pushes blood into the vessels, and the lower, or diastolic, pressure occurs when the heart rests between beats. In a blood pressure reading of 120/80, 120 is the systolic pressure and 80 is the diastolic reading. A reading of 120/80 is said to be normal. High blood pressure can lead to heart disease and strokes.

Blood urea nitrogen (BUN): A waste product of the kidneys. Increased BUN levels in the blood may indicate early kidney disease.

Blood vessels: Tubes that carry blood to and from all parts of the body, including arteries, veins, and capillaries. The heart pumps blood through these vessels so that the blood can carry oxygen and nutrients the cells need, or take away waste that the cells do not need.

Body mass index (BMI): A ratio of weight to height, which can accurately determine whether a person is obese. The BMI is determined by multiplying your weight in pounds by 703, multiplying your height in inches by itself, then dividing the first number by the second one. A BMI reading from 19 to 20 is considered a healthy weight.

Brittle diabetes: A term used when a person's blood sugar level often swings quickly from high to low and from low to high. Also called labile or unstable diabetes.

Bronze diabetes: A genetic disease of the liver in which the body takes in too much iron from food. Also called hemochromatosis.

C

Calorie: A nutritional calorie is calculated as the amount of heat necessary to raise 1 kg of water 1 degree C.

Capillary: The smallest of the body's blood vessels.

Capsaicin: A topical ointment made from chili peppers that is used to relieve the pain of peripheral neuropathy.

Carbohydrates: Starches and sugars in foods.

Cardiomyopathy: Heart damage.

Cardiovascular disease: A variety of heart and blood vessel diseases that include heart attack, stroke, hardening of the arteries, and congestive heart failure.

Cataracts: Condition in the eyes that reduces lens transparency and results in a loss of visual acuity.

Celiac disease: A malabsorption disorder that brings malnutrition, edema, abnormal stools, anemia, and peripheral neuropathy. These abnormalities in the intestinal tract require a gluten-free diet, which involves the avoidance of wheat, rye, oats, barley, and several other grains and grasses.

Cerebrovascular disease: Damage to the blood vessels in the brain, which can cause a stroke. Sometimes the blood vessels can burst, resulting in a hemorrhagic stroke. Diabetics are at high risk for this condition.

Charcot's foot: A deformity of the bones in the feet caused by diabetic nerve damage. It can cause foot ulcers.

Cholecalciferol: Vitamin B_3/D_3.

Cholesterol: A fat found in foods of animal origin and also produced inside the body. It is needed for the production of certain hormones as well as obtaining vitamin D from the sun. Large amounts can cause a narrowing of the arteries in susceptible people.

Choline: A vitamin-like substance related to the B-complex of vitamins.

Chronic: Long-standing or frequently recurring.

Cirrhosis: A severe liver disease characterized by the replacement of the liver cells with scar tissue.

Clinical trial: A scientifically controlled study using people, usually to test the effectiveness of a new treatment.

Cobalamin: Vitamin B_{12}.

Coenzyme: A necessary nonprotein component of an enzyme, most often a vitamin or a mineral.

Congenital defects: Problems that are present at birth.

Congestive heart failure: Chronic disease that develops when the heart is not capable of supplying the oxygen demands of the body.

Contraindication: A condition that makes a treatment not helpful or possibly harmful.

Coronary artery disease: A condition that develops when the heart does not get an adequate supply of blood and oxygen due to hardening of the arteries.

Cortisol: A stress hormone that raises blood glucose levels.

Coxsackie B4 virus: An agent that has been shown to damage the beta cells of the pancreas in lab tests. This virus may be one cause of Type 1 diabetes.

C-peptide: A substance that the pancreas releases into the bloodstream in equal amounts to insulin. A test of C-peptide levels will show how much insulin the body is making.

Creatinine: A chemical in the blood that is passed in the urine. A test of the amount of creatinine in blood or in blood and urine shows if the kidney is working right or if it is diseased.

D

d-alpha tocopherol: Natural vitamin E.

dl: Deciliter; 0.18 pint dry; 0.21 pint liquid.

dl-alpha tocopherol: Synthetic vitamin E.

Delta cell: A cell in the pancreas in the islets of Langerhans. These cells make somatostatin, a hormone that is thought to control how the beta cells make and release insulin and how the alpha cells make and release glucagon.

Dextrose: Also called glucose; it is a simple sugar found in the blood. It is the main source of energy in the body.

Diabetic amyotrophy: A disease of the nerves leading to the muscles. This condition affects only one side of the body and occurs most often in older men with mild diabetes (see **neuropathy**).

Diabetic coma: A severe emergency in which a person is not conscious because the blood glucose is too low or too high. If the level is too low, the person has hypoglycemia; if too high, the patient has hyperglycemia and may develop ketoacidosis.

Diabetic ketoacidosis (DKA): Out-of-control diabetes with high blood sugar; this needs emergency treatment. Blood sugar levels may get too high because of illness, taking too little insulin, or getting too little exercise. The body begins using stored fat for energy, and ketone bodies (acids) build up in the blood.

Signs of DKA include nausea and vomiting, which can lead to loss of water from the body, stomach pain, and deep and rapid breathing. Other signs include a flushed face, dry skin and mouth, fruity breath odor, a rapid or weak pulse, and low blood pressure. If the patient is not given fluids and insulin immediately, ketoacidosis can lead to coma and even death.

Diabetic myelopathy: Damage to the spinal cord found in some diabetics.

Diabetic retinopathy: Disease of the small blood vessels of the eye.

Diabetogenic: Causing diabetes. Some drugs cause blood glucose levels to rise, causing diabetes.

Diabetologist: A doctor who specializes in treating diabetes.

Dialysis: A procedure that substitutes for kidney function by filtering toxic chemicals from the blood and maintaining blood pressure and blood chemical balances.

Diastolic pressure: Blood pressure when the heart is resting between beats.

Disaccharide: Any sugar—lactose, maltose, sucrose—that yields to two monosaccharides when hydrolyzed.

Diuretic: A substance that increases urine output.

DNA: Abbreviation for deoxyribonucleic acid, a chemical substance in plant and animal cells that tells the cells what to do and when to do it. DNA is the information about what each person inherits from his/her parents.

Double-blind, crossover study: In a double-blind study, none of the participants or scientists knows which group of subjects is getting which medication (or placebo). In a crossover study, each group is later switched to the medication (or placebo) they have not been getting. Between the switches may be a "washout" period in which neither group gets any medication for a week or weeks.

Duodenum: Upper portion of the small intestine.

Dupuytren's contracture: This affects the fingers and palm. It is more common in diabetics and may precede diabetes.

Dyslipidemia: High levels of cholesterol and triglyc-erides, which puts patients at risk for hardening of the arteries.

Dyspnea: Labored breathing.

E

Edema: A swelling or puffiness of some part of the body. Water or other body fluids collect in the cells and cause the swelling.

Eicosapentaenoic acid (EPA): A fatty acid found mostly in cold-water fish, such as salmon and sardines.

Endocrine glands: Glands that release hormones into the bloodstream. They affect how the body uses food (metabolism). One endocrine gland is the pancreas, which releases insulin so the body can use sugar for energy.

Endogenous: Grown or made inside the body. Insulin made by the pancreas is endogenous insulin. Insulin made from beef or pork pancreas or derived from bacteria is exogenous, since it is derived from outside the body and must be injected.

End-stage renal disease: A final phase of kidney disease which requires dialysis or kidney transplant.

Enzyme: A special type of protein. Each enzyme usually has its own chemical job to do, such as helping to change starch into glucose (sugar).

Epidemiology: The study of a disease that deals with how many people have it, where they are, how many new cases develop, and how to control the disease.

Epinephrine: One of the secretions of the adrenal glands. It helps the liver release glucose and limit the release of insulin. It also makes the heart beat faster and can raise blood pressure. Also called adrenalin.

Epithelium: Cells that line most of the internal organs.

Essential fatty acids: Fatty acids such as linoleic and linolenic, which the body cannot make.

Essential hypertension: High blood pressure for which a cause has not been found.

Etiology: The study of what causes a disease.

Euglycemia: A normal level of sugar in the blood.

Exchange list: A grouping of foods by type to help people on special diets stay on the diet. Each group lists food in serving sizes. A person can exchange, trade, or substitute a food serving in one group for another food serving in the same group. The lists categorizes foods as: 1) starch/bread; 2) meat; 3) vegetables; 4) fruit; 5) milk; or 6) fats. Within a food group, each serving has about the same amount of carbohydrates, protein, fat, and calories.

Exogenous: Grown or made outside the body.

Extracellular: The space outside a cell.

F

Fasting blood glucose test: A method for finding out how much glucose (sugar) is in the blood. The test can show if a person has diabetes. A blood sample is taken in the lab or doctor's office. The test is usually done in the morning before a person has eaten.

The normal, nondiabetic range for blood glucose is from 70 to 100 mg/dl, depending on the type of blood being tested. A level over 140 mg/dl usually means the person has diabetes, except for newborns and some pregnant women.

Fats: One of the three main classes of foods and a source of energy in the body. Fats help the body use some vitamins (A, D, E, and K) and keep the skin healthy. Saturated fats are solid at room temperature and come chiefly from animal sources. Examples are butter, lard, meat fat, solid shortening, palm oil, and coconut oil. These fats can raise cholesterol levels.

Unsaturated fats, which include monounsaturated fats, are liquid at room temperature and come from plant oils, such as olive, canola, peanut, corn, cottonseed, sunflower, safflower, and soybean. These fats tend to lower cholesterol levels; however, too many unsaturated fats in relation to saturated fats can cause some health problems.

Fatty acids: A basic unit of fats. When insulin levels are too low or there is not enough glucose to use for energy, the body burns fatty acids for energy. The body then makes ketone bodies, which are waste products that cause acid levels in the blood to become too high. This can lead to ketoacidosis, a serious problem.

Fiber: A substance found in foods that come from plants. Fiber helps in the digestive process and is thought to lower cholesterol and help control blood glucose. Soluble fiber, found in beans, fruits, and oat products, dissolves in water and is thought to help lower blood fats and blood sugar. Insoluble fiber, found in whole-grain products and vegetables, passes directly through the digestive system, helping to rid the body of waste products.

Flavonoid: A group of flavone-containing compounds found in nature. These include many of the plant pigments, such as anthocyanins, flavonols, bioflavonoids, anthoxanthins, epigenins, flavones, and others.

Folacin: Folic acid, a B vitamin.

Folic acid: A B vitamin.

Free radicals: Highly unstable molecules, characterized by an unpaired electron, which can bind to and destroy cellular compounds.

Fructose: A type of sugar found in fruits, vegetables, and honey. It is considered a nutritive sweetener since it has calories. It is also called levulose or fruit sugar.

Fundus of the eye: The back or deep part of the eye, including the retina.

G

Galactose: A type of sugar found in milk products and sugar beets. It is also made in the body.

Gangrene: The death of body tissue, usually caused by a loss of blood flow, notably in the legs and feet.

Gastroparesis: A form of nerve damage that affects the stomach, in which food is not digested properly and does not move through the stomach in a normal way. This causes vomiting, nausea, or bloating and interferes with diabetes management. Also see **autonomic neuropathy**.

Gestational diabetes mellitus: A type of diabetes that occurs in pregnancy. In the second half of the pregnancy, the woman may have glucose in the blood at a higher than normal level. When the pregnancy is terminated, blood glucose levels return to normal in about 95% of the cases.

Gingivitis: An inflammation of the gums. If left untreated it can lead to periodontal disease. Typical signs are bleeding gums and inflammation.

Gland: A group of cells that make substances so the other parts of the body can work. As an example, the pancreas is a gland that releases insulin so other body cells can use glucose for energy.

Glaucoma: An eye disease caused by increased pressure in the eye. It can damage the optic nerve and cause impaired vision and blindness.

Glomerular filtration rate: A measure of the kidneys' ability to filter and remove waste products.

Glomeruli: Tiny blood vessels in the kidneys where the blood is filtered and waste products are removed.

Glucagon: A hormone that raises the level of glucose (sugar) in the blood. The alpha cells of the pancreas (in the islets of Langerhans) make glucagon when the body needs to put more sugar into the blood. An injectable form is often used to treat insulin shock. Also see **alpha cell**.

Glucose: A simple sugar found in the blood. Also known as dextrose, it is the body's main source of energy.

Glucose tolerance test: A test to see if a person has diabetes. The test is given in a lab or doctor's office in the morning before the patient has eaten. A first sample of blood is taken, then the person drinks a liquid that has sugar in it. After one hour, a second blood sample is drawn, and after another hour, a third sample is taken. The idea is to see how well the body deals with the glucose in the blood over time.

Gluten: A protein found in certain grains that gives dough its elastic character.

Gluten intolerance: See **celiac disease**.

Glycemic index: Refer to the chapter in the book.

Glycemic response: The effect of different foods on blood glucose levels over time. Researchers have discovered that some kinds of foods may raise blood glucose levels more quickly than other foods containing the same amount of carbohydrates.

Glycogen: A substance made up of sugars. It is stored in the liver and muscles and releases glucose into the blood when needed by the cells. Glycogen is the chief source of stored fuel in the body.

Glycogenesis (glucogenesis): The process in which glycogen is formed from glucose.

Glycolysis: A breakdown of glucose into carbon dioxide and water.

Glycosuria: Having glucose in the urine.

Glycosylated hemoglobin (glycated hemoglobin): The attachment of glucose (sugar) to the hemoglobin protein in red blood cells, and the medical test for this process. The amount of glucose attached to hemoglobin goes up when blood glucose levels are chronically high.

Glycosylated hemoglobin test: A blood test that measures a person's average blood glucose (sugar) level for the two- to three-month period before the test. Also see **hemoglobin A1C**.

Gram: A unit of weight in the metric system. There are 28 grams in 1 ounce. In some diet plans for diabetics, the suggested amounts of food are given in grams. A typical serving size is 100 grams.

Gram-molecule: The amount of a substance with a mass in grams equal to its molecular weight. For example, a molecule of hydrogen weighs 2.016 g. A molecule of water weighs 18.015 g.

H

Hemochromatosis: Iron overload or bronze diabetes.

Hemodialysis: A method of cleaning the blood for those with kidney disease. Also see **dialysis**.

Hemoglobin A1C (HbA1C): The substance of red blood cells that carries oxygen to the cells and sometimes joins with glucose. Because the sugar stays attached for the life of the cell (about four months), a test to measure hemoglobin A1C shows what the person's average blood glucose level was for that period of time.

Hepatic: Pertaining to the liver.

High blood pressure: When the blood flows through the vessels at a greater-than-normal force. High blood pressure strains the heart, harms the arteries, and increases the risk of heart attack, stroke, and kidney problems. Also called hypertension.

High-density lipoprotein cholesterol (HDL): The beneficial kind. These protein particles in the blood transport cholesterol from the blood to be broken down by the liver and help to reduce the risk of heart disease.

HLA antigens: Proteins on the outer part of the cell that help the body fight illness. These proteins vary from person to person. Scientists think that those with certain types of HLA antigens are more likely to develop Type 1 diabetes.

Hormone: A chemical released by special cells to tell other cells what to do. For example, insulin is a hormone made by the beta cells in the pancreas. When released, insulin tells other cells to use glucose for energy.

Hypercholesterolemia: Large amounts of cholesterol in the blood.

Hyperglycemia: Too high a level of glucose in the blood. It's a sign that diabetes is out of control. It occurs when the body does not have enough insulin or cannot use the insulin it does have to turn glucose into sugar. Signs of hyperglycemia are a great thirst, dry mouth, and a need to urinate often. For those with Type 1 diabetes, this may lead to diabetic ketoacidosis.

Hyperinsulinism: Too high a level of insulin in the blood. This generally means that the body produces too much insulin. Researchers believe that this condition may play a role in the development of Type 2 diabetes and hypertension. Also see **Syndrome X**.

Hyperlipidemia, hyperlipemia: Too high a level of fats (lipids) in the blood. Also see **Syndrome X**.

Hyperkalemia: Large amounts of potassium in the blood.

Hypertension: High blood pressure.

Hypoglycemia: Too low a level of sugar in the blood. This occurs when a person with diabetes has injected too much insulin, eaten too little food, or exercised without extra food. The person may feel nervous, shaky, weak, or sweaty and have a headache, blurred vision, and hunger. Taking small amounts of sugar, sweet juice, or food with sugar, cheese, or other food will usually help the person feel better within ten to fifteen minutes. Also called low blood sugar. Also see **insulin shock**.

Hypotension: Low blood pressure or a sudden drop in blood pressure. A person rising quickly from a sitting or reclining position may have a sudden fall in blood pressure, causing dizziness or fainting.

I

Iatrogenic: A condition caused by a physician or other health care provider.

IDDM: Insulin-dependent diabetes. Now called Type 1 diabetes.

Idiopathic: A disease of unknown origin.

Ileum: Lower part of the small intestine, between the jejunum and the cecum.

Impaired glucose tolerance: Blood glucose levels higher than normal but not high enough to be called diabetes. Those with IGT may or may not develop diabetes. Names for IGT no longer used include borderline, subclinical, chemical, or latent diabetes.

Impotence: Loss of a man's ability to have an erect penis and to emit semen. Some men may become impotent after having diabetes for a long time because the nerves or blood vessels to the penis have been damaged. If the problem is psychological, it may be treated with counseling.

Infarction: A quick drop in blood supply to an organ. A myocardial infarction is a heart attack.

Inositol: A vitamin-like substance associated with the B-complex of vitamins.

Insulin: A hormone that helps the body use glucose (sugar) for energy. The beta cells of the pancreas (in the islets of Langerhans) make the insulin. When the body cannot make enough insulin, a diabetic must inject insulin from other sources (beef, pork, human insulin—recombinant DNA origin—or human insulin—pork-derived, semisynthetic).

Insulin allergy: When a person's body has an allergic or bad reaction to taking insulin made from pork, beef, or bacteria, or because the insulin is not exactly the same as human insulin, or because it has impurities. A local allergy results when the skin becomes red and itchy around the place where the insulin is injected. In a systemic allergy, a person's whole body can have a bad reaction, in which the person can have hives or red patches all over the body or may feel changes in the heart rate and in the rate of breathing.

Insulin antagonist: Something that opposes the action of insulin. Insulin lowers the level of glucose in the blood, whereas glucagon raises it. Therefore, glucagon is an antagonist of insulin.

Insulin binding: This happens when insulin attaches itself to something else. When a cell needs energy, insulin can bind with the outer part of the cell. The cell then can bring glucose inside and use it for energy. With the help of insulin, the cell can do its work very well. However, sometimes the body acts against itself.

In this case, insulin binds with the proteins that are supposed to protect the body from outside substances (antibodies). If the insulin is an injected form and not made by the body, the body sees the insulin as an outside or foreign substance. When the injected insulin binds with the antibodies, it does not work as well as when it binds directly to the cell.

Insulin-dependent diabetes: Now called Type 1 diabetes.

Insulin reaction: Hypoglycemia.

Insulin receptors: Areas on the outer part of the cell that allow the cell to bind with insulin that is in the blood. When the cell and insulin bind together, the cell can take sugar from the blood and use it for energy.

Insulin resistance: Many people with Type 2 diabetes produce enough insulin, but their bodies do not respond to the action of insulin. This may happen if the person is overweight and has too many fat cells, which do not respond well to insulin. As people age, their body cells lose some of the ability to respond to insulin.

Insulin resistance is linked to high blood pressure and high levels of fat in the blood. Insulin resistance may happen in those who take insulin injections. They may have to take high doses of insulin daily (200 units or more) to bring their blood sugar down to the normal range. This is also called insulin insensitivity.

Insulin sensitivity: This is said to be the normal state in which the cells of the body are receptive to the action of insulin.

Insulin shock: This occurs when the level of blood sugar drops quickly. The signs are shaking, sweating, dizziness, double vision, convulsions, and collapse. Insulin shock may occur when an insulin reaction is not treated quickly enough. Also see **hypoglycemia** and **insulin reaction**.

Intermittent claudication: Pain in the muscles of the leg that occurs off and on, usually while walking or exercising, and results in lameness (claudication). The pain results from a narrowing of the blood vessels feeding the muscle.

Intramuscular injection: Putting a fluid into a muscle with a needle or syringe.

Intravenous injection: Putting a fluid into a vein with a needle or syringe.

In vitro: A process carried out in lab glassware.

In vivo: A process carried out in a living organism.

Ischemia: A deficiency of blood due to an obstruction of a blood vessel.

Ischemic stroke: Caused by a lack of blood supply to the brain.

Islets of Langerhans: Special group of cells in the pancreas. They make and secrete hormones that help the body break down and use food. Named after Paul Langerhans, the German scientist who discovered them in 1869, these cells sit in clusters in the pancreas. There are five types of cells in an islet: beta cells, which make insulin; alpha cells, which make glucagon; delta cells, which make somatostatin; and PP and D cells, about which little is known.

J

Jejunum: Middle part of the small intestine, between the duodenum and the ileum.

Juvenile onset diabetes: Now referred to as Type 1 diabetes.

K

Ketone bodies: Chemicals that the body makes when there is not enough insulin in the blood and it must break down fat for its energy. Ketone bodies can poison and even kill body cells. When the body does not have the help of insulin, the ketones build up in the blood and then spill over into the urine so that the body can get rid of them. The body can also rid itself of one type of ketone, called acetone, through the lungs. This gives the breath a fruity odor. Ketones that build up in the body for a long time lead to serious illness and coma. Also see **diabetic ketoacidosis**.

Ketonuria: Having ketone bodies in the urine, which is a sign of diabetic ketoacidosis (DKA).

Ketosis: A condition of having ketone bodies build up in the body tissues and fluids. Signs of ketosis are nausea, vomiting, and stomach pain. Ketosis can lead to ketoacidosis.

Kidney disease: Any one of several chronic conditions that are caused by damage to the cells of the kidney. Those who have had diabetes for an extended period may have kidney damage. Also called nephropathy.

Kidney threshold: The point at which the blood is holding too much of a substance, such as glucose, and the kidneys spill the excess sugar into the urine.

Kimmelstiel-Wilson syndrome: Lesions formed on the tubules of the kidneys, which are caused by blood-vessel degeneration related to poorly controlled diabetes. Paul Kimmelstiel was a twentieth-century German pathologist. Clifford Wilson was a twentieth-century English physician.

Korsakoff's disease: Found in alcoholics and others with B-vitamin deficiencies, this syndrome is characterized by amnesia, confusion, and apathy. Sergei Korsakoff was a twentieth-century Russian neurologist.

Kussmaul breathing: A rapid, deep, and labored breathing in those with ketoacidosis or who are in a diabetic coma. It is named after Adolph Kussmaul, the nineteenth-century German doctor who discovered it. Also called air hunger.

L

Labile diabetes: A term that is used to indicate when a person's blood sugar level swings quickly from high to low and from low to high. Also called brittle diabetes.

Lactic acidosis: The buildup of lactic acid in the body. The cells make lactic acid when they use sugar for energy. If too much lactic acid stays in the body, the balance tips and the person begins to feel ill. The signs of lactic acidosis are deep and rapid breathing, vomiting, and abdominal pain. This condition may be caused by diabetic ketoacidosis or liver or kidney disease.

Lactose: A sugar found in milk and milk products (cheese, butter, etc.). Also called milk sugar.

Lactose intolerance: Those who cannot metabolize lactose because they do not have the enzyme lactase.

Lancet: A fine, sharp-pointed blade or needle for pricking the skin.

Latent diabetes: Former term for impaired glucose tolerance.

Lente insulin: A type of insulin that is intermediate-acting. It begins working within four to six hours and stops after about twelve hours. It is a mixture of 30% Semilente and 70% Ultralente insulin.

Leukocytes: White blood cells.

Leukotrienes: Inflammatory substances that are produced when oxygen combines with polyunsaturated fatty acids.

Lipid: Another term for fat, such as cholesterol, triglycerides, and phospholipids. The body stores fat as energy for future use. When the body needs energy, it can break down the lipids into fatty acids and burn them like glucose (sugar).

Lipoatrophy, lipodystrophy: Lumps or small dents in the skin that form when a person keeps injecting the needle in the same spot. Avoid the problem by changing the injection sites.

Lipogenesis: The formation of fats.

Lipoprotein: A complex of fat and protein found in blood and responsible for the transportation of fats in the bloodstream.

Lipotrophic: Substances that prevent the accumulation of fat in the liver.

Low-density lipoprotein cholesterol (LDL): The bad kind. These protein particles help cholesterol and triglycerides to build up in artery walls and can lead to heart disease.

M

Macrosomia: The development of abnormally large babies in some women with diabetes.

Macrovascular disease: Disease of the large blood vessels that can occur when a person has had diabetes for a long time. Fat and blood clots build up in the large blood vessels and stick to the vessel walls. Three kinds of macrovascular disease are coronary disease, cerebrovascular disease, and peripheral vascular disease.

Macula: Center of the retina.

Macular degeneration: A disorder of the eye in which central vision is impaired.

Macular edema: A swelling in the macula, an area near the center of the retina of the eye that is responsible for fine or reading vision. This is a common complaint associated with diabetic retinopathy.

Malondialdehyde: A marker for fatty acid oxidation.

Maturity-onset diabetes: Former term for Type 2 diabetes.

Megaloblast: An immature red blood cell.

Meta-analysis: A compilation of various published studies.

Metabolism: The term for the way cells chemically change food so that it can be used to keep the body alive. One part is called catabolism, when the body uses food for energy, and the other part is called anabolism, when the body uses food to build or mend cells. Insulin is necessary for the metabolism of food.

Mg/dl: Milligrams per deciliter. Term used to describe how much glucose is in a specific amount of blood. In self-monitoring of blood glucose (sugar), test results are given as the amount of glucose in milligrams per deciliter of blood. A fasting reading of 70 to 110 mg/dl is considered in the normal (nondiabetic) range.

Micelle: A microscopic amount of fats and bile salts.

Microaneurysm: A small swelling on the side of tiny blood vessels. They may break and bleed into nearby tissue. Diabetics sometimes get these swellings in the retina of the eye.

Microvascular disease: Disease of the smallest blood vessels that sometimes occurs when a person has had diabetes for a long time. The walls of the vessels become abnormally thick but weak, and tend to bleed, leak protein, and slow the flow of blood through the body.

Millimole: One-thousandth of a gram-molecule.

mmol: Millimole.

Mononeuropathy: A form of diabetic neuropathy affecting a single nerve, often in the eye.

Monosaccharide: A simple sugar, such as fructose or glucose.

Monounsaturated fat: Found in olive oil, canola oil, and nuts, this is considered a heart-healthy fat.

Morbidity rate: The number of people who are sick or have a disease compared with the number who are well.

Mortality rate: The number of people who die of a certain disease compared to the total number of people. Mortality is often stated as deaths per 1,000, 10,000, or 100,000.

Myocardial infarction: Heart attack. It results from permanent damage to an area of the heart muscle. This happens when the blood supply to the area is interrupted because of a narrowed or blocked blood vessel.

Myocardium: Heart muscle.

Myoglobin: Hemoglobin that is found in muscle.

Myoinositol: A substance in the cell that is thought to play a role in helping the nerves to work. Low levels of the substance may be involved in diabetic neurology.

N

Necrobiosis lipoidica diabeticorum: A skin condition usually on the lower part of the legs. The lesions can be small or extended over a large area. They are usually raised, yellow, and waxy in appearance and often have a purple border. Young women are most often affected. It occurs in people with and without diabetes.

Neovascularization: The term used when new, tiny blood vessels grow in a new place, such as from the retina.

Nephropathy: Disease of the kidneys caused by damage to the small blood vessels or to the units in the kidneys that clean the blood. People who have had diabetes for a long time may have kidney damage.

Neuritis: Inflammation of the nerves.

Neuropathy: Disease of the nervous system. Those with long-standing diabetes have nerve damage. The three major forms of nerve damage are peripheral neuropathy, autonomic neuropathy, and mononeuropathy. The most common form is peripheral neuropathy, which mainly affects the feet and legs.

Neurotransmitters: Substances that transmit nerve impulses.

Niacin: Vitamin B_3. Also niacinamide and nicotinic acid.

Nitric oxide: A potentially toxic compound of oxygen and nitrogen that is also a beneficial free radical. It relaxes blood vessels and may play a key role in penile erections and impotence.

Non-essential amino acids: Amino acids necessary for human health, but which can be synthesized by the body.

Non-insulin-dependent diabetes: Now called Type 2 diabetes.

Non-ketonic coma: A type of coma caused by a lack of insulin. A non-ketonic crisis means: 1) very high levels of sugar in the blood; 2) absence of ketoacidosis; 3) great loss of body fluid; 4) a sleepy, confused, or comatose state. This coma often results from some other problem, such as a severe infection or kidney failure.

Norepinephrine: A nerve transmitter derived from tyrosine, the amino acid.

Nucleic acids: Molecular structures, such as DNA, that carry the cell's genetic code or are necessary for protein synthesis.

O

Obesity: When people have 20% or more extra body fat for their age, height, sex, and bone structure. Fat works against the action of insulin. Extra body fat is thought to be a risk factor for diabetes.

Oral hypoglycemic agents: Pills or capsules that lower the level of sugar in the blood.

Overt diabetes: Diabetes in those who show clear signs of the disease, such as great thirst and urgent need to urinate.

Oxalic acid: A dicarboxylic acid found in spinach, chard, rhubarb, and other foods. Spinach, a good source of iron, is a poor source of calcium, since the oxalic acid in the spinach converts the calcium to calcium oxalate and removes large amounts from the body.

Oxidation: A chemical reaction in which a substance combines with oxygen, often to the detriment of health, such as oxygen free radicals.

P

Pancreas: An organ behind the lower part of the stomach that is about the size of a human hand. It makes insulin so that the body can use glucose for energy. It also makes enzymes that help the body digest food. Spread over the pancreas are areas called the islets of Langerhans. The cells in these areas have a special purpose. The alpha cells make glucagon, which raises the level of glucose in the blood. The beta cells make insulin. The delta cells make somatostatin. Little is known about PP and D cells.

Pancreatin: An extract from pork pancreas.

Pantothenic acid: A B vitamin. Sometimes called B$_5$.

Para-amino-benzoic acid (PABA): A vitamin-like substance associated with the B-complex of vitamins.

Parathyroid hormone: A hormone secreted by the parathyroid gland. It is necessary for the regulation of blood calcium levels.

Pathogen: A microorganism that causes infection or disease.

Periodontal disease: Damage to the gums.

Peripheral neuropathy: Nerve damage, usually affecting the feet and legs. It causes pain, numbness, or a tingling feeling. Also called somatic neuropathy or distal sensory polyneuropathy.

Peripheral vascular disease: Disease in the large blood vessels of the arms, legs, and feet. People who have had diabetes for a long time may develop this because major blood vessels in the extremities are blocked and these limbs do not receive enough blood. The signs of PVD are aching pains in the arms, legs, and feet–especially when walking–and foot sores that heal slowly. This can best be avoided by taking good care of the feet, not smoking, and keeping blood pressure and diabetes under control.

Peroxide: The oxide that contains the most oxygen.

Pituitary gland: An endocrine gland in the small, bony cavity at the base of the brain. Often called "the master gland," it serves the body in many ways–in growth, in food use, and in reproduction.

Placebo: A dummy or look-alike pill used in double-blind studies. Neither the volunteers nor the scientists know the testing medication or the placebo until the code is broken at the end of the study.

Platelets: Cell fragments found in the blood.

Polycythemia: An excess of red blood cells.

Polydipsia: Great thirst, often a sign of diabetes.

Polyphagia: Great hunger, often a sign of diabetes. People with great hunger often lose weight.

Polysaccharide: A molecule containing many sugar molecules linked together.

Polyunsaturated fats: A type of fat that comes from vegetables, such as vegetable oils. These are omega-3 oils.

Polyuria: A need to urinate often, a common sign of diabetes.

Preeclampsia: A condition that some women with diabetes have during the late stages of pregnancy. Signs of this disorder include high blood pressure and swelling (edema) because the body cells are holding extra water.

Prostaglandins: Hormone-like substances from linoleic and linolenic acids that help in the contraction of smooth muscle and dilation of blood vessels.

Protein: One of the three main classes of food. Proteins are made of amino acids, which are called the building blocks of the cells. The cells need proteins to grow and to mend themselves. Main sources are meat, fish, poultry, and eggs.

Proteinuria: Too much protein in the urine. It may be a sign of kidney damage.

Prothrombin: A protein in the blood that is necessary for blood clotting.

Pruritus: Itching skin, often a symptom of diabetes.

Pyridoxine: Vitamin B$_6$.

R

Reagents: Strips or tablets that people use to test the level of glucose in blood and urine, or the level of acetone in the urine.

Rebound: A swing to a high level of sugar in the blood after having a low level. Also see **Somogyi effect.**

Receptors: Areas on the outer part of a cell that allow the cell to join or bind with insulin that is in the blood. Also, insulin receptors.

Recommended Daily Allowance (RDA): Suggested amounts of nutrients needed daily by individuals. This particular guide is being phased out, but it is best known to laymen.

Regular insulin: An insulin that is fast acting.

Renal: Pertains to the kidneys.

Renal threshold: When the blood is holding so much of a substance, such as sugar, that the kidneys allow the excess glucose to spill into the urine. Also called kidney threshold, spilling point, and leak point.

Respiratory distress syndrome: Difficulty in breathing.

Retina: Center part of the back lining of the eye that senses light. It has many small blood vessels that are sometimes harmed when a person has had diabetes for a long time.

Retinol: Vitamin A.

Retinopathy: A disease of the small blood vessels in the retina of the eye. Also see **diabetic retinopathy**.

Riboflavin: Vitamin B_2.

Risk factor: Anything that raises the chance that a person will get a disease. With Type 2 diabetes, people have a greater risk of getting the disease if they weigh more (20% or more) than they should.

S

Saccharide: Sugar molecule.

Satiety: A feeling of fullness.

Saturated fat: A type of fat that is usually solid at room temperature. Usually derived from animal sources.

Secondary diabetes: When a person develops diabetes because of another disease or because of taking certain drugs or chemicals.

Serotonin: A neurotransmitter formed from tryptophan, the amino acid. It regulates pain, mood, sleep, and appetite.

Serum: The fluid portion of blood that remains after clotting.

Shock: A person with diabetes can go into shock when the level of blood sugar drops suddenly. Also, insulin shock.

Somatostatin: A hormone made by the delta cells of the pancreas. It may control how the body secretes two other hormones, insulin and glucagon.

Somogyi effect: A swing to a high level of glucose in the blood from an extremely low level, usually occurring after an untreated insulin reaction during the night. The swing is caused by the release of stress hormones to counter low glucose levels. People who experience high levels of blood sugar in the morning may need to test their blood glucose levels in the middle of the night. If blood sugar levels are falling or low, adjustments in evening snacks or insulin doses may be recommended. The condition is named after Dr. Michael Somogyi, an American biochemist who first identified it. Also called rebound.

Sorbitol: A sugar in alcohol.

Spilling point: When the blood is holding so much of a substance, such as glucose, that the kidneys allow the excess to spill into the urine. Also, renal threshold.

Statins: Drugs used to lower LDL-cholesterol.

Steatorrhea: Excess fat in the stool.

Stiff hand syndrome: Thickening of the skin of the palm that results in loss of ability to hold the hand straight. This condition occurs only in diabetics.

Stroke: Disease caused by damage to blood vessels in the brain. Depending on the part of the brain affected, a stroke can cause a person to lose the ability to speak or move a part of the body, such as an arm or leg. Usually only one side of the body is affected. Also, cerebrovascular disease.

Subclinical deficiency: A deficiency of various nutrients that do not result in overt physical symptoms. You might have a vitamin C deficiency but not sufficient to cause scurvy.

Subcutaneous: Below the skin.

Sucrose: Table sugar. A form of sugar that the body must break down into a more simple form before the blood can absorb it and take it to the cells.

Sugar: A class of carbohydrates that taste sweet. Sugar is a quick and easy fuel for the body to use. Types of sugar are lactose, glucose, fructose, and sucrose.

Sulfonylureas: Pills or capsules people take to lower the level of glucose (sugar) in the blood. Also, oral hypoglycemic agents.

Symptom: A sign of disease. Having to urinate often is often a symptom of diabetes.

Syndrome: A set of signs or a series of events occurring together to make up a disease or health problem.

Syndrome X: A term describing a combination of health conditions that place a person at high risk for heart disease. These conditions are Type 2 diabetes, high blood pressure, high insulin levels, and high levels of fat in the blood.

Systemic: A term used to describe conditions that affect the entire body. Diabetes is a systemic disease because it involves many parts of the body, such as the pancreas, eyes, kidneys, heart, and nerves.

T

Tachycardia: Unusually fast heart beat.

Thiamine: Vitamin B_1.

Thrombus: A blood clot that forms within an artery wall or cavity of the heart.

Tocopherol: Vitamin E.

Toxemia of pregnancy: A condition in pregnant women in which poisons such as the body's own waste products build up and may cause harm to mother and fetus. The first signs of toxemia are swelling near the eyes and ankles (edema), headache, high blood pressure, and weight gain that the mother might confuse with the normal weight gain during pregnancy. The mother may have sugar and acetone in the urine.

Toxic: Harmful, having to do with poison.

Trans fatty acid: A type of fat found in margarine.

Transient ischemic attack (TIA): Temporary problem, such as slurred speech, or numbness of the arm, due to partial blockage of arteries to the brain.

Trauma: A wound, hurt, or injury to the body. Trauma can also be mental, such as when a person is under stress.

Triglyceride: A type of blood fat. The body needs insulin to remove this type of fat from the blood. When diabetes is under control and a person's weight is what it should be, the level of triglycerides in the blood is usually what it should be. Triglyceride levels around 100 mg/dl are considered normal.

Type 1 diabetes mellitus: Formerly called insulin-dependent diabetes.

Type 2 diabetes mellitus: Formerly called non-insulin-dependent diabetes.

U

Ubiquinone: A fat-soluble compound also called coenzyme Q. It is involved in the production of energy from carbohydrates. Coenzyme Q10 is being used to treat heart disease.

Ulcer: A break in the skin or a deep sore.

Ultralente insulin: A type of insulin that is long acting.

Unit of insulin: U-100 insulin means 100 units of insulin per milliliter (ml) or cubic centimeter (cc) of solution. Most insulin made in the U.S. is U-100.

Unsaturated fats: A type of fat, such as those from fish oils and vegetable oils.

Unstable diabetes: A type of diabetes when a person's blood sugar level often swings quickly from high to low and low to high. Also called brittle diabetes and labile diabetes.

Urea: One of the chief waste products of the body. When the body breaks down food, it uses what it needs and throws the rest away as waste. The kidneys flush the waste from the body in the form of urea, which is in the urine.

Uremia: Urine in the blood.

Uric acid: The end product in the metabolism of purines, which is excreted in the urine. Excess blood levels are found in gout.

UTI: Urinary tract infection.

V

Vascular: Pertaining to the body's blood vessels; namely, arteries, veins, and capillaries.

Vasoconstriction: A constriction of blood vessels.

Vasodilation: A dilation or expansion of blood vessels.

Vein: A blood vessel that carries blood to the heart.

Ventricle: One of the two lower chambers of the heart.

Visceral fat: Fat in the abdomen that may be a risk factor for diabetes and heart disease.

Vitrectomy: Removing the gel from the center of the eyeball because it has blood and scar tissue in it that blocks sight. An eye surgeon replaces the clouded gel with a clear fluid. Also see **diabetic retinopathy**.

Vitreous humor: The clear jelly (gel) that fills the center of the eye.

Void: To empty the bladder in order to obtain a urine sample for testing.

Index

acetylcholine, 247
N-acetylcysteine, 134, 315–316
acidophilus, 126
acne vulgaris, 249
Acpr30, 49
acupuncture, 338
adenosine triphosphate (ATP), 315
adiponectin, 49
adrenal glands, 247
adult-onset diabetes. *See* Type 2 diabetes
  (adult-onset)
African-Americans
  blood pressure reductions in, 61
  cardiovascular risk among, 60
  diabetes risk among, 60
  diet quality and, 60
  Type 2 diabetes among, 61
  Vitamin C levels in, 61
  Vitamin E levels in, 61
Agent Orange, 9–10
aggression, 156–157
aging, 314
albumin
  above-normal, 260
  defined, 110
  excretion of, Vitamin E and, 299
  levels in child diabetics, 291
  levels, selenium deficiency and, 298
  mode of detection, 250
albuminuria, 133, 249
alcohol consumption
  beta-carotene supplements and, 275
  diabetes risk and, 64
  fat oxidation and, 188
  magnesium deficiency and, 60, 291
  Syndrome X and, 190
  without eating, *xiii*, 149
aldose reductase inhibitors, 259
alpha cells, 14
alpha-lipoic acid
  antioxidant action of, 313–316, 318
  blood glucose control and, 188, 318
  cataract and, 86
  defied, 313
  excretion of, Vitamin E and, 299
  free radical damage to cholesterol and,
    318
  functions of, 213
  glucose transport and, 315–316, 318–319
  heart disease and, 316
  kidney disease prevention in rats and,
    317–318
  liver disease and, 316
  nerve function in rats and, 317
  oxygen transport and, 316
  peripheral neuropathy and, 316–317
  polyneuropathy and, 315–316
  tyrosine metabolism and, 84
Alzheimer's disease, 21–22
amino acids
  defined, 320
  essential, 320
  isomerism of, 321–322

non-essential, 320
  proportions in food, 321
amniocentesis, 78
amputation, 3, 5, 102
amylose, 52, 164
anemia
  iron-deficiency, 311
  megaloblastic, 229, 241, 242
  pernicious, 229–230
angina pectoris
  coenzyme Q10 and, 326, 327
  hypoglycemia and, 152, 156, 158
  magnesium sulfate for, 292
  preventing, 158
anthocyanins, 55
antibiotics, 245, 246
antidiabetic medication, chromium and,
  285–286
antioxidants
  as treatment after heart attacks, 299
  benefits of, 41
  cataracts and, 262
  defined, 271
  eye-protective, 8–9, 93
  infectious disease and, 262
  vitamins as, 219
antipsychotic agents, 146
apolipoprotein-a, 140
apolipoprotein-b, 140, 179, 180, 272
apolipoproteins, 140
apples, 28
aqueous humor, 81
arachnoid, 275
arginine, 170, 189, 320, 322
arterial disease, magnesium and, 292–293
arterial thrombosis, 278
arteries, 184
arteriosclerosis
  diabetic incidence of, 38
  sugar consumption and, 44
asthma
  magnesium deficiency and, 60
  supplementation and, 89–90, 300
atherosclerosis
  diabetes and, 27
  diabetic incidence of, 38
  high insulin levels and, 145
  homocysteine and, 244
  lipoprotein-A and 183
  magnesium deficiency and, 292
  pectins and, 208
  preventing, 208, 258, 332
  sugar and, 193
  Vitamin E and, 41
ATP (adenosine triphosphate), 315
autoimmune disease, 73, 77
avidin, 245
avocados, 29
B-complex vitamins
  See also specific B vitamins and biotin;
    choline; folic acid; inositol; inositol
    hexaniacinate; pantothenic acid
  glutathione concentrations and, 275

ingestion mode recommended, 226, 227
  summary of, 226–227
balsam pear (bitter melon), 332
bananas, 29
barley, 207, 286
basal body temperature test, 115
beans, green, 28
beets, 28
berries, 28
beta-blockers, 146, 147
beta-carotene
  See also carotenoids
  dietary, 222
  disease risk reduction and, 222
  dosages, 221, 262
  supplements, 275
  Vitamin A activity of, 221
beta cells
  autoimmunity to, 73, 77, 78
  damage to, 19, 268
  defined, 14, 77, 235, 274
  function impairment of, 144
  gurmar (*Gymnema sylvestre*) and, 334
  magnesium and, 292, 293
  nicotinamide and, 232
  preventing destruction of, 313
  protecting, 234, 235, 274
  viruses and, 268
beta-glucan, 205
betaine, 134, 249, 250
betaine hydrochloride, 92
biotin
  dosages of, 331
  food sources of, 245
  functions of, 228, 245
  glucose utilization and, 246
  neuropathy and, 246
  supplementation, 245–246
birth control pills, 65, 147, 238
bitter gourd, 330
bitter melon, 332
blood clots, 134
blood clotting, 272
blood glucose
  alpha-lipoic acid and, 188, 318
  bitter melon and, 332
  control of, 39, 154, 322
  defined, 18
  drugs which elevate, 146, 147
  fasting
    chromium and, 282, 283, 284
    Vitamin C and, 293
  fenugreek and, 139, 331, 332
  ginseng and, 333
  guar gum and, 208
  high levels of, 5, 38, 145, 147
  ivy gourd and, 331
  jackass bitters (*Neurolaena lobata*) and,
    334
  marshmallow (*Althaea officinalis*) and,
    334
  milk thistle (*Silybum Marianum*) and, 334
  niacin and, 234, 236

359